Fatigue Science for Human Health

Y. Watanabe, B. Evengård, B.H. Natelson,
L.A. Jason, H. Kuratsune
Editors

Fatigue Science for Human Health

Springer

Yasuyoshi Watanabe, M.D., Ph.D.
Program Director, Molecular Imaging Research Program, RIKEN, 6-7-3 Minatojima-minamimachi, Chuo-ku, Kobe 650-0047, Japan;
Professor, Department of Physiology, Osaka City University Graduate School of Medicine, 1-4-3 Asahi-machi, Abeno-ku, Osaka 545-8585, Japan

Birgitta Evengård, M.D.
Professor, Senior Consultant
Division of Clinical Microbiology, Department of Laboratory Medicine, Karolinska Institutet at Karolinska University Hospital Huddinge, SE-141 86 Stockholm, Sweden;
Division of Infectious Diseases, Department of Clinical Microbiology, Umeå University, SE-901 85 Umeå, Sweden

Benjamin H. Natelson, M.D.
Professor of Neurosciences, University of Medicine and Dentistry, New Jersey Medical School, Newark, NJ 07103, USA

Leonard A. Jason, Ph.D.
Professor and Director, Center for Community Research, DePaul University, 990 West Fullerton, Suite 3100, Chicago, IL 60614, USA

Hirohiko Kuratsune, M.D., Ph.D.
Professor, Department of Health Science, Faculty of Health Science for Welfare, Kansai University of Welfare Sciences, 3-11-1 Asahigaoka, Kashiwara, Osaka 582-0026, Japan

Library of Congress Control Number: 2007938889

ISBN 978-4-431-73463-5 Springer Tokyo Berlin Heidelberg New York

Springer is a part of Springer Science+Business Media
springer.com

Printed in Japan

Typesetting: SNP Best-set Typesetter Ltd., Hong Kong
Printing and binding: Hicom, Japan

Printed on acid-free paper

Preface and Mini-review: Fatigue Science for Human Health

Yasuyoshi Watanabe

What is fatigue? Why do we feel tired sometimes or seemingly all of the time? What is the physiological role or meaning of the sensation of fatigue? How is chronic fatigue related to various diseases? How can we prevent chronic fatigue and exhaustion?

In the past we really did not know very much about the mechanisms of fatigue. Fatigue or tiredness is really an important bio-alarm, without which we might drop into an unrecoverable exhaustive state and in the most severe case even die, referred to in Japanese as *karoshi*. As compared with the mechanisms of other bio-defense systems such as pain and fever, little is known regarding molecular/neuronal mechanisms of fatigue. Cytokine-prostaglandin systems are involved as the major factors in the induction and/or mediation of pain and fever. Although some pre-inflammatory cytokines may be the central mediator(s) in fatigue (see the chapters by Katafuchi and the one by Inoue et al.), the prostaglandin systems are probably not involved in the mechanisms of fatigue because cyclooxygenase inhibitors, both COX-1 and COX-2 ones, could not reduce the hypo-activity caused by poly I:C injection in rats, although they are quite effective as anti-febrile drugs (Matsumura K et al, unpublished data). Lactate, which was previously considered to be a candidate fatigue-inducing substance accumulating during severe exercise, is no longer thought to be a causative substance of fatigue (see the chapter by Tanaka and Watanabe).

Figure 1 shows the statistics on fatigue in Japan in 2004. Although surprisingly a lot of people are suffering from chronic fatigue lasting longer than 6 months (more than one-third of the Japanese population), integrated research on fatigue had not been organized until quite recently. Fatigue is a sensation that probably all people have experienced and is therefore quite familiar to all of us, but its molecular and neural mechanisms have not been elucidated yet, probably because of the complicated nature of the causes. However, we know that fatigue definitely

---

Program Director, Molecular Imaging Research Program, RIKEN;

Professor, Department of Physiology, Osaka City University Graduate School of Medicine

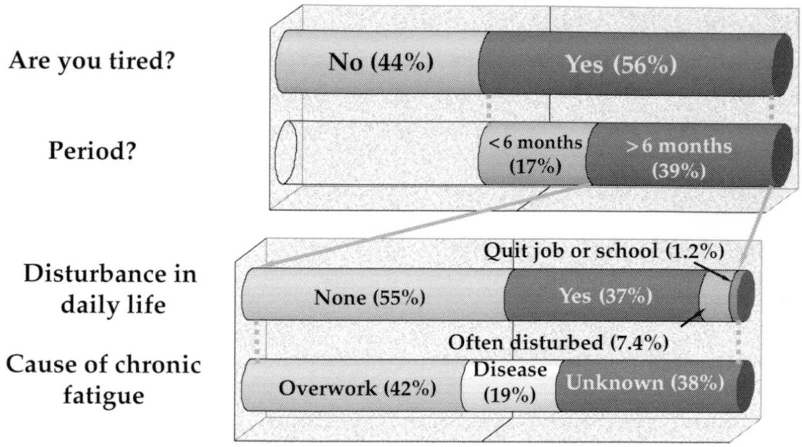

Fig. 1. Statistics in Japan in 2004. The research project under Ministry of Education, Culture, Sports, Science, and Technology, the Japanese Government made the questionnaire-based search with 2,742 answers from the citizens in Osaka area

decreases the efficiency with which we perform our daily tasks or studies. Thus it is of great value to our modern society for scientists to extensively analyze the causes of fatigue and to develop methods to quantify fatigue, with the goal of developing methods or therapies to afford better recovery from and perhaps even avoidance of severe chronic fatigue. The economic gain would be really quite large if chronic fatigue could somehow be cured. To our regret and surprise, almost all commercially available means for recovery from fatigue are not yet based upon scientific and medical evidence.

In light of the situation outlined above, Watanabe and Kuratsune organized an integrated research project entitled "The molecular/neural mechanisms of fatigue and fatigue sensation and the way to overcome chronic fatigue" under the aegis of the Ministry of Education, Culture, Sports, Science, and Technology, Japan, and carried it out from 1999 to 2005. The project was conducted by 26 laboratories in various universities and institutions with Yasuyoshi Watanabe as the chief researcher. The project made the following major contributions to our knowledge of fatigue: 1) Elucidation of the brain regions and their neurotransmitter systems responsible for fatigue sensation and chronic fatigue; 2) development of a variety of methods and scales to quantitatively evaluate the extent of fatigue; 3) development of animal models based on different causes of fatigue; 4) elucidation of molecular/neural mechanisms of fatigue in humans and animals; and 5) invention of various methods or therapies to treat chronic fatigue and chronic fatigue syndrome (CFS).

As can be seen in several chapters of this book, the pathogenesis of CFS is becoming a little clearer than before through the cooperation and findings of many investigators internationally from such fields as virology, immunology, endocrinology, physiology, biochemistry, psychiatry, and neuroscience.

In order to develop the foods and drugs to help overcome fatigue, we have been making efforts through the anti-fatigue project, organized by Soiken Co., Ltd., (2003–2007)(see the chapter by Kajimoto), and through the 21st Century COE Program called the "Establishment of the center of excellence (COE) to overcome fatigue (2004–2009)." More recently, the research has been directed not only toward foods and drugs to overcome fatigue but also toward various aspects of the environment, such as air-conditioning; the interior design of homes, hotel rooms, and offices; aromas; music; city design; and vehicular traffic. Although fatigue is a problem of individuals, it is also one of civilized societies, and we should therefore investigate and analyze the social aspects of fatigue, especially in terms of modern city life (see the chapter by Evengård). The contents of this book summarize our fatigue researchers' achievements, and present the status of research on fatigue and the perspectives on remedies for chronic fatigue and chronic fatigue syndrome. To generate international discussion, we organized The International Conference on Fatigue Science—the first in 2002 in Sandhamn, Sweden, and a second in 2005 in Karuizawa, Japan. As a consequence, the editors and contributors decided to collect the papers presented at these two conferences and incorporate them in this book entitled *Fatigue Science for Human Health*.

Concerning the molecular mechanisms of chronic severe fatigue addressed in this book, the only ones clearly involved are the following:

1. Oxidative stress: its prolongation or poor elimination
2. Pro-inflammatory cytokines: their central role in fatigue mediation
3. Less energy reservoir state, especially for repair of damaged intracellular and intercellular components (e.g. carbonyl proteins)
4. Neuro-immune-endocrine dysfunction and characteristic autonomic nerve dysfunction

In this context, some possible bio-toxins and lowered detoxification capacities are highlighted.

Recent progress in the neuroscience field has been marked (see also the chapter by Natelson and the one by Chaudhuri et al). Particularly, I would like to introduce our hypothesis on brain dysfunction in chronic fatigue. The team with Watanabe and Kuratsune investigated the brain regions responsible for the fatigue sensation by using positron emission tomography (PET), and found the regions in Brodmann's area 10/11 well correlated with the fatigue sensation, areas in which motivation and evaluation of perceived information are organized (Tajima, S. et al., manuscript in preparation). Recent single-photon emission computed tomography (SPECT) studies [1–3] using ^{99m}Tc-hexamethyl-propylene-amine oxime revealed that most CFS patients showed cerebral hypoperfusion in a variety of brain regions such as the frontal, temporal, parietal, and occipital cortices; anterior cingulate; basal ganglia; and brain stem. Furthermore, they suggested that central nervous system (CNS) dysfunction may be related to the neuropsychiatric symptoms of CFS patients. To confirm these findings, we studied the regional cerebral blood flow (rCBF) in 8 CFS patients and 8 age- and sex-matched controls by use of ^{15}O-labeled water ($H_2{}^{15}O$) and PET, and found that the rCBF was lower in the CFS patient group than in the control group in the brain regions including the frontal, temporal, and occipital cortices; anterior cingulate; basal ganglia; and brain stem [4]. These brain regions correspond to various neuropsychiatric complaints: autonomic imbalance, sleep disturbance, many kinds of pain, and the loss of concentration, thinking, motivation, and short-term memory. Therefore, our results from the first quantitative rCBF study done on CFS patients with PET are in good agreement with the data from the previous SPECT studies, and indicate that various neuropsychiatric complaints found in CFS patients might be related to dysfunction in these regions of the CNS.

Furthermore, when we studied the cerebral uptake of [2-^{11}C] acetyl-L-carnitine in the same 8 CFS patients and 8 age- and sex-matched normal controls by using PET, a significant decrease in uptake was found in several brain regions of the patient group, namely, in the prefrontal (Brodmann's area 9/46d) and temporal (BA21 and 41) cortices, anterior cingulate (BA24 and 33), and cerebellum [4]. These findings suggest that the levels of neurotransmitters biosynthesized through acetyl-L-carnitine may be reduced in some brain regions of chronic fatigue patients and that this abnormality may be one of the keys to unveil the mechanisms underlying chronic fatigue sensation.

More recently, using magnetic resonance imaging (MRI), we found that patients with CFS have reduced gray matter (GM) volume in their bilateral prefrontal cortices.[5] Furthermore, right-hemisphere GM volume correlated negatively with the subjects' fatigue ratings [5]. This is consistent with the above-mentioned result that showed decreased uptake of acetyl-L-carnitine, perhaps indicating a decrease in the biosynthesis of glutamate, in the prefrontal cortex. The prefrontal cortex may therefore be part of the neural underpinnings of fatigue.

Much more striking, we demonstrated by functional MRI studies the vulnerability of the neuronal activity in task-unrelated brain regions in CFS patients, although in the healthy subjects decreased neuronal activity was seen only in task-related brain regions [6]. Apparently, a system guarding against further exhaustion may be built into the brain.

We also studied 5-HT transporter (5-HTT) density in 10 patients with CFS and 10 age-matched normal controls by using PET with the radiotracer [^{11}C](+)McN5652. Analysis using a statistical parametric mapping software (SPM99; The Wellcome Department of Cognitive Neurology, London, UK) revealed that the density of 5-HTTs in the rostral subdivision of the anterior cingulate was significantly reduced in CFS patients [7]. In addition, the density of 5-HTTs in the dorsal anterior cingulate was negatively correlated with the pain score [7]. Therefore, an alteration in the serotoninergic neurons in the anterior cingulate plays a key role in the pathophysiology of CFS.

Apparently, these PET results on 5-HTT density seem to be inconsistent with our results regarding the 5-HTT gene promoter polymorphism [8], where CFS patients could have a greater frequency of the L allele, which affords greater transporter efficiency. However, it might be the case that the reduction in 5-HTT density in CFS patients with L and XL allelic variants is less than that in CFS patients with S allelic variants. Because 5-HT biosynthesis in the brain is thought to deteriorate

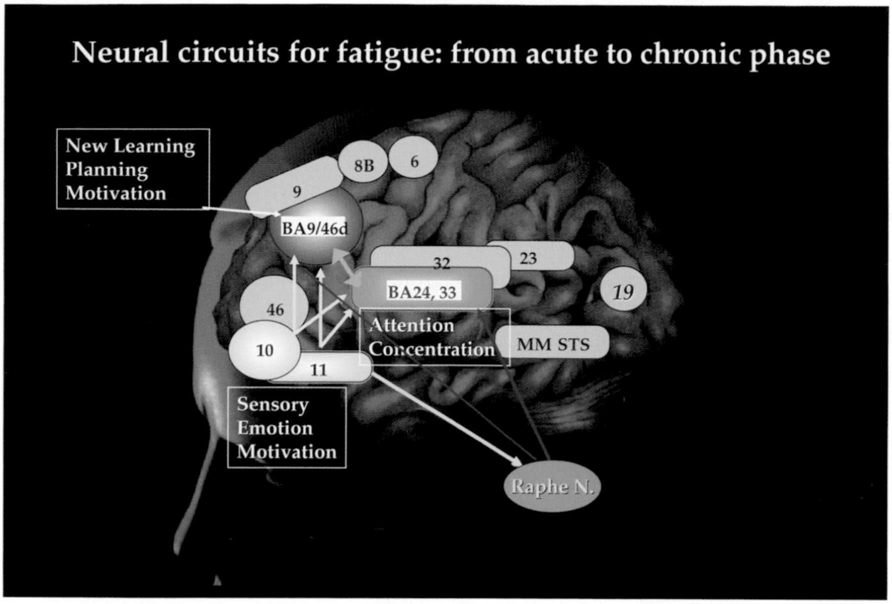

Fig. 2. The working hypothesis in dysfunction of neural circuits from acute to chronic fatigue. Watanabe and colleagues summed up their recent data from PET and fMRI

in patients with CFS, 5-HT deficiency in the synapses might be more serious in patients with L and XL allelic variants. If so, it is consistent with the finding that selective serotonin re-uptake inhibitor (SSRI) treatment is effective for some patients with CFS. To clarify the full particulars of brain dysfunction in patients with CFS, we are now studying 5-hydroxy-L-tryptophan (5-HTP) uptake, L-DOPA uptake, and muscarinic acetylcholine receptor density by using PET. We plan to report the results of these studies concerning brain dysfunction found in patients with CFS in the near future. So far, however, we propose the working hypothesis on this dysfunction in chronic fatigue, as shown in Fig. 2.

Quantification of fatigue or invention of fatigue scales specific for the induced load (physical load, mental load, or mixed ones) is also a central issue to be developed in fatigue science (Lists 1 and 2; see also the chapter by Kajimoto and the one by Kondo). For this purpose, we developed a new clinical scale based on the results of a 64-item questionnaire (see the chapter by Fukuda et al.). Also, nonverbal scales to assess frontal lobe function (see the chapter by Mizuno et al.), behavior amount (by using an actigraph), and autonomic function (by using acceleration plethysmography) have been developed. Blood and saliva samples from CFS patients and from individuals with induced fatigue (physical and mental) were analyzed, and we found a specific pattern or spectrum of the components [9]. By using these physiological and biochemical (including immunological and viral) biomarkers (see the chapter by Kajimoto), we started a project to develop evidence-based anti-fatigue foods, especially those foods that can prevent fatigue (Soiken

List 1. Evaluation protocol for the extent of fatigue

Questionnaire, VAS, Face scale
- fatigue, sleep, life trends, temperament and character investment (TCI), food intake

Physiological biomarkers
- autonomic, cognitive, sleep diagram, activity, working memory, fatigability

Biochemical biomarkers
- virological, immunological, endocrinological, energy substrates, redox

Doctor interview
- motivation, vividness?

List 2. Scales/Biomarkers for quantification of fatigue

- **Cortical function: attention, concentration, and working memory**
  - Advanced Trail Making Test (ATMT)
  - Dual Task Test (DTT), n-back task
- **Evaluation by behavioral measures**
  - motion capture, actigraph (gyroscope-type)
- **Autonomic nerve function**
  - acceleration plethysmography (APG), ECG
- **Biochemical markers in the plasma and saliva**
  - immune and endocrine biomarkers, amino acids, iron, heme, vitamins, viruses and near infrared-factors

Project). In 2007, or by the beginning of 2008, we could have the first anti-fatigue product derived from the Soiken Project.

One thing is very clear: if we would like to elucidate the mechanisms of CFS and to devise a systematic remedy for CFS patients, we may learn more by studying both CFS and chronic fatigue. What is specific to CFS? Unfortunately, most studies have merely focused on the differences between CFS patients and healthy volunteers. However, whether factors or treatments relate to CFS or chronic fatigue is at times unclear and leads to confusion. If we could have some means of distinguishing between chronic fatigue and CFS, e.g., as like pre-disease and disease, respectively, we would be able to study at least three conditions (groups), i.e., healthy, chronic fatigue, and CFS. Elsewhere, we should compare healthy, CFS, and chronic fatigue with regard to other causes and diseases. Such studies could help both CFS and chronic fatigue patients. Toward this end, we propose here the promotion of "fatigue science for the benefit of human health." It is our hope that more researchers from various disciplines will join the study of fatigue science after having read this book and the references cited therein.

On behalf of the editors, I would like to thank all the contributors to this book, and also all of their colleagues and collaborators. Some of them could not be included in this book because of a conflict of interest with original papers. I also thank Prof. Osamu Hayaishi, Prof. Hiroo Imura, the late Prof. Yasutomi Nishizuka, Prof. Ryoji Noyori, Dr. Teruhisa Noguchi, Prof. Teruo Kitani, Prof. Yutaka Oomura, and Prof. Nobuya Hashimoto, for their pertinent advice. In addition, many thanks are due to the members and staff of the research project "The molecular/neural mechanisms of fatigue and fatigue sensation and the way to overcome chronic fatigue" under the auspices of the Ministry of Education, Culture, Sports, Science, and Technology, Japan, and also to those of the 21st Century COE Program "Establishment of the center of excellence (COE) to Overcome Fatigue." Finally, I am especially grateful to Dr. Junichi Seki, the Mayor of Osaka City; Prof. Satoru Kaneko, the President of Osaka City University (OCU); Prof. Yoshiki Nishizawa, the Dean of OCU Medical School; the members and colleagues of the anti-fatigue project organized by Soiken Co., Ltd.; Dr. Larry D. Frye for editorial help with this manuscript; and the editorial staff of Springer Japan for the great effort they made for the publication of this book.

References

1. Ichise M, Salit IE, Abbey SE, et al. (1992) Assessment of regional cerebral perfusion by ^{99m}Tc-HMPAO SPECT in chronic fatigue syndrome. Nucl Med Commun 13:767–772.
2. Costa DC, Tannock C, Brestoff J (1995) Brainstem perfusion is impaired in chronic fatigue syndrome. QJM 88:767–773.
3. Fischler B, D'Haenen H, Cluydts R, et al. (1996) Comparison of 99mTc HMPAO SPECT scan between chronic fatigue syndrome, major depression and healthy controls: an exploratory study of clinical correlates of regional cerebral blood flow. Neuropsychobiology 34:175–183.
4. Kuratsune H, Yamaguti K, Lindh G, et al. (2002) Brain regions involved in fatigue sensation: reduced acetyl-carnitine uptake into the brain. Neuroimage 17:1256–1265.
5. Okada T, Tanaka M, Kuratsune H, et al. (2004) Mechanisms underlying fatigue: a voxel-based morphometric study of chronic fatigue syndrome. BMC Neurol 4:14.
6. Tanaka M, Sadato N, Okada T, et al. (2006) Reduced responsiveness is an essential feature of chronic fatigue syndrome: an fMRI study. BMC Neurol 6:9.
7. Yamamoto S, Ouchi Y, Onoe H, et al. (2004) Reduction of serotonin transporters of patients with chronic fatigue syndrome. Neuroreport 15:2571–2574.
8. Narita M, Nishigami N, Narita N, et al. (2003) Association between serotonin transporter gene polymorphism and chronic fatigue syndrome. Biochem Biophys Res Commun 311:264–266.
9. Sakudo A, Kuratsune H, Kobayashi T, et al. (2006) Spectroscopic diagnosis of chronic fatigue syndrome by visible and near-infrared spectroscopy in serum samples. Biochem Biophys Res Commun 345:1513–1516.

Contents

Dimensions and Assessment of Fatigue

Leonard A. Jason and Michelle Choi

Summary

In this chapter, we first review the sources of diagnostic unreliability, otherwise known as variance, which lead to disagreement among clinicians regarding diagnostic decisions. We then review issues related to the assessment of fatigue. We conclude that basic data on scale reliability are often missing, few studies provide information about the cut-off scores that identify clinical cases, and there are few direct comparisons of existing fatigue scales. Fatigue scales used in chronic fatigue syndrome (CFS) studies should have been diagnostically validated in CFS and depression samples, and should represent several factorally distinct dimensions of fatigue. In addition, fatigue scales need to give an accurate assessment of the severe fatigue that is characteristically observed among people with CFS.

Dimensions and Assessment of Fatigue

Fatigue has come to be recognized as a serious symptom of many chronic illnesses that can significantly impair a person's functioning and negatively impact their quality of life [1,2]. These include fatigue after cancer treatment [3,4], systemic lupus erythematosus (SLE) [5], multiple sclerosis [6], HIV infection, viral and cholestatic liver diseases, rheumatoid arthritis [7], and chronic fatigue syndrome (CFS) [8]. Even in conditions where fatigue is considered to be a primary or common symptom, such as multiple sclerosis (MS) or SLE, levels of fatigue may not always correlate with disease status or physiological findings [6,9,10].

In this chapter, we review issues related to the assessment of fatigue. However, before reviewing actual studies or instruments that measure fatigue, it is important to consider sources of diagnostic unreliability, technically known as variance, that can lead to disagreement among clinicians regarding diagnostic decisions [11].

DePaul University, Center for Community Research, 990 West Fullerton, Suite 3100, Chicago, IL 60614, USA

Sources of Diagnostic Unreliability

Sources of variance can be divided into the following five categories: subject variance, occasion variance, information variance, observation variance, and criterion variance [12]. Subject variance occurs when patients have different conditions at different times. For example, a patient may have acute alcohol intoxication on admission to a hospital, but develop delirium tremens several days later. Occasion variance occurs when patients are in different stages of the same condition at different times. An example would be a patient with multiple sclerosis who was in remission during one period of illness and symptomatic during another. Information variance occurs when clinicians have different sources of information about their patients. For example, one clinician may regularly question patients about areas of functioning and symptoms, which another clinician does not assess. Observation variance occurs when clinicians presented with the same signs and symptoms differ in what they detect and perceive. An example of this type of variance would be a disagreement among clinicians as to whether a patient is irritable or depressed. Criterion variance occurs when there are differences in the formal inclusion and exclusion criteria that clinicians use in reaching diagnostic conclusions. An example would be a disagreement as to whether difficulty concentrating is a necessary criterion for the pronouncement of fatigue.

Studies examining sources of diagnostic unreliability have shown that subject, occasion, and information variance account for only a small portion of diagnostic reliability [12]. However, criterion variance, i.e., differences in the formal inclusion and exclusion criteria used by clinicians to classify patients' data into diagnostic categories, accounts for the largest portion of diagnostic unreliability. Therefore, an improvement in diagnostic reliability is primarily dependent on reducing criterion variance as a source of unreliability. Criterion variance is most likely to occur when operationally explicit criteria do not exist for diagnostic categories [12]. In other words, inclusion and exclusion criteria need to be consistent across measures in order to compare fatigue states across patients adequately.

When diagnostic categories lack reliability and accuracy, the validity (i.e., usefulness) of a diagnostic category is inherently limited by its reliability. Therefore, to the extent to which a diagnostic category is unreliable, a limit is placed on its validity for any type of clinical research or administrative use [12]. The reliability of clinical diagnosis is also crucial when conducting assessment studies. If the reliability of the diagnostic groups studied is limited, the results of any study using such diagnostic categories are likely to be unreliable and/or invalid. Issues concerning the reliability of clinical diagnoses are therefore complex, and have important research and practical implications.

The low reliability of routine diagnostic procedures is a crucial problem in the assessment of fatigue, which affects both clinical work and research efforts to improve the management, treatment, and care of patients [13]. Problems regarding diagnostic reliability and validity have been topics of discussion and controversy for many years [14]. As an example, both the first and second editions of the American Psychiatric Association's official publication on nomenclature, the *Diagnostic and Statistical Manual of Mental Disorders* (DSM I, DSM II) [15,16], were predominantly composed of largely unreliable, purely clinical descriptions of psychiatric disorders [13]. The number of researchers who found diagnostic judgments based on clinical interviews to be unreliable out-numbered those who found them to be reliable [17]. The problem of low inter-rater reliability in psychiatric diagnosis was attributable to the inability of two examiners to write down and agree in advance what symptoms needed to be present before a specific diagnosis could be made [17]. In other words, the low rates of inter-rater reliability were due to criterion variance: differences in the formal inclusion and exclusion criteria used by clinicians to classify patients' data into diagnostic categories. Because criterion variance is likely to occur when no operationally explicit criteria exist for diagnostic categories, in 1972 the St. Louis group developed the Fieghner criteria [18]. The Fieghner criteria were operationally explicit criteria for the then 16 diagnostic categories of the DSM II. Use of the Fieghner criteria led to an immediate and dramatic improvement in clinician–clinician diagnostic reliability [18].

By the 1970s, researchers in the field of diagnostics also recognized that the provision of operationally explicit, objectively debatable criteria was not enough to ensure that clinicians would know how to elicit the necessary information from a clinical interview to permit them to apply it to the reliable criteria [19]. These concerns led to the development of a series of structured interview schedules, such as the Structured Clinical Interview for DSM IV Axis 1 [14,17,20,21]. The benefit of structured interview schedules is that they ensure that clinicians in the same or different settings conduct clinical interviews and examinations that maximize the accuracy of clinical diagnoses [19]. The use of structured interview schedules increases the chance that the clinical material needed to apply the diagnostic criteria is elicited by structuring and standardizing the questions asked by each interviewer [19]. Thus, structured interview schedules serve to remove as much as possible of the unreliability in the resulting psychiatric diagnosis introduced by differences in the way clinicians elicit clinical information. Together, the provision of operationally explicit, objectively debatable criteria and standardized interviews was found to significantly improve the reliability of clinical diagnosis for a number of psychological and psychiatric conditions [13]. It is possible that similar strategies might be used to enhance the reliability of assessments of fatigue.

Diagnostic and epidemiological research requires diagnostic categories that are both reliable and valid [22]. Thus, the criteria used to define fatigue must be clearly operationalized. Tucker [23], however, warns that in the contemporary practice of psychiatry, the patient's history and report of functioning is not always considered to be essential to the diagnostic process. Rather, the focus tends to be merely on the symptoms presented, without regard to either the antecedents or consequences of those symptoms [23]. In emphasizing and focusing on a predetermined set of symptoms, the views of the patient may be dismissed, and additional sources of important information, such as the reports of family and friends, tend to be ignored.

Meaningful distinctions between patients within the same diagnostic categories are also likely to be disregarded. For example, in the evaluation of subjective experiences (i.e., complaints of pain, fatigue, etc.), self-reported symptoms cannot be effectively interpreted without careful consideration of the antecedents, consequences, overall context, and fluctuations in intensity over time (i.e., the patient's story) [23].

Cantwell [22] believes that diagnostic criteria should specify which diagnostic instrument to use, what types of informant to interview, and how to determine the presence and severity of the criteria. It is necessary to specify a certain number and type of symptoms that should be present in order to make a particular diagnosis. In addition to the importance of the number and type of symptoms, definitions of fatigue should also include specific guidelines pertaining to the importance of symptom severity in the diagnostic procedure. Given the high variability in symptom severity among people with fatigue, standardized procedures should be employed for determining whether or not a particular symptom is severe enough to qualify as an occurrence of one of the symptoms required for a diagnosis of fatigue. For example, if a patient presents with a symptom such as postexertional malaise, standard questions should include the duration, frequency, and severity of the symptoms, including onset, pattern, intensity, and associated factors.

A final consideration is the use of polythetic criteria (i.e., sets of criteria in which not all the criteria need to be present before making a diagnosis). It is argued that while standardized diagnostic criteria are needed for research, the use of polythetic criteria developed by expert committees (as is the case with CFS) may not be methodologically sound [23]. For example, the use of polythetic criteria may result in a comparison of two different groups of patients within the same diagnostic category, or of similar groups in different diagnostic categories [23]. Research by Kendler and Gardner [24] highlights the arbitrary and varied results that can be found when different polythetic criteria are used. Kendler and Gardner [24] conducted a study to evaluate the DSM IV diagnostic criteria for major depression. The results of their investigation revealed minimal empirical support for the DSM IV requirements of 2 weeks duration, five or more symptoms, and clinically significant impairment, and suggested that most changes in functioning appeared to be continuous. Based on these findings, Kendler and Gardner [24] suggested that major depression, as defined by the DSM IV, may be a diagnostic convention imposed on a continuum of depressive symptoms of varying severity and duration.

The results obtained by Kendler and Gardner [24] are of great importance because they demonstrate that although significant improvements in the classification and diagnosis of psychiatric disorders have occurred through the use of operationalized criteria, the classification methods and the validity of diagnostic criteria are also matters of importance that cannot be ignored. With respect to the development of diagnostic instruments to measure fatigue, the findings of Kendler and Gardner [24] strongly suggest a careful consideration and examination of classification methods.

Classification Methods

At present, a variety of classification methods are used to study individuals with symptoms of fatigue. For example, Fukuda et al. [25] used a clinical approach to the classification of individuals with chronic fatigue syndrome (CFS). Others have provided experimental evidence for the importance of the CFS criteria. For example, Hartz et al. [26] examined people with CFS and compared them with people with other fatigue-related conditions and those with no symptoms of fatigue. They concluded that people with fatigue could be classified according to the degree to which they matched the case definition of CFS [25]. Friedberg et al. [27] found three factors (cognitive problems, flu-like symptoms, and neurological symptoms) in a sample of patients with CFS. Finally, Linder et al. [28] used artificial neural networks to classify patients with chronic fatigue (including CFS and idiopathic chronic fatigue), SLE, and fibromyalgia, and were able to achieve a sensitivity of 95% and a specificity of 85%.

Nisenbaum et al. [29] also conducted an empirical test of the current US case definition of CFS. In this study, they collected data on the occurrence of 30 symptoms commonly experienced by people with CFS in a random sample of people who reported that they were suffering from unexplained fatigue of six months duration or longer, and also in a sample of people who reported that they were suffering from unexplained fatigue of 1–5 months duration. Factor analysis was used to identify underlying relations among the symptom data. They found that three correlated factors ("fatigue–mood–cognition" symptoms, "flu-type" symptoms, and "visual impairment" symptoms) explained a set of correlations between fatigue lasting for 6 months or more and 14 interrelated symptoms. No factor explained the correlations among fatigue lasting for 1–5 months and other symptoms. While the findings of this study do provide empirical support for the interrelations among unexplained fatigue of 6 months duration or longer and symptoms included in the CFS case definition, this type of finding is of interest because it indicates that only fatigue lasting 6 months or more (with at least four additional minor symptoms based on the 1994 CFS criteria [25]) overlaps with published criteria to define CFS.

Haley et al. [30] conducted a study to determine whether Gulf War Syndrome was best characterized as a group of distinct syndromes rather than as one overarching syndrome. To accomplish this task, they developed a standardized survey to measure the myriad symptoms frequently reported by veterans complaining of Gulf War Syndrome. For each symptom endorsed by the survey, a series of follow-up descriptive questions were asked to elucidate the nature of the symptom (e.g., fatigue characterized by excessive daytime sleepiness versus fatigue characterized by excessive muscle exhaustion after exertion). Separate factor analyses were performed on each set of follow-up questions to clarify the various features and meanings of each symptom. For example, for the symptom of fatigue, the following nine descriptions were used to disentangle the different meanings of fatigue: (1) too weak in the hands or arms to complete work; (2) too weak in the legs to complete work; (3) too weak in the body to do normal work; (4) wearing out too quickly to finish work; (5) having too little energy to start work; (6) feeling too sleepy to do normal work; (7) feeling very sleepy most of the day; (8) having to take naps frequently during the day; (9) nodding off to sleep while working or driving. Factor analysis of these nine items revealed the following two factors: excessive muscle exhaustion, with items 1 through 5 loading on this factor, and excessive daytime sleepiness, with items 6 through 9 loading on this factor [30]. After a factor analysis was conducted for individual sets of symptom descriptors, another factor analysis was performed on the factors generated from the analyses of the symptom descriptors to identify clusters of symptoms that might represent hidden syndromes within Gulf War Syndrome. The results of this analysis produced six factors, impaired cognition, confusion ataxia, arthromyoneuropathy, phobia apraxia, fever adenopathy, and weakness incontinence, with each factor representing a syndrome or different cluster of symptoms.

Statistical procedures have also been used by other investigators in an attempt to classify the wide array of patients who present with fatigue as a primary problem or complaint. In a study conducted by Hall et al. [31], cluster analysis was used to identify homogenous subgroups within a sample of fatigued patients in order to facilitate the diagnosis and treatment of the underlying disorder. Data were collected for each patient regarding the presence or absence of 15 symptoms and 3 demographic variables. The results of the cluster analysis revealed the presence of the following four distinct reasons for fatigue within the sample of fatigued patients: organic, anxiety, depression, and mixed anxiety and depression [31]. Factor analytic studies have tended to find multiple factors or clusters of fatigue-related symptoms. Ray et al. [32] factor analyzed a list of symptoms in 208 patients with postviral fatigue, and found that four factors emerged: emotional distress, fatigue, somatic symptoms, and cognitive difficulty. Jason et al. [33] factor analyzed fatigue-related symptoms reported by 780 people with chronic fatigue. They found four factors: lack of energy, physical exertion, cognitive problems, and fatigue and rest.

Reeves et al. [34] recently attempted to use empirical methods to operationalize the CFS criteria [25] using the medical outcomes survey short form 36 (SF-36), the checklist of individual strength (CIS), the multidimensional fatigue inventory (MFI), and the CDC (Centers for Disease Control and Prevention) symptom inventory. On the scales of the SF-36, substantial reductions in occupational, educational, social, or recreational activities were defined as scores lower than the 25th percentile on the physical function (less than or equal to 70), role physical function (less than or equal to 50), social function (less than or equal to 75), or role emotional (less than or equal to 66.7) subscales. Severe fatigue was defined as greater than or equal to 13 on the MFI general fatigue subscale, or greater than or equal to 10 on the reduced activity subscale. Individuals also needed to have four or more symptoms and to score 25 or more on the CDC's symptom inventory case definition (a sum of the products of the frequency and intensity scores of the eight CFS case definition symptoms). Subjects who met the CFS case criteria [25] had significantly worse impairment, more severe fatigue, and more frequent and severe symptoms than other subjects in the study who were ill but who did not meet the CFS definition.

Jason (see http://iacfs.net/p/1,544.html) has recently criticized these criteria as being too broad.

Measures of Fatigue

Friedberg and Jason [35,36] provided a review of some of the more common and well-validated fatigue rating scales (Table 1), and a recent article [37] provided a comprehensive review of 30 published scales. Clearly, at this time there is on no "gold standard" of fatigue severity available. As mentioned in a previous review [35], fatigue scales most frequently involve fatigue intensity and fatigue/function effects, although as Table 1 indicates, some scales also measure fatigue/affect constructs. Most measures of fatigue involve either verbal or numerical ratings, although some have used a visual analogue scale, and each of these methods is described below.

One of the most commonly used techniques to assess subjective symptoms (e.g., pain, nausea, fatigue, dyspnea) is the visual analogue scale (VAS). The VAS is a line of predetermined length (typically 100 mm) that is anchored at both ends with words that are descriptive of the extreme boundaries of the phenomenon being assessed (e.g., "no fatigue at all" and "worst fatigue possible"). Patients are asked to draw a mark through the line to indicate the intensity of the phenomenon being measured. The VAS can then be scored by measuring the distance from one end of the scale to the mark drawn by the patient, thereby providing an objective representation of a previously subjective and unquantified phenomenon [38]. This type of graphic method is quick and simple to construct and administer. However, some populations have difficulty with this technique (e.g., the elderly), reproduction tends to distort the length of the line, there is no "true" equal interval or ratio scale, it cannot be administered over the telephone, and anchoring ideas are often imprecise [38,39].

Owing to the limitations of the VAS technique, researchers have recommended that other measurement techniques be used to assess the subjective symptoms of fatigue [35]. An alternative to the VAS is the verbal rating scale (VRS). The VRS comprises a list of adjectives that describe different levels of intensity of the given phenomenon. Patients are asked to read over the list and select the adjective or descriptive phrase that best describes their level of the phenomenon. The primary advantages of using VRS scales are that they are easy to administer and score, they have demonstrated good evidence of construct validity, and compliance with the measurement task is high [39]. The primary disadvantages include the difficulty of use with populations with limited vocabulary, the fact that patients are forced to choose a word even if no word on the scale appropriately describes the intensity of their symptoms, and that if they are scored using a ranking method, the score represents ordinal data and must be treated as such statistically [39].

Subjective phenomena may also be assessed using numerical rating scales (NRS). This can easily be accomplished by asking patients to rate each of their symptoms on a scale of 0–10 or 0–100, where 0 represents no intensity and 10 or

Table 1. Fatigue rating scales (updated from Friedberg and Jason [35])

Name of scale	Description	Format	No. of items	Strengths/limitations
Fatigue intensity				
Piper fatigue scale [72]	Seven dimensions of fatigue, including 3 intensity dimensions	VAS	42	Multidimensional measure/respondents' difficulty with VAS format/not validated in chronic fatigue patients
Fatigue scale [40]	Measures of mental and physical fatigue	VRS	11	Treatment sensitivity/does not differentiate CFS and primary depression
Energy/fatigue scale [48]	Brief measure of vitality (fatigue and energy level)	VRS	4	Ease of administration/floor effects in severely fatigued patients
VAS-F [73]	Measure of energy and fatigue	VAS	18	Convergent and discriminant validity/fatigue and sleepiness confounded
Rhoten fatigue scale [74]	Single energy/fatigue item	NRS	1	Ease of administration/inadequate validation data/limited information about fatigue states
Fatigue/function				
Fatigue severity scale [49]	Measures effect of activities on functioning	VRS	9	Good validation data with different populations/possible ceiling effects with severe fatigue
Checklist individual strength [75]	Measures fatigue severity, concentration, motivation, and physical activity	VRS	20	Good validation data/unclear whether CIS differentiates CFS and primary depression
Fatigue assessment instrument [76]	Measures effect of activities on functioning	VRS	9	Measures behavioral aspects of fatigue, including consequences of fatigue/limited validation data
Multidimensional assessment of fatigue [77]	Measures 5 dimensions of fatigue, including impact on daily activities	VAS or VRS	16	Brief yet thorough in scope/limited data on construct validity/not validated in chronic fatigue patients
Fatigue impact scale [78]	Measures cognitive, physical, and social functioning in relation to fatigue	VRS	40	Differentiates CFS from MS/considerable overlap with depression symptoms/limited validation data in chronic fatigue patients
Multidimensional fatigue inventory [79]	Measures 5 fatigue dimensions, including reduced activity	VRS	20	One subscale dimension approximates anhedonia, not fatigue/factor structure may be questionable
Fatigue/affect				
Profile of fatigue-related states [70]	Measures 4 fatigue dimensions, including emotional distress	VRS	54	Comprehensive measure of CFS subjective states/discriminant validity of dimensions may be questionable
Profile of mood states [80]	Measures 6 dimensions, including emotional, fatigue and confusion states	VRS	65	Treatment sensitivity/adequate convergent validity of fatigue and vigor subscales/length and poor discriminant validity of dimensions

VAS, visual analogue scale; VRS, verbal rating scale; NRS, numerical rating scale

100 represents the worst intensity possible. The number that the patient chooses is the symptom's intensity score. Numerical rating scales have been shown to be consistently valid measures of symptom intensity, particularly for pain intensity [39]. The primary advantages of using NRS scales are that they are easy to administer and score, they have demonstrated good evidence of construct validity, compliance with the measurement task is high, and the data can be treated as ratio data [39]. The drawbacks of this technique primarily concern the lack of evidence regarding the relative treatment sensitivity of the NRS to that of other measures such as the VAS.

We now describe a few of the more popular and well-validated fatigue scales. A more comprehensive list is given in Table 1 [35]. Many fatigue measures were developed for specific medical conditions, but several have been developed to measure the subjectively experienced fatigue that might occur in varied medical illnesses.

The Fatigue Scale. The fatigue scale [40] is a 14-item verbal rating instrument with a 4-choice format that measures fatigue intensity. This scale was originally used in a hospital-based case control study [41] and also in a study designed to measure responses to treatment [42]. David et al. [43] found a continuous distribution of fatigue scores on this scale in a sample in Great Britain. The fatigue scale produces a total score, a score reflecting mental fatigue, and a score reflecting physical fatigue. The fatigue scale was further refined by Chalder et al. [40]. Despite its brevity, the scale was found to be reliable and valid, and it has good face validity and reasonable discriminant validity. This 11-item scale is commonly scored in one of two ways: continuous scoring code responses according to a four-option continuum, with codes ranging from 0 to 3, and total scores ranging from 0 to 33 (with higher scores signifying greater fatigue). Dichotomous scoring code responses according to a two-option dichotomy, where responses are normally coded as 0 or 1, are represented by a score of 0, and responses normally coded as 2 or 3 are represented by a score of 1. Total dichotomous scores of four or more items coded as 1 characterize cases of significant fatigue [40]. The fatigue scale is commonly used in community-based studies of fatigue, chronic fatigue, and CFS [44,45]. Jason et al. [46] used a receiver operating characteristic curve analysis to differentiate people with CFS from healthy controls, although those with SLE were most similar to those with CFS. Factor analysis has uncovered two dimensions, physical and mental fatigue, although one study has questioned the stability of this factor structure [47]. One limitation of this scale is its inability to distinguish between CFS and primary depression patients.

The Energy/Fatigue Scale. Ware and Sherbourne [48] developed the energy/fatigue scale, which is another verbal rating scale of fatigue intensity. This scale consists of five questions with a five-choice response format. This scale uses adjectives that describe both fatigue (worn out, tired) and energy (pep, energy). This scale was derived from the Rand vitality index, and it has shown good internal consistency [48]. However, the brevity of the energy/fatigue scale may result in scores that do not fully reflect the severity of severely disabling fatigue illnesses [36].

Fatigue Severity Scale. The Krupp fatigue severity scale is an example of a fatigue/function measure, which attempts to capture the relationship between the symptoms of fatigue and the function level. It includes 9 items rated on 7-point scales and is sensitive to different aspects and gradations of fatigue severity. Most items in the Krupp scale are related to the behavioral consequences of fatigue. This scale has the advantages of being both brief and easy to use, although a ceiling effect may limit its ability to assess severe fatigue-related disability. Previous findings have demonstrated the utility of the fatigue severity scale [49] to discriminate between individuals with CFS, MS, and primary depression [50]. In addition, the fatigue severity scale [49] was normed on a sample of individuals with MS or SLE, and healthy controls. A study by Taylor et al. [51] compared the fatigue scale [40] with the fatigue severity scale [49] on a sample of healthy controls and a CFS-like group. Within the CFS-like group, the fatigue severity scale [49] was most closely associated with severity ratings for the eight CFS symptoms [25], as well as with functional outcomes related to fatigue.

Checklist of Individual Strength. The checklist of individual strength (CIS) is a 20-item inventory with four subscales: fatigue severity, reduction in concentration, motivation, and physical activity [52,53]. A score above 36 represents severe fatigue. The CIS asks respondents about the preceding 2 weeks, and interviewees use a 7-point Likert scale ranging from 1 = "Yes, that is true" to 7 = "No, that is not true." A considerable amount of normative data has been collected with reference to both CFS and postcancer patients. This scale has high internal consistency, and can discriminate between healthy individuals, patients with CFS, and patients with multiple sclerosis [52]. While the CIS has shown sensitivity to treatment intervention in patients with CFS [54], it is still unclear whether it can differentiate between CFS and depression.

Somatic and Psychological Health Report. The somatic and psychological health report (SPHERE) is a 36-item instrument that identifies severe and disabling fatigue, and measures accompanying symptoms and somatic distress. The SPHERE allows for concurrent measurements of depression, anxiety, and fatigue as independent constructs, and hence it is useful as a screening instrument [55]. It has been used extensively in studies of primary care patients [56] and patients with postinfective and postcancer fatigue [57]. However, it does not address fatigue in the same detail as other scales mentioned above, and screens only for depression and anxiety [58].

Measures of Physical Activity

At present, levels of physical activity are typically assessed in three ways: by getting individuals to recall and report their physical activity, by asking individuals to maintain activity diaries or records, or by getting individuals to wear a mechanical or electrical monitoring device [59]. Current measures of physical activity can therefore be classified as either direct or indirect measures. Direct measures of physical activity include questionnaire assessment, activity diaries, and mechanical or electrical monitoring devices. Indirect measures of physical activity include dietary assessment, body composition measurement, assessment of physiological fitness, and occupational classification. Although all the assessment methods listed above are useful, questionnaires have become the preferred instrument in surveys assessing physical activity [60].

Activity Logs. A practical alternative, or perhaps supplement, to the questionnaire format is the use of activity logs and records. The NIH (National Institute of Health) activity record, the ACTRE, is an example of a daily self-administered log of physical activity. The ACTRE provides a functional assessment of physical activity through the use of a daily log format that measures the quantity and intensity (e.g., sedentary, active, etc.) of an individual's physical activity [61]. The ACTRE also assesses the more subjective features of each physical activity, such as whether it was associated with pain or fatigue, or perceived as being enjoyable, meaningful, or difficult to perform [61]. A profile of function can then be obtained by establishing a sequence of activity that is quantified in terms of the amount and quality of time spent [61]. In a validation study of the ACTRE, Gerber and Furst [61] found that it provides a valid measure of physical activity by capturing the sequence of activities across a day in an individual's life. Furthermore, data collected on the ACTRE can be totaled, and specific abilities can be rated in terms of associated symptoms. In effect, clinicians are able to obtain a composite picture that represents a comprehensive profile of functioning as well as of areas of dysfunction [61]. For example, using this instrument, King [62] found that, compared with people with major depression or controls, people with CFS spent significantly more time resting, spent significantly more time in low-intensity activities (e.g., activities performed lying down), and reported significantly more time in activities that produced fatigue.

Actigraphy. An actigraph is a small, light-weight, cost-efficient activity monitor that can be worn on the waist, has a long battery life, and can collect data continuously every minute of the day and night for 22 days before the memory is completely full [63]. One important use of the actigraph is to verify self-reported improvements in physical function. Unlike most activity monitoring devices, the actigraph is capable of recording movement intensity [64]. Tryon and Williams [63] demonstrated both within and between device reliability and validity of the actigraph as a monitoring instrument. Data collected by the actigraph can be downloaded to a computer for the purpose of analysis. The CSA (Computer Science and Applications) actigraph transduces activity using an accelerometer. An 8-bit analog-to-digital converter quantifies these measurements into 128 levels of positive acceleration and 128 levels of negative acceleration, called activity units, 10 times each second. The 600 measurements made each minute are averaged and stored in the memory. Averaging over time integrates the acceleration units over time, resulting in average velocity units measured in meters per minute. As an example of the types of finding that emerge when employing this assessment device, Tryon et al.

[65] found that patients with CFS had a blunted circadian rhythm. Continuous actigraphy, augmented with a daily activity diary, could be incorporated into fatigue assessment and treatment in order to collect the necessary data to evaluate circadian rhythm and to follow its changes throughout treatment. Ohashi et al. [66] found that patients with CFS had more abrupt interruptions during voluntary physical activity than healthy controls.

Conclusions and Recommendations

In response to the complex nature of fatigue, most measures of fatigue have moved away from single questions (e.g., "Do you feel tired?") and now employ a multidimensional approach toward fatigue [2]. These measures assess the effects of fatigue on daily activities, mental and physical fatigue, and other fatigue characteristics and related symptoms [40,67,68]. Fatigue has also been described in terms of the level of severity, the level of impairment that it causes, physiological and psychological fatigue (i.e., physical vs. mental), and duration [67,68]. Unfortunately, as indicated in Dittner et al.'s comprehensive review of fatigue scales [37], basic data on the reliability of such scales are rarely available, few provide information on the cutoff scores for identifying clinical cases, and there have been few direct comparisons of different scales.

Recently, several authors have made recommendations about the use of scales to measure fatigue. For example, Friedberg and Jason [36] suggested that the fatigue scales used in CFS studies should employ those that have been diagnostically validated in CFS and depression samples, and which also assess several factorally distinct dimensions of fatigue. They concluded that the Krupp fatigue severity scale would be the easiest to use and score, because it also provides a rapid assessment of fatigue-related impairments. Reeves et al. [58] also reviewed fatigue scales that have been used in studies of CFS, and they recommended that in future such studies should consider using the more extensive checklist of individual strength, but that shorter instruments such as the Chalder and Krupp scales were also appropriate. They also recommended that investigators should use the somatic and psychological health report as a screening instrument for potential study participants. As Stouten [69] correctly notes, some fatigue scales (e.g., Krupp, CIS, Chalder) do not accurately represent the severe fatigue that is characteristics of CFS (with the exception of the profile of fatigue-related symptoms [70]).

While some researchers have proposed a categorical classification of fatigue (i.e., the absence or presence of fatigue), several other studies have suggested that fatigue is best conceptualized on a continuum [44,45,71], with the variability of fatigue reflecting the difference in degree of severity [44]. Despite these more recent attempts to understand the phenomenon of fatigue, the major problem with such self-reporting measures is that they remain largely subjective. In research investigations, it would be prudent to use at least two fatigue instruments, which would provide a more thorough description of the fatigue experience and the opportunity for concurrent validation of each scale, as well as convergent validation with other measures [36].

Acknowledgments. Parts of this paper were presented at the NIH Workshop on the Role of Fatigue in Rheumatic Diseases, September 9, 2004, Warrenton, VA, USA. The authors appreciate the funding provided by NIAID (grant number AI 49720).

References

1. Chaudhuri A, Behan PO (2004) Fatigue in neurological disorders. Lancet 363:978–988
2. Torres-Harding S, Jason LA (2005) What is fatigue? History and epidemiology. In: DeLuca J (ed) Fatigue as a window to the brain. MIT Press, Boston
3. Bartsch HH, Weis J, Moser MT (2003) Cancer-related fatigue in patients attending oncological rehabilitation programs: prevalence, patterns, and predictors. Onkologie 26:51–57
4. Smets EMA, Garssen B, Schuster-Uitterhoeve ALJ, de Haes JCJM (1993) Fatigue in cancer patients. Br J Cancer 68:220–224
5. Jacobson DL, Gange SJ, Rose NR, Graham NM (1997) Epidemiology and estimated population burden of selected autoimmune diseases in the United States. Clin Immunol Immunopathol 84:223–243
6. Schwid SR, Covington M, Segal BM, Goodman AD (2002) Fatigue in multiple sclerosis: current understanding and future directions. J Rehabil Res Dev 39:211–224
7. Swain MG (2000) Fatigue in chronic disease. Clin Sci 99:1–8
8. Jason LA, Fennell P, Taylor RR (eds) (2003) Handbook of chronic fatigue syndrome. Wiley, New York
9. Wang B, Gladman DD, Urowitz MB (1998) Fatigue in lupus is not correlated with disease activity. J Rheumatol 25:892–895
10. Omdal R, Waterloo K, Koldingsnes W, Husby G, Mellgren SI (2003) Fatigue in patients with systemic lupus erythematosus: the psychosocial aspects. J Rheumatol 30:283–287
11. Jason LA, King CP, Richman JA, Taylor RR, Torres SR, Song S (1999) US case definition of chronic fatigue syndrome: diagnostic and theoretical issues. J Chronic Fatigue Syndrome 5:3–33
12. Spitzer R, Endicott J, Robins E (1975) Clinical criteria for psychiatric diagnosis and DSM-III. Am J Psychiatry 132:1187–1192
13. Leckliter IN, Matarazzo JD (1994) Diagnosis and classification. In: Van Hasselt VB, Hersen M (eds) Advanced Abnormal Psychology. Plenum, New York, pp 3–18
14. Garfield S (1993) Methodological problems in clinical diagnosis. In: Sutker PB, Adams HE (eds) Comprehensive handbook of psychopathology. Plenum, New York
15. American Psychiatric Association (1952) Diagnostic and statistical manual of mental disorders. American Psychiatric Association, Washington, DC
16. American Psychiatric Association (1968) Diagnostic and statistical manual of mental disorders, 2nd edn. American Psychiatric Association, Washington, DC
17. Matarazzo J (1983) The reliability of psychiatric and psychological diagnosis. In: Hooley J, Neale J, Davidson G (eds) Readings in abnormal psychology. Wiley, New York, pp 36–65
18. Helzer J, Robins L, Taibleson M, Woodruff R, Reich T, Wish E (1977) Reliability of psychiatric diagnosis. Arch Gen Psychiatry 34:129–133
19. Endicott J, Spitzer RL (1977) A diagnostic interview. The schedule for affective disorders and schizophrenia. Paper presented at the American Psychiatric Association, Toronto, Canada
20. American Psychiatric Association. (1994) Diagnostic and statistical manual of mental disorders, 4th edn. American Psychiatric Association, Washington, DC

21. First MB, Spitzer RL, Gibbon M, Williams JBW (1995) Structured clinical interview for DSM-IV axis disorders. Patient edition. Biometrics Research Department, New York State Psychiatric Institute, New York
22. Cantwell DP (1996) Classification of child and adolescent psychopathology. J Child Psychol Psychiatry 37:3–12
23. Tucker G (1998) Putting DSM-IV in perspective. Am J Psychiatry 155:159–161
24. Kendler K, Gardner C (1998) Boundaries of major depression. An evaluation of DSM-IV criteria. Am J Psychiatry 155:172–177
25. Fukuda K, Straus SE, Hickie I, Sharpe MC, Dobbins JG, Komaroff A (1994) The chronic fatigue syndrome: a comprehensive approach to its definition and study. Ann Intern Med 121:953–959
26. Hartz A, Kuhn EM, Levine PH (1998) Characteristics of fatigued persons associated with features of chronic fatigue syndrome. J Chronic Fatigue Syndrome 4:71–97
27. Friedberg F, Dechene L, McKenzie M, Fontanetta R (2000) Symptom patterns in long-term chronic fatigue syndrome. J Psychosom Res 48:59–68
28. Linder R, Dinser R, Wagner M, Krueger GRF, Hoffmann A (2002) Generation of classification criteria for chronic fatigue syndrome using an artificial neural network and traditional criteria set. In vivo 16:37–44
29. Nisenbaum R, Reyes M, Mawle AC, Reeves W (1998) Factor analysis of unexplained severe fatigue and interrelated symptoms. Am J Epidemiol 148:72–77
30. Haley RW, Kurt TL, Hom J (1997) Is there a Gulf War syndrome? Searching for syndromes by factor analysis of symptoms. J Am Med Assoc 277:215–222
31. Hall DG, Sanders SD, Replogle WH (1994) Fatigue: a new approach to an old problem. J Miss State Med Assoc 35:155–160
32. Ray C, Weir RC, Cullen S, Phillips S (1992) Illness perception and symptom components in chronic fatigue syndrome. J Psychosom Res 36:243–256
33. Jason LA, Taylor RR, Kennedy CL, Jordan K, Huang CF, Torres-Harding S, Song S, Johnson D (2002) A factor analysis of chronic fatigue symptoms in a community-based sample. Soc Psychiatry Psychiatric Epidemiol 37:183–189
34. Reeves WC, Wagner D, Nisenbaum R, Jones JF, Gurbaxani B, Solomon L, Papanicolaou D, Unger ER, Vernon SD, Heim C (2005) Chronic fatigue syndrome: a clinical empirical approach to its definition and study. BMC Med 3:19; doi:10.1186/1741-7015-3-19 (available at: http://www.biomedcentral.com/content/pdf/1741-7015-3-19.pdf)
35. Friedberg F, Jason LA (1998) Understanding chronic fatigue syndrome: an empirical guide to assessment and treatment. American Psychological Association, Washington, DC
36. Friedberg F, Jason LA (2002) Selecting a fatigue rating scale. CFS Res Rev 3:5–7, 11
37. Dittner AJ, Wessely SC, Brown RG (2004) The assessment of fatigue. A practical guide for clinicians and researchers. J Psychosom Res 56:157–170
38. Miller M, Ferris D (1993) Measurement of subjective phenomena in primary care research: the visual analogue scale. Fam Pract Res J 13:15–24
39. Jensen M, Karoly P (1992) Self-report scales and procedures for assessing pain in adults. In: Turk D, Melzack R (eds) Handbook of Pain Assessment. Guildford Press, New York
40. Chalder T, Berelowitz G, Pawlikowsy J, Watts L, Wessely D (1993) Development of a fatigue scale. J Psychosom Res 37:147–153
41. Wessely S, Powell R (1989) Fatigue syndromes: a comparison of chronic "postviral" fatigue with neuromuscular and affective disorders. J Neurol Neurosurg Psychiatry 52:940–948
42. Butler S, Chalder T, Ron M, Wessely S (1991) Cognitive behavior therapy in chronic fatigue syndrome. J Neurol Neurosurg Psychiatry 54:153–158
43. David AS, Pelosi A, McDonald E, Stephens D, Ledger D, Rathbone R, Mann A (1990) Tired, weak, or in need of rest: fatigue among general practice attenders. Br Med J 301:1199–1202
44. pawlikowska T, Chalder T, Hirsch SR, Wallace P, Wright DJM, Wessely SC (1994) Population-based study of fatigue and psychological distress. Br Med J 308:763–766
45. Loge JH, Ekeberg O, Kaasa S (1998) Fatigue in the general Norwegian population: normative data and associations. J Psychosom Res 45:53–65

46. Jason LA, Ropacki MT, Santoro NB, Richman JA, Heatherly W, Taylor RR, Ferrari JR, Haney-Davis TM, Rademaker A, Dupuis J, Golding J, Plioplys AV, Plioplys S (1997) A screening scale for chronic fatigue syndrome: reliability and validity. J Chronic Fatigue Syndrome 3:39–59
47. Morriss RK, Wearden AJ, Mullis R (1998) Exploring the validity of the Chalder fatigue scale in chronic fatigue syndrome. J Psychosom Res 45:411–417
48. Ware JE, Sherbourne CD (1992) The MOS 36-item short form health survey (SF-36). I. Conceptual framework and item selection. Med Care 30:473–483
49. Krupp LB, LaRocca NG, Muir-Nash J, Steinberg AD (1989) The fatigue severity scale: application to patients with multiple sclerosis and systemic lupus erythematosus. Arch Neurol 46:1121–1123
50. pepper CM, Krupp LB, Friedberg F, Doscher C, Coyle PK (1993) A comparison of neuropsychiatric characteristics in chronic fatigue syndrome, multiple sclerosis, and major depression. J Neuropsychiatry Clin Neurosci 5:200–205
51. Taylor RR, Jason LA, Torres A (2000) Fatigue rating scales: an empirical comparison. Psychol Med 30:849–856
52. Vercoulen JHMM, Hommes OR, Swanink CMA, Jongen PJ, Fennis JF, Galama JM, van der Meer JW, Bleijenberg G (1996) The measurement of fatigue in patients with multiple sclerosis: a multidimensional comparison with chronic fatigue syndrome and healthy subjects. Arch Neurol 53:642–649
53. Beursken AJHM, Bultmann U, Kant I, Vercoulen JHMM, Bleijenberg G, Swaen GMH (2000) Fatigue among working people: validity of a questionnaire measure. Occup Environ Med 57:353–357
54. Prins JB, Bleijenberg G, Bazelmans E, Elving LD, de Boo TM, Severens JL, van der Wilt GJ, Spinhoven P, van der Meer JWM, Prins JWM (2001) Cognitive behaviour therapy for chronic fatigue syndrome: a multicentre randomised controlled trial. Lancet 357:841–847
55. Koschera A, Hickie I, Hadzi-Pavlovic D, Wilson A, Lloyd A (1999) Prolonged fatigue, anxiety and depression: exploring relationships in a primary care sample. Aust N Z J Psychiatry 33:545–552
56. Hickie IB, Davenport T, Hadzi-Pavlovic D, Koschera A, Naismith S, Scott EM, Wilhelm K (2001) Development of a simple screening tool for common mental disorders in general practice. Med J Aust 175:S10–S17
57. Bennett BK, Hickie IB, Vollmer-Conna US, Quigley B, Brennan CM, Wakefield D, Douglas MP, Hansen GR, Tahmindjis AJ, Lloyd AR (1998) The relationship between fatigue, and psychological and immunological variables in acute infectious illness. Aust N Z J Psychiatry 32:180–186
58. Reeves WC, Lloyd A, Vernon SD, Klimas N, Jason L, Bleijenberg G, Evengard B, White PD, Nisenbaum R, Unger ER (2003) Identification of ambiguities in the 1994 chronic fatigue syndrome research case definition and recommendations for resolution. BMC Health Serv Res 3:25 (http://www.biomedcentral.com/content/pdf/1472-6963-3-25.pdf)
59. Cartmel B, Moon T (1992) Comparison of two physical activity questionnaires, with diary for assessing physical activity in an elderly population. Clin Epidemiol 45:877–883
60. paffenbarger R, Blair S, Lee I, Hyde R (1993) Measurement of physical activity to assess health effects in free-living populations. Med Sci Sports Exercise 25:60–70
61. Gerber LH, Furst G (1992) Validation of the NIH activity record. A quantitative measure of life activities. Arthritis Care Res 5:81–86
62. King CP (2001) The development of a diagnostic instrument for chronic fatigue syndrome. Unpublished doctoral dissertation, DePaul University, Chicago
63. Tryon WW, Williams R (1996) Fully proportional actigraphy: a new instrument. Behav Res Methods Instrum Comput 28:392–403
64. Jason LA, King CP, Frankenberry EL, Jordan KM, Tryon WW, Rademaker F, Huang C-F (1999) Chronic fatigue syndrome: assessing symptoms and activity level. J Clin Psychol 55:411–424

65. Tryon WW, Jason LA, Frankenberry E, Torres-Harding S (2004) Chronic fatigue syndrome impairs circadian rhythm of activity level. Physiol Behav 82:849–853
66. Ohashi K, Bleijenberg G, van der Werf S, Prins J, Amaral LAN, Natelson BH, Yamamoto Y (2004) Decreased fractal correlation in diurnal physical activity in chronic fatigue syndrome. Methods Inf Med 43:26–29
67. Barofsky I, West Legro M (1991) Definition and measurement of fatigue. Rev Infect Dis 13: S94–S97
68. Cope H (1992) Fatigue: a non-specific complaint? Int Rev Psychiatry 4:273–280
69. Stouten B (2005) Identification of ambiguities in the 1994 chronic fatigue syndrome research case definition and recommendations for resolution. BMC Health Serv Res 5:37 (doi:10.1186/1472-6963-5-37)
70. Ray C, Weir WRC, Phillips S, Cullen S (1992) Development of a measure of symptoms in chronic fatigue syndrome: the profile of fatigue-related symptoms (PFRS). Psychol Health 7:27–43
71. Wessely S (1998) The epidemiology of chronic fatigue syndrome. Epidemiol Psychiatr Soc 7:10–24
72. piper B, Lindsey A, Dodd M, Ferketich S, Paul S (1989) The development of an instrument to measure the subjective dimension of fatigue. In: Funk S, Tornquist E, Champagne M, Copp L, Wiese R (eds) Key aspects of comfort: management of pain, fatigue, and nausea. Springer, New York, pp 199–207
73. Lee KA, Hicks G, Nino-Murcia G (1991) Validity and reliability of a scale to assess fatigue. Psychiatry Res 36:291–298
74. Rhoten D (1982) Fatigue and the post-surgical patient. In: Norris DM (ed) Concept clarification in nursing. Aspen, Rockville, pp 277–300
75. Vercoulen JHMM, Swanink CMA, Fennis JFM, Galama JMD, van der Meer JWM, Bleijenberg G (1994) Dimensional assessment of chronic fatigue syndrome. J Psychosom Res 38:383–392
76. Schwartz JE, Jandorf L, Krupp LB (1993) The measurement of fatigue: a new instrument. J Psychosom Res 37:753–762
77. Belza B, Henke C, Yelin E, Epstein W, Gillis C (1993) Correlates of fatigue in older adults with rheumatoid arthritis. Nurs Res 42:93–99
78. Fisk JD, Ritvo PG, Ross L, Haase DA, Marrie TJ, Schlech WF (1994) Measuring the functional impact of fatigue: initial validation of the fatigue impact scale. Clin Infect Dis 18 (Suppl 1):S79–83
79. Smets EMA, Garssen B, Bonk B, Haes JCJM (1995) The multi-dimensional fatigue inventory (MFI): psychometric qualities of an instrument to assess fatigue. J Psychosom Res 39:315–325
80. McNair D, Lorr R, Droppleman L (1992) Edits manual for the Profile of Mood States. Educational and Industrial Testing Services, San Diego

Fatigue: Epidemiology and Social/Industrial Aspects

Birgitta Evengård

Summary

There is no doubt that the symptoms of fatigue are costly for both society and for the individual. Fatigue is found in a spectrum of diseases and illnesses caused by pathology in biological systems, but also by environmental factors which directly or indirectly influence biological systems in the human body. Although it has been known for a long time that more women than men suffer from this group of illnesses, little research has focused on the influence of gender, e.g., the circumstances which women and men live under, on the outcome of fatigue-related health problems. The complex interaction between different regulatory systems connecting body, soul, and mind is clearer today as molecular techniques are being developed. Data on a genetic linkage to chronic fatigue have also been established.

The evaluation of huge data sets evolving from molecular epidemiological studies and successfully integrating sets of data from other studies covering many dimensions of human life has the potential to improve the general health of the community and promote the prevention of illness.

The need to include social dimensions such as gender, e.g., the social constructs of the roles and behavior of women and men, girls and boys, and also other groups with less influence in a particular society, e.g., immigrants, refugees, the handicapped, and other groups characterized by some sort of stigma, when working toward improved health is widely understood today and possible in practise. The main issue remains whether or not the politics of the day will let it happen, whether appropriate policy documents will be published, and above all whether money for research and development will be distributed.

Chronic illnesses are a major part of the burden of ill health in modern society. To be able to prevent, bring relief to, and to cure these conditions would be a major

---

Division of Infectious Diseases, Department of Clinical Microbiology, Umeå University, SE-901 85 Umeå, Sweden

achievement with impacts on the level of individual health and economy, as well as at the societal level. A study from the Centre for Disease Control (CDC), Atlanta, USA, has estimated the national costs for chronic fatigue syndrome (CFS) alone to represent an annual productivity loss of US $9.1 billion [1]. In Sweden, since the end of the 1990s, there have been many people on sick leave or taking early retirement. Many of the causes for this have fatigue as a dominant symptom. The cost for sick leave and early retirement in Sweden alone is more than US $17 billion annually.

First, one needs to agree what fatigue is, as it is not defined by a numeric value [2,3]. One definition accepted by an international network of researchers [4] in the field is as follows:

> ". . . fatigue is a lack of energy that affects mental and physical activity, which differs from sleepiness and lack of motivation, and which may be aggravated by, but is not primarily attributable to, minor exercise or diagnosable diseases."

There is no doubt that it is not a symptom that is considered to have much value in medical education, and thus by the medical profession. However, among patients, it is a symptom of primary concern.

To date, there are have been few publications on the epidemiology of the various forms of chronic fatigue throughout the world [5,6,7,8,9]. It is important to differentiate studies performed within clinical samples (primary care, tertiary reference centres) from those performed at the population level, which present little selection bias.

Within our research group in Sweden, ongoing work is focusing on describing the epidemiological patterns and the role of genes and the environment in the most severe phenotype of fatigue illnesses, chronic fatigue syndrome (CFS), in a representative sample of the Swedish population, the Swedish Twin Registry [9]. In this project, the collection of epidemiological data, clinical and biological data, and psychological and sociodemographic data are included, and most are evaluated from a gender perspective. Although most studies report that a majority of patients are women, to date there are few if any studies presenting data with a gender perspective. We think this is an important aspect of research design for a condition of unknown origin, which entails high costs both for the individual and for society. We also believe that an integrated approach is the solution, and may be the only one to approach the true cause of this illness.

We describe the prevalence of conditions characterized by chronic fatigue and their risk factors in patients and affected twins, and in particular in an affected twin in comparison to their healthy co-twin [10]. This population-based design gives us the possibility of evaluating the validity of the CFS definition and later, through molecular epidemiology, identifying biological determinants which may be of potential value for diagnosis [11,12]. These data were also analyzed from a gender perspective. Through the collection of different kinds of environmental data, social and psychological influences can also be described [13]. This opens up discussion into future avenues of investigation on the best treatment schemes. In this chapter, some of our findings will be presented and discussed, together with a review of other reports.

Background to CFS

The signs and symptoms which provide the basis for any definition of a chronic fatigue state have been described in the literature since the end of the 19th century. At that time the condition was labeled *neurasthenia*, but during the last three decades, several alternative terms have been introduced, such as postviral fatigue syndrome, myalgic encephalomyelitis, and Iceland disease [14,15]. Since 1994, there has been an agreement to use the term chronic fatigue syndrome in the clinical setting, and the diagnostic criteria published by the CDC are to be applied for research purposes [16]. Nowadays, CFS can be summarized as a severe fatigue experience with a minimal duration of 6 months, involving physical, emotional, and cognitive impairment in daily life activities, and showing at least four of the eight ancillary symptoms defined (presence of sore throat, tender lymph nodes, muscle pain, multi-joint pain, headache with new onset, unrefreshing sleep, postexertional malaise, and impaired memory and/or concentration). However, this definition has been challenged by some researchers and the ambiguities which arise can only be resolved in an international study, since different influences (biological, social, cultural, environmental) will influence the subjective criteria included [17].

Etiological Debate

There is no predominant explanatory model for the origin and development of CFS [18,19,20]. An array of biological hypotheses regarding the causative mechanisms has been promulgated, including immune dysfunction, body dysfunction following infection, neuroendocrine dysfunction, and cardiorespiratory and sleep abnormalities [21,22,23,24,25a,25b,26]. In parallel, psychological and psychosocial factors have also been considered, either for their direct involvement or in conjunction with biological factors [27a,27b,28,29,30]. Extensive discussions have considered the possible role of psychiatric conditions, such as depression and anxiety disorders, in the differential diagnosis or as co-morbid conditions [11,31,32,33]. Adding to this is a growing bulk of work on the possible genetic background of CFS. CFS is a complex illness, where genetic and environmental factors may possibly interact in the susceptible individual [34].

We designed a study using the Swedish Twin Registry (STR), which to date is the largest in the world to perform a population-based study [9]. This was also a nation-wide study, because we know that the geographical spread of twins represents the Swedish population as seen in other contexts. In short we screened 31 405 individuals (aged 42–65 years) for symptoms of fatiguing illness via a telephone questionnaire. We refined these self-reported symptoms via data from several national registries (registries for death, Swedish national cancer register, and in-patient hospitalization), and from a physicians' review of all available medical records (n = 2489) in order to reach a close approximation to the dominant case definition of CFS.

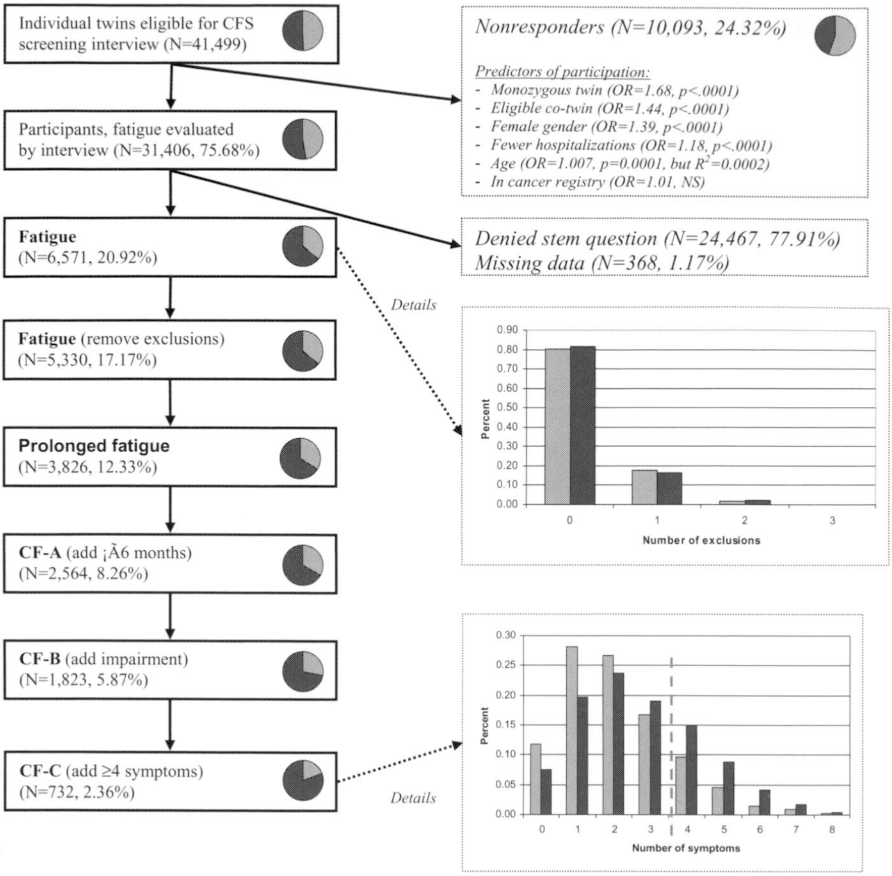

Fig. 1. Flowchart depicting the definitions of fatigue-related variables. As data were available on all twins regardless of participation, we could evaluate the predictors of participation. The small pie charts in each box show the proportions of males (*light grey*) and females (*dark grey*). Details regarding reliability, a symptom histogram, and the numbers of exclusionary conditions are also shown. CFS, chronic fatigue syndrome. From Evengard et al 2005 with permission

This study revealed four striking findings:

1. the high prevalence of CFS-like illness;
2. the arbitrariness of the cut-off point chosen for the number of symptoms in the current CFS definition;
3. the influence of gender;
4. the lack of a predictive effect of education or occupation.

The prevalence of CFS is described in Fig. 1, together with results from other population-based studies shown as sex-disaggregated data. We started by asking about fatigue during the last 6 months, and then asked the twins many more stringent questions. From Fig. 1, it is clear that the prevalence and gender composition

Table 1. Epidemiology of chronic fatigue (CFS-like illness) and chronic fatigue syndrome (CFS) studied in population-based samples, showing gender distribution

Year of study	Study site	Point prevalence of CFS-like illness	Ratio ♀/♂	Point prevalence of true CFS	Reference
1995–1997	Chicago, Illinois	1.42%	ND	0.42%	Jason et al. 1999
1997	Wichita, Kansas	0.98%	2 : 6	0.23%	Reyes et al. 2003
1998	Iceland	1.4%	3 : 5	ND	Lindal et al. 2002
1998–2002	Sweden	2.36%	4 : 2	ND	Evengard et al. 2005

change as the definition becomes more stringent. CF-A means fatigue with a duration of more than 6 months, CF-B is the same as CF-A plus impairment, and CF-C also adds the presence of more than four of the eight symptoms in the current definition.

Over one-fifth of the sample (21%) declared that they had suffered fatigue during the last 6 months. When we removed the data on twins who had plausible explanations for their fatigue (which we found by comparisons with registries and with medical records), the prevalence was 18%. When we asked about fatigue lasting more than 1 month the prevalence sank to 12%, and with the inclusion of a CFS-like illness (CF-C) the prevalence was 2.4%. This estimate is considerably higher than that found in the population interview studies of CFS-like illness in the United States (0.007% and 0.23%), but is comparable to population questionnaire surveys in the USA and Iceland [7,8] (Table 1).

The prevalence of CFS could not be estimated as no clinical evaluation was performed. The two population studies that estimated the prevalence of CFS (0.42% and 0.24%) had low participation rates in the clinical examination phase (41% and 54%) and could have underestimated the prevalence of CFS. Thus, the results of our study suggest that the prevalence of current CFS might be considerably higher than has previously been recognized.

Current Definition of CFS

In the current internationally accepted definition of CFS there are eight symptoms. This definition implies the presence of a qualitative difference between individuals with 0–3 symptoms and those with 4–8 symptoms. However, the lack of discontinuity between three and four symptoms in either men or women, as seen in Fig. 1, suggests the arbitrariness of the cut-off point. The ambiguities with this definition can be resolved by using a different type of study design, i.e., population-based, including latent class analysis and cluster analysis of symptoms. The great expense and labour involved stress the need for a study with global involvement.

Demographic Data

Demographic data from our study are presented in Table 2.

Gender. As shown in Table 2, the preponderance of females increased (to nearly four times more than males) and the total prevalence decreased with increasingly restrictive definitions of the illness. The nature and source of the profound impact of gender on the risk of fatigue is unknown, but it is likely to be highly complex as it could be the result of factors that operate from the genetic to the sociological level. Future studies should benefit from the inclusion of this perspective in an all-time integrated manner [35].

Education. Sweden is a country with equal access to medical care and basic education for both sexes. Thus, it is not surprising that there were no differences in educational attainment between fatigued and nonfatigued subjects. Two community-based studies and one nation-wide study from the USA all demonstrated that CFS patients had lower educational levels than nonfatigued individuals. Our study, which also represents full coverage of an entire country, demonstrates no such differences in risk, despite known inequalities in health status as a function of socioeconomic status. Therefore, there is little evidence to support the supposition that fatigue is a malady of the educated as previously thought.

Occupation. Much of the attention to societal costs related to sick leave involving fatigue and CFS has focused on the influence of the working environment. Poorly structured working environments, unemployment, and insecure jobs have been put forward as an explanation for the large-scale deterioration of psychological well-being in the population in Sweden. In our data, there was a strong relationship between occupation and CFS-like illness (when the analysis was not substantially confounded by the influence of gender). Our findings underscore the need to evaluate risk factors separately by gender. Despite the fact that 79% of Swedish women and 84% of Swedish men are in the work force, 44% of women work in areas which are dominated (>60%) by women, such as service-related professions. The clear female preponderance with increasingly restrictive criteria for CFS-like illness could well reflect specific working-life inequalities, but not occupational categories per se. In Sweden, parts of the work force dominated by women (with the public as the employer) were the target for thorough structural changes and cut-downs before the onset of the ongoing epidemic of high rates of sick leave. It is plausible that this has had an impact of the poorer level of health in the country. Thus, despite the uneven distribution of occupation by gender, fatigue is not predicted by occupation. Other environmental factors, and the biological consequences of the female gender in this context, should be further explored.

Health Status. As expected, in this study fatiguing illness was strongly associated with a greater likelihood of poorer health status and greater health-related impairment (Table 2). The debilitating effects of CFS-like illness are notable, as reflected by clear increases in reports of poorer health, and increasing number of days of

Table 2. The relationships between increasingly stringent definitions of fatiguing illness, and demography and health status[a]

Variable	Entire sample (N = 31 406)	CF-A (N = 2564)	CF-B (N = 1823)	CF-C (N = 732)	Statistical comparisons CF-A	CF-B	CF-C
Females	47.51%	66.89%	71.97%	80.87%	1.92 (1.76–2.09)	2.43 (2.19–2.70)*	3.92 (3.24–4.72)*
Age at interview (years, mean (SD))	53.7 (5.8)	53.2 (5.5)	53.0 (5.5)	52.7 (5.3)	0.99 (0.98–0.99)	0.99 (0.98–0.99)*	0.99 (0.99–1.00)*
Years of education (mean (SD))	11.1 (3.1)	11.1 (3.0)	11.3 (3.0)	11.1 (2.9)	1.00 (1.00–1.00), NS	1.00 (1.00–1.00), NS	1.00 (1.00–1.00), NS
Occupation (%)					Total, χ^2 = 73.0*	Total, χ^2 = 93.0*	Total, χ^2 = 33.0*
Legislators, senior officials,	7.00	4.96	4.52	4.34	Male, χ^2 = 15.2, NS	Male, χ^2 = 13.2, NS	Male, χ^2 = 16.3, 0.03
managers	15.72	14.63	15.97	12.75			
Professionals	18.41	18.87	19.93	17.09	Female, χ^2 = 11.2, NS	Female, χ^2 = 13.9, NS	Female, χ^2 = 10.1, NS
Technicians, associated	10.97	11.86	12.34	12.61			
professionals	18.66	23.35	24.23	29.69			
Clerks	2.98	2.54	2.01	1.82			
Service workers, shop sales	11.33	9.32	7.93	7.00			
workers	10.16	8.88	7.59	8.40			
Skilled agricultural or fishery	4.76	5.59	5.47	6.30			
workers							
Craft, related trade workers							
Machine operators, assemblers							
Elementary occupations							
Health status (%)							
General health excellent/good	53.98	57.66	52.31	45.21	1.17 (1.08–1.27)*	0.92 (0.84–1.01), NS	0.69 (0.60–0.80)*
Better/same health as 5 years	76.68	47.45	41.71	35.76	0.24 (0.22–0.26)*		0.16 (0.14–0.19)*
earlier	73.31	40.70	30.82	17.81	0.22 (0.20–0.24)*	0.19 (0.18–0.21)*	0.08 (0.06–0.09)*
Health does not limit activities	87.81	69.11	61.88	53.69	0.27 (0.24–0.29)*	0.14 (0.13–0.16)*	0.15 (0.13–0.18)*
Days when health limited activities (0–7)						0.20 (0.18–0.22)*	

[a] See text for definitions of CF-A, CF-B, and CF-C. For age, the odds ratios are per decade. For occupation, the χ^2 statistics have 8 df. The statistical comparisons for the four health status variables show the odds ratios and 95% confidence intervals (via generalized estimating equations) for health status as the dependent variable and fatigue as the independent variable. (From Evengard et al 2005 with permission)

* $P < 0.0001$

health-related impairment in normal activities. As shown in Table 2, the most severely fatigued subjects (CF-C) report significant impairment in perceived health status. Moreover, these effects are generally evident for less severe definitions of fatiguing illness (CF-A and CF-B). The impact of the symptom of chronic fatigue from the subject's perspective is of great significance. In contrast, the medical records rarely mentioned fatigue (data not shown). Thus, there is a discrepancy between the subject's experience of the impact of chronic fatigue and its salience in the medical sphere. Medical education in the Western world does not include these aspects, and thus the medical profession is, in general, not attentive to the symptom of fatigue.

Heterogeneity of Patients According to the Current Definition

During the last decade, all research has been based on the criteria set up by the international consensus meeting in 1994 [16]; the symptoms included represent a consensus derived from several older criteria. This historical fact illustrates the heterogeneity of the clinical cases of CFS, ranging from obviously more postinfectious, acute cases, to prolonged suffering with psychosocial hallmarks. In order to address this debate, we have performed a latent class analysis of all symptoms reported by Swedish twins recognizing prolonged fatigue [36]. The results are summarized in Table 3. The five distinguishable subtypes obtained show that the distribution of symptoms between groups is skewed, as well as the impact on gender proportion. It is very interesting that 14% of this population has been classified in this context to be "CFS-like." This class most probably includes patients with ME = myalgic encephalopothy; a diagnosis put forward by patients organisations. Experienced clinicians know that there are patients who fit no other classification. However, the use of the current definition, which results from studies focusing on causalities, will be blurred by the heterogeneity of the subjects studied. The other classes were dominated by men (residual) or by women (rheumatic, depressive, and acute physical syndrome). Of course the criteria in the definition have importance both from a clinical point of view and for research and development of treatment schemes. The need for a definition based on results from designed studies is illustrated by articles highlighting ambiguities in the current definition and stressing the need for subtypes [37].

Genetics in Twins

When symptoms were compared between female and male monozygotic and dizygotic twins, no trait of heritability could be found [38]. When using twin statistics, and looking into additive genetic effects, shared environmental effects, and individual-specific environmental effects, no difference was found between women and men.

We found that despite substantial differences in prevalence, the relative importance of genes and environment was similar in both genders. However, there are modest genetic effects for most definitions of fatigue in females and for the first three in males. Otherwise individual-specific effects were the predominant source of variation. In addition, a small but conceptually important contribution of shared environmental effects was found. In theory, genetic variation can also be a host factor of importance in the causality behind CFS. The results indicate that it should be relevant to search for genes that confer vulnerability to CFS-like illness. Interestingly, the results from a population-based study in the USA designed by the Center for Disease Control (CDC) included the finding that the patterns of expression of about two dozen genes are different in CFS patients [39]. These results are discussed in more detail below.

Stress and Personality

In a case-controlled study assessing the prospective association of premorbid self-reported stress and personality using the data from the investigation of twins, and comparing these with data collected 25 years earlier, it was found that elevated premorbid stress is a significant risk factor for CFS-like illness, the effect of which may be buffered by genetic influences [40].

Emotional instability assessed 25 years earlier is associated with chronic fatigue through genetic mechanisms, which contribute to both personality style and expression of the disorder. These are plausible mechanisms for chronic fatiguing illness. To date, these data have not been analyzed in a sex-disaggregated manner.

Other gender differences have been found, not in the twin population but in a cohort of CFS patients at a tertiary clinic. Comparisons were made with healthy controls and patients with diabetes mellitus (unpublished data). Patients with CFS reported more negative life events than healthy controls, and women with CFS reported more negative life events than men. Women with CFS differed from healthy women in that they had experienced significantly more negative life events (in clusters of loss, work, and bullying). When a symptom check list reflecting the psychopathology (the internationally validated SCL-90) was used, it was found that both females and males with CFS had significantly more symptoms of somatization, obsessive–compulsive disorder, depression, and anxiety than the healthy women and men. There was also a strong correlation between negative life events and symptoms in the SCL-90 for both sexes when patients with CFS were compared with healthy controls.

Clearly it is unlikely that analyzing one or just a few variables will explain such a complex illness as CFS. To be able to analyze large amounts of data in an integrative manner should be a way to move forward in this field of science.

"High-throughput 'omic' technology is increasingly used in clinical and epidemiological studies but our ability to analyze and interpret high-content and complex databases has not kept pace. This is not because the mathematical and

Table 3. Latent class analysis of 11 fatigue-related characteristics with gender distribution

	Fatigued sample	Class 1	Class 2	Class 3	Class 4	Class 5
Class probability	1.00	0.14	0.29	0.17	0.35	0.05
Class label/mnemonic	—	CFS-like	Residual	Rheumatic	Depressive	Acute physical syndrome
Female	0.62	0.87 ↑	0.44 ↓	0.65	0.65	0.61
Memory deterioration	0.49	0.98 ↑	0.09 ↓	0.33 ↓	0.74 ↑	0.33 ↓
Sore throat	0.12	0.27 ↑	0.04	0.03	0.05	0.94 ↑
Tender lymph nodes	0.07	0.22 ↑	0.00	0.03	0.02	0.51 ↑
Muscle pain	0.38	0.95 ↑	0.09 ↓	0.79 ↑	0.14 ↓	0.69 ↑
Multijoint pain	0.29	0.75 ↑	0.05 ↓	0.79 ↑	0.04 ↓	0.40
Headache	0.11	0.35 ↑	0.02	0.07	0.11	0.19
Unrefreshing sleep	0.80	0.97 ↑	0.56 ↓	0.85	0.91	0.81
Postexertional malaise	0.16	0.55 ↑	0.02	0.14	0.12	0.26
Impairment	0.61	0.99 ↑	0.16 ↓	0.64	0.84 ↑	0.57
Duration ≥6 months	0.49	0.87 ↑	0.25 ↓	0.67 ↑	0.51	0.17 ↓
Fatigue classification						
Prolonged fatigue	0.73	0.94	0.54	0.83	0.78	0.51
CF-A	0.49	0.87	0.25	0.67	0.51	0.17
CF-B	0.36	0.86	0.02	0.44	0.44	0.08
CF-C	0.14	0.86	0.00	0.11	0.01	0.04
Mean number of symptoms	2.4 (1.6)	5.03 (1.01)	0.86 (0.69)	3.03 (0.89)	2.14 (0.82)	4.13 (1.20)
Mean months of fatigue (SD)	27.3 (60.5)	62.1 (84.8)	10.2 (36.6)	38.8 (69.8)	24.2 (55.3)	7.65 (29.1)
Validators						
Mean age at interview (years (SD))	52.5 (5.6)	52.2 (5.35)	52.9 (5.81)	53.4 (5.44)	51.9 (5.53)	52.7 (5.43)
Major depressive episode in lifetime	0.37	0.57	0.20	0.35	0.44	0.31
Chronic widespread pain	0.08	0.30	0.01	0.12	0.03	0.04

The top panel shows the class–item probabilities from a 5 latent class solution. The lower two panels show potential validators of the latent class solution relating to fatigue (middle panel), and characteristics of relevance to chronic fatigue (lower panel), where the values shown are proportions of the class or mean (SD), as appropriate (From Sullivan et al. 2005, with permission)

computational means do not exist. Rather, it is because optimal understanding of complex diseases requires an integrated perspective of several disciplines." This quote is from an article by Vernon & Reeves [39], and it really emphasizes that complex illnesses represent alterations in homeostatic systems arising from the combined action of several factors, such as genes, behavior and environment. Now we are starting to use molecular methods to analyze these factors, and considerable amounts of data are being generated [31,32]. However, we also need to develop the tools to analyze this data.

It really seems as if we are at a moment when huge transitions can take place in the realm of research. Today, biological and psychological data can be co-analyzed with social data and environmental factors of potential influence for the pathology.

To talk about a shift of paradigm might be a little premature but a movement toward an integrative approach to research into the complex conditions of unhealthy people is certainly a change for many researchers educated in the old-fashioned academic way.

Recently, data on a genetic linkage to chronic fatigue have come from several research groups [31,34]. As mentioned above, at CDC, CFS has been linked to five mutations in three genes that are related to the body's ability to handle stress. Also, people with the syndrome have differences in genetic activity levels that affect the way they respond to stress accumulated over a lifetime. CDC Director Julie Gerberding said, this research "is really the first credible evidence of the biological basis for chronic fatigue syndrome".

These findings arose from a longitudinal population-based study in Wichita, from 1997 to 2000. The data gathered from the 227 participants, at a cost of about US $2 million, included a full clinical evaluation, electrophysiological measurements of sleep physiology, cognitive function, and autonomic nervous system function, and detailed blood work that included DNA and gene activity analysis. About 50 genes were targeted, as well as 500 polymorphisms in genes that are active in the hypothalamus–pituitary–adrenal (HPA) axis [39].

Of importance were five single nucleotide polymorphisms (SNPs) in three genes: those coding for the glucocorticoid receptor, for serotonin, and for tryptophan hydroxylase. These are of importance in the function of the HPA, which is the body's stress response system. The effect of the variations appears to be that people with these polymorphisms are less able to cope with stress.

In one of the many reports coming out of this study, three distinct fatigued groups were identified: those with extreme fatigue, those with symptoms such as heart-rate variability and cortisol disturbances, and a group that was primarily menopausal women. Again, the importance of sex-disaggregated data is highlighted.

The growing body of evidence that patients with CFS have abnormalities in gene expression was reinforced by the findings of Kerr et al [11]. Immune activation and mitochondrial dysfunction was confirmed when more than 9000 genes were analyzed in 25 patients and 25 controls. In 16 genes, reproducible alterations in gene regulation were detected.

Gräns et al. (2005) reported from the patient cohort in Stockholm that three genes (CD83, NRK1, BOLA1) were activated in women who had a noninfectious and slow onset of the illness [31]. Again, this points to the importance of the subgrouping of patients when analyzing data.

However, all of these findings in small cohorts should be interpreted with care, and more studies including a higher number of patients need to be done before these findings are established.

Estrogen and Estrogen Receptors—A Recent Field of Research

The sex difference observed for CFS indicates a role for estrogen and estrogen receptors (ERs) in disease development. Estrogen is a steroid hormone that plays important roles in various physiological processes, including sexual development and the reproductive cycle.

Furthermore, an immunomediated pathogenesis has been suggested for CFS which provides an additional connection to estrogen, a hormone which displays immunomodular functions. Several autoimmune diseases such as rheumatoid arthritis (RA) and multiple sclerosis (MS) afflict more women than men. Also, MS and RA usually improve during pregnancy, suggesting that estrogen could play an immunosuppressive role in these contexts. Estrogen exerts its effects by binding to the estrogen receptors (ERs). Both CFS and estrogen have been linked to a Th2-type response of the immune system. Frequency differences between patients and control groups in naturally occurring base-pair changes, referred to as single nucleotide polymorphisms (SNPs), indicate a linkage of the particular genomic region and the disease under study. An association of SNPs in ER-β with disease has been reported in, e.g., anorexic and bulimic patients. These diseases also occur predominantly in women.

We investigated a possible association of ER mRNAs and two ER-β single nucleotide polymorphisms (SNPs) with CFS [41]. Messenger RNA levels of ER-α, ER-βwt, and ER-βcx were investigated in peripheral blood mononuclear cells (PBMCs) from 30 CFS patients and 36 healthy controls by quantitative real-time polymerase chain reaction (PCR). Two ER-β SNPs were scored in the same material.

The CFS patient group showed significantly lower mRNA expression levels of ER-βwt compared with the healthy control group. No differences were observed for ER-α or ER-βcx between patients and controls. There were no significant differences in frequency of the ER-β SNPs investigated between patients and controls.

The reduced ER-βwt expression levels observed in this study are consistent with an immune-mediated pathogenesis of CFS. In addition, the observation that ER-βwt expression is decreased in CFS could provide an entry point for identifying interesting and potentially disease-causing candidate molecules for further study. A possible connection between estrogen, ERs, and CFS should be further evaluated.

Based on the unequal sex distribution for CFS and the reported improvement in health status after estrogen treatment, we hypothesized that differential expression of ERs could occur in CFS. In this study, we investigate this hypothesis by exploring possible associations between ER mRNA expression levels and/or genetic variants and CFS.

Some studies have indicated an association of CFS with de-regulation of immune functions and hypothalamic–pituitary–adrenal (HPA) axis activity. In studies reported from CDC [42,43], the association of sequence variations in the glucocorticoid receptor gene (NR3C1) with CFS was examined, since NR3C1 is a major effector of the HPA axis. There were 137 participants in the study. Nine single nucleotide polymorphisms (SNPs) in NR3C1 were tested for an association of polymorphisms and haplotypes with CFS. An association of multiple SNPs with chronic fatigue was observed compared with nonfatigued (NF) subjects ($P < 0.05$), and similar associations were found with quantitative assessments of functional impairment (by the SF-36), with fatigue (by the multidimensional fatigue inventory), and with symptoms (assessed by the Center for Disease Control Symptom Inventory). Subjects homozygous for the major allele of all associated SNPs were at increased risk of CFS, with odds ratios ranging from 2.61 (Cl 1.05–6.45) to 3.00 (Cl 1.12–8.05). These results demonstrate that NR3C1 is a potential mediator of chronic fatigue, and implicate variations in the 5′ region of NR3C1 as a possible mechanism through which the alterations in HPA axis regulation and the behavioral characteristics of CFS may be manifest. Existing treatment schemes [44,45] will possibly be modified by, or exchanged for biological manipulations.

Obviously, with new techniques which are capable of detecting pathology in the genome in patients suffering from disease and complex illnesses, CFS science has moved forward toward an increased understanding of the mechanisms involved in the pathology. The evaluation of huge data sets evolving from molecular epidemiological studies, which successfully integrate sets of data from other studies covering many dimensions of human life, has the potential to provide better health care and promote the prevention of illness.

The need to include social dimensions such as gender, e.g., the social constructs of the roles and behavior of women and men, girls and boys, and also other groups with less influence in a particular society, e.g., immigrants, refugees, the handicapped, and other groups characterized by some sort of stigma, when working towards improved health is today widely understood and possible in practise. The main issue remains whether or not the politics of the day will let it happen, whether appropriate policy documents will be published, and above all whether money for research and development will be distributed.

References

1. Reynolds KJ, Vernon SD, Bouchery E, et al. (2004) The economic impact of chronic fatigue syndrome. Cost Eff Resour Alloc 2:4

2. Asbring P, Narvanen AL (2003) Ideal versus reality: physicians perspectives on patients with chronic fatigue syndrome (CFS) and fibromyalgia. Soc Sci Med 57:711–720
3. Bottiger LE (1967) [Fatigue: the incapacity to continue]. Lakartidningen 64:984–992
4. Jones JF, Kohl KS, Ahmadipour N, Bleijenberg G, Buchwald D, Evengard B, Jason LA, Klimas NG, Lloyd A, McCleary K, Oleske JM, White PD; The Brighton Collaboration Fatigue Working Group (2007) Fatigue: Case definition and guidelines for collection, analysis, and presentation of immunization safety data. Vaccine. March 12: Epub ahead of print
5. Lewis G, Wessely S (1992) The epidemiology of fatigue: more questions than answers. J Epidemiol Community Health 46:92–97
6. Jason LA, Richman JA, Rademaker AW, et al. (1999) A community-based study of chronic fatigue syndrome. Arch Intern Med 159:2129–2137
7. Reyes M, Nisenbaum R, Hoaglin DC, et al. (2003) Prevalence and incidence of chronic fatigue syndrome in Wichita, Kansas. Arch Intern Med 163:1530–1536
8. Lindal E, Stefansson JG, Bergmann S (2002) The prevalence of chronic fatigue syndrome in Iceland: a national comparison by gender drawing on four different criteria. Nord J Psychiatr 56:273–277
9. Evengard B, Jacks A, Pedersen NL, et al. (2005) The epidemiology of chronic fatigue in the Swedish Twin Registry. Psychol Med 35:1317–1326
10. Demitrack MA (1997) Neuroendocrine correlates of chronic fatigue syndrome: a brief review. J Psychiatr Res 31:69–82
11. Kerr JR, Christian P, Hodgetts A, et al. (2006) Current research priorities in chronic fatigue syndrome/myalgic encephalomyelitis (CFS/ME): disease mechanisms, a diagnostic test and specific treatments. J Clin Pathol Aug 25, Epub ahead of print
12. Steinau M, Unger ER, Vernon SD, et al. (2004) Differential-display PCR of peripheral blood for biomarker discovery in chronic fatigue syndrome. J Mol Med 82:750–755
13. Evengard B, Jonzon E, Sandberg A, et al. (2003) Differences between patients with chronic fatigue syndrome and with chronic fatigue at an infectious disease clinic in Stockholm, Sweden. Psychiatr Clin Neurosci 57:361–368
14. Beard GM (1869) Neurasthenia, or nervous exhaustion. Boston Med Surg J 80:217–221
15. Holmes GP, Kaplan JE, Gantz NM, et al. (1988) Chronic fatigue syndrome: a working case definition. Ann Intern Med 108:387–389
16. Fukuda K, Straus SE, Hickie I, et al. (1994) The chronic fatigue syndrome: a comprehensive approach to its definition and study. International Chronic Fatigue Syndrome Study Group. Ann Intern Med 121:953–959
17. Reeves WC, Lloyd A, Vernon SD, et al. (2003) Identification of ambiguities in the 1994 chronic fatigue syndrome research case definition and recommendations for resolution. BMC Health Serv Res 3:25
18. Evengard B, Schacterle RS, Komaroff AL (1999) Chronic fatigue syndrome: new insights and old ignorance. J Intern Med 246:455–469
19. Evengard B, Klimas N (2002) Chronic fatigue syndrome: probable pathogenesis and possible treatments. Drugs 62:2433–2446
20. Wessely S (1997) Chronic fatigue syndrome: a 20th century illness? Scand J Work Environ Health 23 Suppl 3:17–34
21. Klimas NG, Salvato FR, Morgan R, et al. (1990) Immunologic abnormalities in chronic fatigue syndrome. J Clin Microbiol 28:1403–1410
22. Krupp LB, Jandorf L, Coyle PK, et al. (1993) Sleep disturbance in chronic fatigue syndrome. J Psychosom Res 37:325–331
23. Lloyd AR, Wakefield D, Boughton C, et al. (1988) What is myalgic encephalomyelitis? Lancet 1:1286–1287
24. Abbey SE, Garfinkel PE (1991) Neurasthenia and chronic fatigue syndrome: the role of culture in the making of a diagnosis. Am J Psychiatr 148:1638–1646
25a. Sharpe MC, Archard LC, Banatvala JE, et al. (1991) A report. Chronic fatigue syndrome: guidelines for research. J R Soc Med 84:118–121

25b. Theorell T, Blomkvist V, Lindh G, et al. (1999) Critical life events, infections, and symptoms during the year preceding chronic fatigue syndrome (CFS): an examination of CFS patients and subjects with a nonspecific life crisis. Psychosom Med 61:304–310
26. White PD, Thomas JM, Amess J, et al. (1995) The existence of a fatigue syndrome after glandular fever. Psychol Med 25:907–916; www.scb.se
27a. Fischler B (1999) Review of clinical and psychobiological dimensions of the chronic fatigue syndrome: differentiation from depression and contribution of sleep dysfunctions. Sleep Med Rev 3:131–146
27b. Katon WJ, Buchwald DS, Simon GE, et al. (1991) Psychiatric illness in patients with chronic fatigue and those with rheumatoid arthritis. J Gen Intern Med 6:277–285
28. Lindal E, Bergmann S, Thorlacius S, et al. (1997) Anxiety disorders: a result of long-term chronic fatigue. The psychiatric characteristics of the sufferers of Iceland disease. Acta Neurol Scand 96:158–162
29. Skapinakis P, Lewis G, Meltzer H (2003) Clarifying the relationship between unexplained chronic fatigue and psychiatric morbidity: results from a community survey in Great Britain. Int Rev Psychiatr 15:57–64
30. Wessely S, Powell R (1989) Fatigue syndromes: a comparison of chronic "postviral" fatigue with neuromuscular and affective disorders. J Neurol Neurosurg Psychiatr 52:940–948
31. Grans H, Nilsson P, Evengard B (2005) Gene expression profiling in the chronic fatigue syndrome. J Intern Med 258:388–390
32. Kaushik N, Fear D, Richards SC, et al. (2005) Gene expression in peripheral blood mononuclear cells from patients with chronic fatigue syndrome. J Clin Pathol 58:826–832
33. Vernon SD, Unger ER, Dimulescu IM, et al. (2002) Utility of the blood for gene expression profiling and biomarker discovery in chronic fatigue syndrome. Dis Markers 18:193–199
34. Whistler T, Unger ER, Nisenbaum R, et al. (2003) Integration of gene expression, clinical, and epidemiologic data to characterize chronic fatigue syndrome. J Transl Med 1:10
35. Richman JA, Jason LA, Taylor RR, et al. (2000) Feminist perspectives on the social construction of chronic fatigue syndrome. Health Care Women Int 21:173–185
36. Sullivan PF, Pedersen NL, Jacks A, et al. (2005) Chronic fatigue in a population sample: definitions and heterogeneity. Psychol Med 35:1337–1348
37. Jason LA, Corradi K, Torres-Harding S, et al. (2005) Chronic fatigue syndrome: the need for subtypes. Neuropsychol Rev 15:29–58
38. Sullivan P, Evengard B, Jacks A, Pedersen N (2005) Twin analysis of chronic fatigue in a Swedish national sample. Psychol Med 35:1327–1336
39. Vernon SD, Reeves WC (2006) The challenge of integrating disparate high-content data: epidemiological, clinical, and laboratory data collected during an in-hospital study of chronic fatigue syndrome. Pharmacogenomics 7(3):345–354
40. Kato K, Sullivan PF, Evengård B, Pedersen NL. Premorbid predictors of chronic fatigue. Arch Gen Psychiatr, in press
41. Gräns H, Nilsson M, Dahlman-Wright K, Evengard B (2006) Levels of estrogen receptor alpha, beta and betacx mRNA in Swedish patients with chronic fatigue syndrome. J Clin Pathol May 26, Epub
42. Rajeevan MS, Smith AK, Dimulescu I, Unger ER, Vernon SD, Heim C, Reeves WC (2006) Glucocorticoid receptor polymorphisms and haplotypes associated with chronic fatigue syndrome. Genes Brain Behav Jun 1, Epub
43. Gupta S, Aslakson E, Gorbaxani BH, Vernon SD (2002) Inclusion of the glucocorticoid receptor in a hypothalamic pituitary adrenal axis model reveals bistability. Theor Biol Med Model Feb 14;4:8
44. Surawy C, Hackmann A, Hawton K, et al. (1995) Chronic fatigue syndrome: a cognitive approach. Behav Res Ther 33:535–544
45. Rimes KA, Chalder T (2005) Treatments for chronic fatigue syndrome. Occup Med (London) 55:32–39; Science (2006) 312:669–671

Development of a Method of Evaluation of Fatigue and Its Economic Impacts

Osami Kajimoto

Summary

If a method for the qualitative and quantitative evaluation of fatigue can be developed, it will be useful not only as a means of self-monitoring by individuals and improving occupational health, but also for facilitating the development and commercialization of antifatigue medications and food supplements. Although it is difficult to determine with precision the economic loss caused by fatigue, there is no question that the successful suppression of chronic fatigue (which is one factor responsible for the onset or exacerbation of lifestyle-related chronic diseases) will greatly contribute to decreasing medical expenditure. It is known that major signs of fatigue, which appear in the form of compromised physical and mental function, are closely related to the function of the frontal lobes (which may be the center for fatigue recognition) and of the autonomic nervous system. For this reason, the quantification of fatigue requires the development of biomarkers capable of objectively and sensitively evaluating changes in frontal lobe function (working memory, etc.) and autonomic nervous system function (pulse waves, etc.). Qualitative and quantitative evaluations of fatigue will be possible by meta-analyses of changes in biochemical, immunological, and physiological markers in blood, saliva, and urine, as well as changes in brain function imaging in the presence of mental or physical stress.

Quantification of Fatigue

Significance of the Quantification of Fatigue

According to the definition proposed by Kitani [1], fatigue is a state of compromised physical and mental function, accompanied by unique pathological discomfort and the desire for rest, and arising from excessive physical and/or mental

Department of Biomarker and Molecular Biophysics, Osaka City University Graduate School of Medicine, Osaka, Japan activity. This definition suggests that the quantification of fatigue will require the development of biomarkers capable of objectively assessing discomfort and the desire for rest, as well as the degree to which physical and mental functions are compromised.

As noted in the definition provided above, "discomfort and the desire for rest" occur in "fatigue." During hard exercise, the muscles, bones, and tendons are used excessively, and the resultant fatigue is perceived by the brain. The perception of fatigue by the brain involves the transmission of fatigue-related information from peripheral tissue (muscle, etc.) to the brain, and the transduction of such information within the brain by various substances and signals. These substances and signals can thus be expected to serve as biomarkers for the quantification of fatigue.

The objective quantification of the degree of fatigue using biomarkers is of great importance. It is known that an accumulation of fatigue or stress can increase adrenocortical hormone releasing factor (CRF) and reduce splenic NK cell activity (through the activation of noradrenaline), resulting in compromise of the immune function [2]. It is also known that fatigue increases the risk of lifestyle-related diseases by reducing oxygen radical scavenging activity [3]. Therefore, if biomarkers of fatigue can be developed and a method of quantification of fatigue established, they will facilitate the prevention of fatigue due to excessive training or work, and thus contribute to the preservation and promotion of health, and control of medical expenditure. They will also allow the development of effective antifatigue medications, foods, etc., and the means to verify their efficacy, and will greatly contribute to improving the comfort of living environments (housing, etc.).

Quantification of Fatigue and Frontal Lobe Function

Previous studies of patients with chronic fatigue syndrome (CFS) revealed that the sites of the brain perceiving fatigue are probably the prefrontal area (Brodmann 9/46d) and the anterior cingulate gyrus, where reduced biosynthesis of glutamic acid (a neurotransmitter) has been noted in patients with CFS. In a study of healthy individuals exposed to mental stress, analyses of changes in brain activity using positron emission tomography (PET) following extended performance of the advanced trail-making test (ATMT) (described below) revealed the appearance of a significant increase in signals in the orbitofrontal area (Brodmann 11), the medial prefrontal area (Brodmann 10), and the anterior cingulate cortex (Brodmann 24) [4]. In a study of rats with fatigue induced by rearing them for 5 days in a cage placed in water at a depth of 1.5 cm and a water temperature of 23°C, Mizokawa et al. [5] reported reduced uptake of [^{18}F] FDG by the frontal lobe and anterior cingulate gyrus.

The prefrontal area (Brodmann 9/46d) has also been called the "superfunctioning area," and serves as the "command center" controlling volition and behavioral planning by individuals. It can also be viewed as the "center of strategy" for improving the efficiency of information processing in the brain. The anterior cingulate gyrus is known to be involved in the regulation of the sense of pain, concentration, and the autonomic nervous system. The compromised physical and mental function observed during fatigue is often identical to the symptoms observed during dysfunction of the prefrontal area or the anterior cingulate gyrus, suggesting that the prefrontal area and anterior cingulate gyrus play important roles in the mechanism of the expression of fatigue. A reduction in work efficiency, a reduction in volitional activity, a disturbance of circadian rhythms, and slow adaptation to the environment are examples of this condition.

It has been reported that injury of the prefrontal area can lead to serious impairment of the working memory, i.e., the short-term memory needed for efficient behavior and judgment [6]. Studies using PET and fMRI demonstrated that implementing tasks involving the working memory increased the activity in the prefrontal areas (area 46, among others). These findings suggest that the degree of mental fatigue, in the form of reduced work efficiency, can be quantified using working memory, which reflects prefrontal function.

Based on this hypothesis, we have developed the advanced trail-making test (ATMT), which is capable of objectively assessing changes in working memory function. The ATMT is a test to measure fatigue, and was jointly developed by Osaka University (Laboratory of Psychophysiology, Department of Psychiatrics, Osaka University School of Medicine) and Soiken. It features a visual task involving connecting the numbers 1 through 25, in order, as presented on a touch panel display. The task was developed by modifying the conventional trail-making test (which has been used in departments of neurology since the 1950s) to allow it to be used on personal computers. In the conventional trail-making test, the task is to connect the targets with a single stroke of a brush on an A4 size sheet of paper. With our modified version of the test, this task is implemented on a computer display, allowing the time required for each reaction to be measured. With the ATMT, it is also possible to present new targets by erasing targets that have been touched, and also to randomly change the location of targets. In this fashion, the ATMT allows subjects to be exposed to continuous mental stress under identical conditions, and makes it possible to measure fatigue during the task. If the results are compared between tasks which involve a change in the target arrangement each time and those which keep the target arrangement constant, it is possible to assess the extent to which a subject utilizes their memory of the arrangement during the test and, based on the results of this assessment, to evaluate their working memory.

The ATMT is composed of two tasks (F and R) with different target arrangement patterns (Fig. 1). In task F, pushing the first target (1) results in the disappearance of that target and the appearance of a new target (26), in a random location, without changing the arrangement of the other targets. In task R, pushing the first target results in the disappearance of that target and the appearance of a new target (26), in a random location, accompanied by a change in the arrangement of the other targets (2–25). During task F, the subject can decrease their reaction time by memorizing the arrangement of the other targets. During task R, on the other hand, the

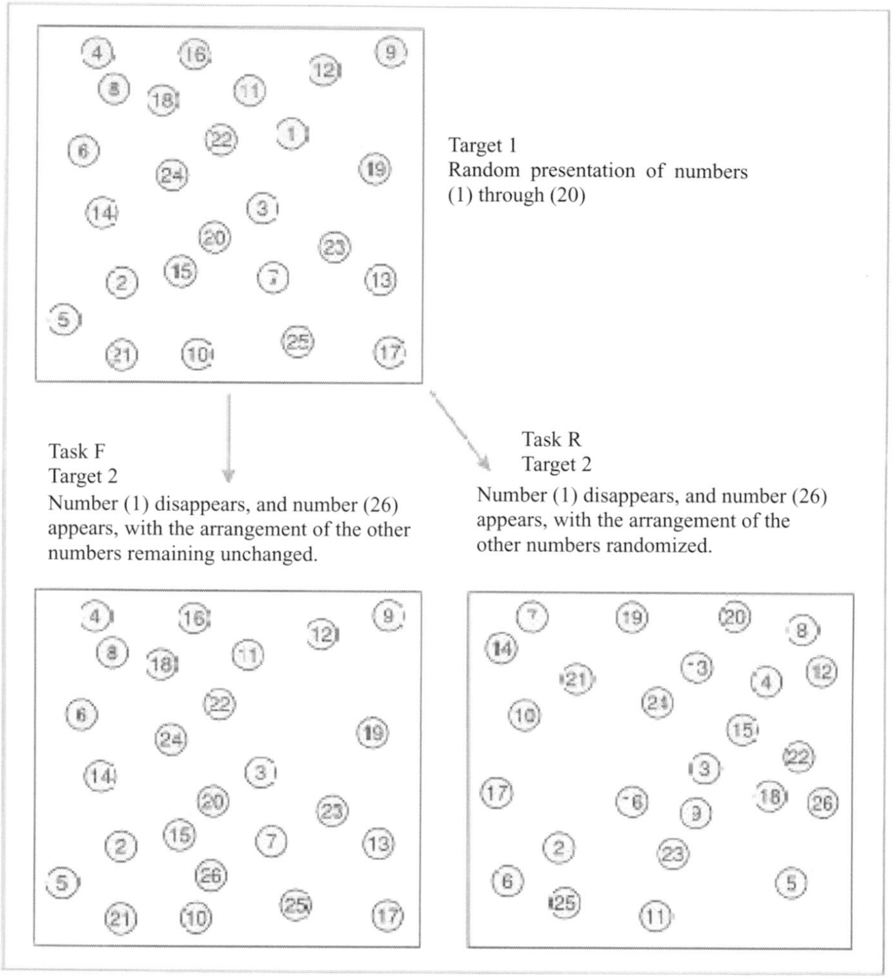

Target 1
Random presentation of numbers
(1) through (20)
Task F
Target 2
Number (1) disappears, and number (26) appears, with the arrangement of the other numbers remaining unchanged.
Task R
Target 2
Number (1) disappears, and number (26) appears, with the arrangement of the other numbers randomized.

Fig. 1. Differences between tasks F and R in the advanced trail-making test (ATMT)

subject cannot memorize the target arrangement. Thus, the functioning level of the working memory can be assessed by comparing the reaction time in task F (which allows efficient information processing via the use of working memory) with that in task R (which does not permit the use of working memory).

Figure 2 shows the reaction time for each target in tasks F and R. During task F the target arrangement is fixed, allowing the subject to memorize the target positions and to gradually decrease their reaction time. During task R the target arrangement is changed each time a target is reached, requiring the subject to locate the next target from among a new arrangement of 25 numbers after each target number is reached. During this task, all targets (1–25) are of identical design, making it

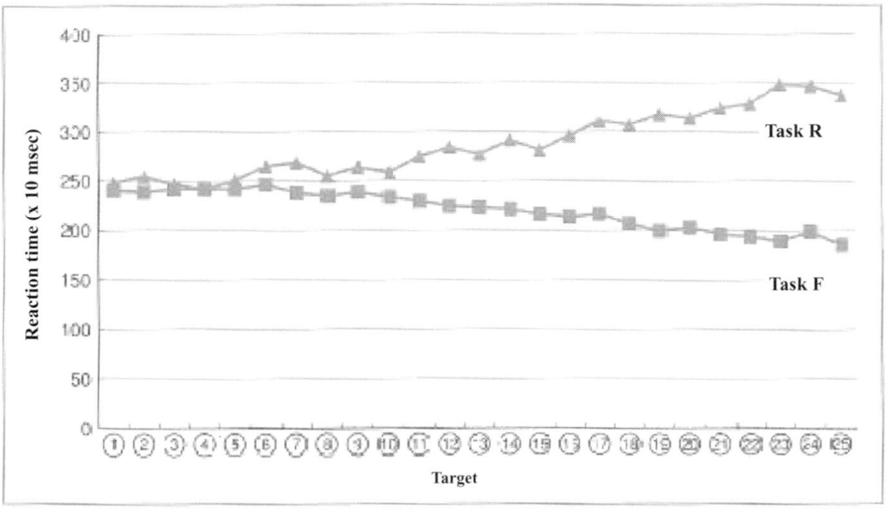

Fig. 2. Patterns of reaction times in the ATMT for healthy individuals

impossible for the subject to utilize their working memory. Therefore, during task R, the reaction time from target to target will not decrease, and instead tends to become longer during the latter half of the test. A comparison of reaction times between these two tasks allows an evaluation of the level of functioning of the subject's prefrontal area on the basis of the extent of the use of working memory.

Unlike the difference in reaction time between task F and task R, the prolongation of reaction time during the latter half of task R seems to reflect a narrowing of the field of fixation due to fatigue. This is because the amount of information processed by the visual system is quite large in humans, and considerable degrees of attention and neural resources are required for processing visual information. Once fatigue has developed, the field of fixation will probably be narrowed protectively and unintentionally in order to reduce the amount of visual information supplied, causing delays in reaction during task R. The prolongation of the reaction time during task R can thus serve as a physiological marker of fatigue.

At present, the ATMT is being used in clinical studies of fatigue at several medical facilities such as the Outpatient Fatigue Clinic of Osaka City University Hospital. Because the ATMT does not involve an assessment of knowledge, its results are not related to the level of education of the subject. Very little learning takes place with respect to the outcome of this test, making it possible to repeat it many times. Therefore the ATMT has been applied to the self-monitoring of fatigue, and the evaluation of the efficacy of antifatigue medications and food supplements.

Quantification of Fatigue and Autonomic Nervous System Function

A number of experiments have been reported concerning the effects of mental fatigue (including emotional stress), physical fatigue, and compound fatigue (e.g., driving automobiles) on the function of the autonomic nervous system of healthy individuals. Previous studies of chronic fatigue syndrome demonstrated disturbances of functions associated with the autonomic nervous system, such as heart rate, pulse waves, blood pressure, autonomic reflexes, homeostasis, immune function, and hormone regulation [7,8]. Many studies have determined the coefficients of variance of changes in heart rate R–R interval, power spectral analysis, pulse wave frequency analysis, etc., which are associated with the autonomic nervous system, for an evaluation of fatigue not only in patients with CFS, but also in healthy individuals [9–11].

Yamaguchi et al. [12] analyzed the accelerated pulse waves and found that the amplitude of the pulse waves was significantly different during mental stress from the amplitude before and after the period of stress, and that the amplitude of the pulse waves decreased in the presence of fatigue. Yamaguchi et al. [12] also conducted a cross-over controlled study on mental stress in humans using the fragrance of some green leaves which had been shown to have marked antifatigue effects in a previous study in monkeys exposed to a sustained task. These leaves were composed of *trans*-2-hexenal, *cis*-hexenol, etc. That study revealed that after mental stress, the degree of fatigue, rated on the visual analog scale (VAS), rose in both the fragrance-treated group and the control group, with no significant intergroup difference, but that the reaction time in the ATMT and the DPG (Derivative of plethysmogram) amplitude differed significantly between the two groups. This finding is important because it reflects success in detecting a difference in degree of fatigue, which is not detectable with the VAS with use of a physiological indicator. The development of biomarkers based on chaotic analysis of accelerated pulse waves is ongoing. It is expected that a more sophisticated method of quantification of fatigue will be established in the near future.

Quantification of Fatigue and Biomarkers

In previous studies of changes in physiological functions associated with fatigue, the delayed recovery of heart rate and respiratory rate, elevation of the stimulatory threshold for tendon reflexes, a reduction in the blood pressure-adjusting function following postural change, a dilation of the distance between two points on the skin, a reduction in the ability to discern flashing lights, and other changes have been found. In hematological testing, elevations in blood lactic acid and pyruvic acid levels and reductions in pH have been demonstrated. In addition, reduced salivary pH and increased urinary protein level have been reported, among other changes.

Table 1. Immunological and biochemical markers of fatigue

(1)	Blood gas and electrolytes Blood gas analysis (BE), pH, electrolytes, Fe, Cu, Mg
(2)	Metabolism Glucose, lactic acid, pyruvic acid, uric acid, amino acids, plasma protein fraction, albumin, ketone bodies, free fatty acids, T-Ch, TG, LDL, HDL, creatinine, acylcarnitine, carnitine, ATP/ADP/AMP
(3)	Growth factors TGF-β, BDNF (brain-derived neurotropic factor), NT-4, FGF, EGF
(4)	Oxidative stress Glutathione (oxidized, reduced), SH group-containing substances, ascorbic acid turnover, oxidized bilirubin, NO metabolites, lipid peroxide
(5)	Vitamins Vitamin B (B1, B6, B12), vitamin C, vitamin E, folic acid
(6)	Neuroendocrine peptides Cortisol, ACTH, DHEAS, DHEA, TSH, T3, T4, insulin, IGF, secretin, renin-angiotensin system, ACE, vanylmandelic acid (VMA), catecholamines, manserin
(7)	Neurotransmitters Monoamine metabolites, tetrahydrobiopterin (BH4), taurine, GABA, choline turnover
(8)	Enzymes 2-5-olligoadenylaye synthetase, RNase-L, muscle enzymes (CPK, LDH, aldolase)
(9)	Immunity, cytokines, and viral markers IFN-α, IL-1β, IL-6, TNF-α, viral markers, NK cell activity, virus reactivation factor, lymphocyte subsets (CD4, CD8, CD19, etc.), IgE

Possible biomarkers of fatigue caused by physical exercise include a reduction of ATP, an elevation of lactic acid level, and accompanying acidosis, among others. Lactic acid is formed by the glial cells around the neurons in the brain, and is utilized effectively as a source of energy by neurons when their supply of glucose is insufficient. It therefore seems unlikely that an elevation of the blood lactic acid level by exercise affects neuronal activity in the brain. Furthermore, fatigue has not been found to be induced by treatment with lactic acid. Together, these and other findings suggest that lactic acid is not useful as a biomarker of fatigue.

A comprehensive analysis of changes in biomarkers of fatigue in blood and saliva following a period of mental or physical stress is now ongoing, primarily at Soiken, Ltd (Table 1). It is empirically known that herpes zoster and herpes labialis tend to appear during fatigue, and an immunological study designed to evaluate the degree of fatigue on the basis of an analysis of virus reactivation factors is now ongoing. A close involvement of fatigue with the immune function is already evident in view of the findings that fatigue alters the levels of cytokines such as TGF-β, IL-6, and IFN-α.

Apart from studies involving the induction of fatigue, attempts at identifying fatigue-related factors in patients with CFS have also been made by Kuratsune et al. [13] and other study groups. For example, the blood level of acylcarnitine, which is known to be involved in mitochondrial energy production and to play a significant role in brain nerve activities, was shown to be persistently low in patients with CFS [13], and a reduced uptake of acylcarnitine in specific areas of the brain has been reported [14]. Fatigue appears to be closely related to changes in hypothalamic–pituitary–adrenal axis (HPA axis) activity. It has been reported that patients with CFS exhibited decreased blood levels of dehydroepiandrosterone sulfate (DHEAS), an adrenocortical hormone [15]. Furthermore, European investigators have reported that the treatment of healthy individuals with adrenocorticotropic hormone (ACTH) reduced the ratio of dehydroepiandrosterone (DHEA) to cortisol, while the treatment of CFS patients with ACTH did not alter this ratio [16]. These findings suggest that the measurement of blood levels of ACTH, DHES, and DHEAS may be useful for evaluating the degree of fatigue. Tetrahydrobiopterin (BH4), a coenzyme involved in the biosynthesis of various neurotransmitters, has been shown to stimulate the release of the neurotransmitters dopamine, serotonin, and noradrenaline [17]. Following the administration of 5,7-dihydroxytriptamine (DHT) into the cerebral ventricle, the administration of BH4 stimulated the recovery of spontaneous activity in rats [18].

In the Soiken Project for Fatigue Quantification, 18 leading pharmaceutical and food companies in Japan, the Osaka City Government, and 7 Japanese universities are working together to develop a method of quantifying fatigue by making use of physiological, biochemical, and immunological markers. It is expected that a method of self-monitoring of fatigue by a simple measurement of saliva or another type of sample will be established in the near future, and this will contribute to the preservation and promotion of the health of individuals.

Economic Losses Due to Fatigue in Japan, and Economic Impacts of Quantification of Fatigue

According to an epidemiological survey conducted in Japan in 1999 by the Ministry of Health, Labour, and Welfare (MHLW) Study Group on Fatigue, about 60% of working individuals experienced fatigue (4.72 million people), and more than 50% of these individuals (2.96 million people) had suffered from chronic fatigue lasting for at least 6 months [19]. In these circumstances, the annual sales of tonic beverages that are intended to replenish nutrition for the purpose of reducing fatigue have amounted to about 260 billion yen [20]. However, none of these beverages have been shown in scientific clinical studies to be useful for reducing or preventing fatigue. If biomarkers of fatigue can be developed and a method of quantitative evaluation of fatigue established, they will facilitate the scientifically valid development of antifatigue medications and food supplements. If medications and food supplements with reliable efficacy can be marketed, they will contribute to reducing the economic losses due to fatigue in workers in various industrial sectors, and also to enlarging the market for these products. They will also facilitate self-medication by individuals suffering from fatigue. Large economic impacts can thus be anticipated, including decreases in national medical expenditure, which is currently about 30 trillion yen per year [21], and increased control of Japan's financial deficits caused by over-expenditure on the national health insurance system.

Current Status of Fatigue in Society

As the Japanese social structure becomes increasingly more complex, health hazards (fatigue, stress, etc.) are also increasing. This change is closely related to the recent changes in the industrial structure and work style in Japan. According to a report from the Labor Health Research and Strategy Council for the 21st Century [22], the total number of individuals working in Japan increased from 50.94 million in 1970 to 64.62 million in 1999. A comparison of the number of individuals working in each industrial sector between 1970 and 1999 shows that the ratio is 0.36 for agriculture and forestry (a marked decrease), but 2.25 for the service sector (a large increase). In an analysis of work style, diverse changes were noted during this period, e.g., the adoption of new working time systems (laying emphasis on the discretion of individual workers, the adoption of flexible working hours, etc.), a diversification of night work and work shifts, changes in the types of employment (increases in part timers, contract-based workers, etc.), increases in new forms of business (24-h stores, daily care assistance businesses, etc.), increased globalization of enterprises, intensified information systems in the work place, and so on. These changes have resulted in increased levels of physical and mental fatigue in various sectors, including those in which workers have less access to labor health services. Regarding working hours, a stress factor common to all these sectors, 5.77 million people worked 60 h or more per week in sectors other than agriculture and forestry in 1999, and 6.70 million people worked night shifts (2200 hours to 0500 hours). In these circumstances, the number of individuals who are unable to continue work due to illness caused by mental or occupational stress, and also the number of people who commit suicide, have been increasing. According to a survey on workers' health in 2002 [23], about 62% of all workers suffered intense anxiety, problems, or stress related to their work or occupation. This percentage is approximately equal to that (ca. 63%) found in the same survey in 1997, but about 1.2 times greater than that found in 1982, indicating that the percentage of these workers has not decreased after the marked increase found previously. The percentage of workers taking time off work because of injury or sickness due to stress (as a cause or precipitating factor) was as high as 45.6%. Psychological disorders were the reason for taking time off for about 15% of all workers who took holidays of 1 month or longer. About 13 000 workers committed suicide in 1998. According to one estimate, depression is responsible for about 70% of all suicides committed by workers. It has also been reported that stress in the workplace has increased the percentage of workers visiting psychiatric clinics by 1.4–2.4-fold, and increased the incidence of depression by 5–14-fold. Industrial stress and the illnesses associated with it have thus become serious social issues.

Economic Losses Due to Fatigue

Psychological disorders and industrial stress can cause personal, social, and economic losses in businesses because they reduce productivity, increase the incidence of labor accidents, reduce worker satisfaction, and reduce the quality of products and services. The loss in the labor force due to these factors is reported to account for at least 10%–20% of the total labor cost (about 60 billion yen per year in Japan). Furthermore, exposure to industrial stress increasingly causes long-term absence in workers, psychological problems in workers, and labor accidents. This type of stress is thus becoming a significant problem in company management. According to the Assurance Section of the Labor Accident Compensation Division of MHLW, the numbers of applications for, and certifications of, labor accidents were only 2 and 0, respectively, in 1991, but were 341 and 100, respectively, in 2002. Therefore, the prevention of industrial stress is now an important concern in company management. In 2000, the Ministry of Labor (later renamed the MHLW) published Guidelines for Promotion of Mental Health of Workers in Workshops ("Mental Health Guidelines"). Efforts have since been made to improve the welfare of workers (e.g., establishing mental health care facilities) at individual enterprises, primarily via health insurance unions and labor unions. However, in the survey of workers' health in 2002 cited above, 65.1% of workers reported that they were aware of some problems related to health management and antistress measures which should be improved in their company. This percentage indicates that the efforts of businesses to cope with industrial stress have not been adequate, possibly because of the investment costs required.

Markets for Antifatigue Medications and Food Supplements Among Health Promotion Products

Because workplace environments have not been adequately improved to cope with industrial stress, the workers themselves have recently begun to pay close attention to health care, and in many cases have actively committed themselves to self-medication and the use of alternative medicines for the purpose of recovering from physical or mental fatigue caused by such stress. Recent trends in these markets include those described below. In the market for health-promoting products (food supplements, health-promoting apparatus, etc.), products which were designed primarily for business use in the past, have recently been distributed as home-use products, and products targeted to narrow segments of the community have recently begun to be sold to consumers in general. The size of this market has been increasing steadily despite the unfavorable economic status of consumers in the Japanese economic slump. According to a questionnaire survey published in the Government's Monthly Economic Report in April 2003 [24], more than 70% of consumers were interested in health promotion products, and 43.9% of all households reported that their purchase of products of this kind had increased from 5 years previously. Thus, the strong interest of consumers in health promotion products has been accompanied by increased purchasing of such products. When the future intentions of consumers were investigated, 29.0% of households indicated that they planned to increase their expenditure on health-promoting products. This markedly exceeded the percentage of households planning to decrease such expenditures (4.9%), and suggests that this market will continue to grow in the future. When the increases in the purchase of health-promoting products were investigated, the category consisting of food supplements, herbal medicines, tonic beverages, and related products was found to account for the highest percentage (62.6%). This finding probably reflects the fact that new distribution routes (supermarkets and convenience shops where consumers can buy products after checking them visually, in addition to the conventional mail-order distribution system) have become available, and that these products are now easier to ingest than before. These findings also suggest that the market for health-promoting products will continue to grow steadily. In these circumstances, tonic beverages (including products classified as medicines or quasi-medicines, in addition to nonmedical products) advertised as being useful for reducing fatigue have formed a large section of the market, with total annual sales amounting to about 260 billion yen since 1999, when restrictions on this type of product were relaxed. If new distribution routes, which may be difficult to develop for tonic beverages, are developed for antifatigue medications and food supplements, and if these medications and supplements are offered in formulations which are easier to ingest, the market for antifatigue medication and food supplements should continue to grow.

Antifatigue Food Supplements as Food for Specified Health Use (FOSHU)

The Government's Monthly Economic Report in April 2003 [6] presented data on the expectations of consumers regarding health-promoting foods. The most frequent requests were "easy-to-understand labeling regarding quality and efficacy" (62.4%) and "inspection and evaluation by public institutions" (53.3%). These results indicate that consumers are demanding an evaluation of the efficacy and safety of foods based on scientific evidence, and clear labeling to convey that information. In 1991, the Specific Health Promotion Foods System was started in Japan. This system pertains to governmental permits and approval of health-promoting foods and their labeling pursuant to the Ministerial Ordinance on Amendment of the Rules for Enforcement of the Nutrition Improvement Act (Ministry of Health and Welfare Ordinance No. 41). In 2001, the System on Foods with Health Promoting Functions came into effect. Under this system, foods meeting certain criteria related to vitamins and minerals can be labeled as foods with health-promoting functions, while labeling as food for specified health use (FOSHU) is permitted for foods which have passed the MHLW's inspection and evaluation of a scientific demonstration of efficacy (related to physiological functions and health promotion) and safety (pursuant to Article 26 of the Health Promotion Act). Thus, consumers in Japan can now select health-promoting foods using known criteria for efficacy and safety thanks to the System on Foods with Health Promoting Functions. This trend in administration appears to be useful, since it satisfies the expectations of consumers.

The Biotechnology Strategy Conference (chairman T. Kishimoto, ex-president of Osaka University) has set the goal of increasing the market for food for specified health use (FOSHU) to 3 trillion yen by 2010. The Economic and Financial Advisory Council (chairman J. Koizumi, Prime Minister), organized in 2003, made clear its policy of lifting the ban on mixed use of insurance-based health care and non-insurance-based health care services. It is very likely that foods with specific functions, such as food for specified health use (FOSHU), will increasingly be utilized clinically, sometimes in place of ethical medicines. A high demand is expected for the development of specific health-promoting foods that can stimulate recovery from fatigue or alleviate fatigue. The MHLW has also provided examples of labeling for food for specified health use (FOSHU), e.g., "This food is suitable (useful) for people experiencing physical fatigue," suggesting that antifatigue effects can be referred to in labeling which emphasizes the health effects of food for specified health use (FOSHU). However, no such foods have yet been approved. Consumers have strong needs and high expectations regarding food for specified health use (FOSHU) which is effective against fatigue, and it is desirable that such foods be commercialized as soon as possible.

Development of Antifatigue Medications and Food Supplements

At present, no foods for specified health use (FOSHU) which are effective against fatigue are available on the market, because no method for the quantification of fatigue has been established. Although many tonic beverages are advertised as being effective against fatigue (including those classified as medications or quasi-medications), none have demonstrated their efficacy scientifically. In these circumstances, the Study Group on Fatigue, organized under MEXT (Ministry of Education, Culture, Sports, Science and Education) using the budget for the promotion of science and technology, conducted a "Study on the molecular and neuronal mechanism of fatigue and the sensation of fatigue—a study tailored to the needs of citizens" in 1999. In that study, the results of previous noncomprehensive studies on the molecular and neuronal mechanisms of fatigue were combined, and new methods (e.g., brain function imaging, gene analysis, etc.) were used to further research into fatigue and the recovery from, and prevention of, fatigue. Furthermore, in November 2003, the Project for Fatigue Quantification and the Development of Antifatigue Medications and Food Supplements was organized as a joint industrial–governmental–academic project, with Soiken Ltd. serving as a core member. This project is planned to continue for 3 years (October 2003 to September

2006). During the first phase (November 2003 to September 2005), a technique for fatigue quantification based on biomarkers will be developed, and indicators of fatigue will be explored. During the second phase (October 2005 to September 2006), the efficacy of antifatigue products will be tested. It is expected that the results of these studies will be further verified in clinical studies designed to develop antifatigue medications and food supplements with scientifically demonstrated efficacy.

Economic Impacts of Antifatigue Medications and Food Supplements

Antifatigue medicines and food supplements are expected to have various economic impacts. Industrially, these products will reduce economic losses arising from fatigue-related problems (reduced productivity, increased accidents and illnesses, deterioration of human relationships, etc.). If workers practice self-medication using antifatigue treatments and food supplements, national medical expenditure, which is currently 30 trillion yen per year (229 000 yen per head) [3] will be reduced, and control of the financial deficits resulting from national health insurance may be possible. It has also been reported that fatigue is closely related to the regulation of the endocrine and immune systems. For example, it is known that stress due to fatigue activates cytokines involved in immune regulation, causing Th2 bias in the Th1/Th2 balance [25]. If the relationship between this alteration and immune diseases can be clarified, it will be possible to use antifatigue medication and food supplements to prevent and treat immune diseases. It seems likely that the market size for antifatigue medicines and food supplements will be comparable to, or larger than, the current market for tonic beverages (260 billion yen) if products with scientifically demonstrated efficacy are commercialized. It has been estimated that the market for food for specified health use (FOSHU) will grow to about 34.5 billion yen in 2003 from 24 billion yen in 2002, following governmental approval of new products in this category. The antifatigue effect is a completely new concept in the health-promoting food industry. If foods for specified health use (FOSHU) with this effect are approved, their market size may well surpass expectations. In conclusion, the development of antifatigue medications and food supplements can be expected to have economic impacts on diverse aspects of society (industry, national health care policy, and the creation of new markets), and it is desirable that the first such products be commercially available in 3–5 years.

References

1. Kitani T (2001) Fatigue science. Kodansha, Tokyo, 2–4
2. Hayaishi O (1991) Stress society and mental health. Sekai Hoken Tsushinsha, Tokyo

3. Helmut S, Inoue M (2000) Antioxidants in disease mechanisms and therapy. Iyaku (Medicine and Drug) Journal, Tokyo
4. Onoue H, Tajima Y, Yamamoto S, Watanabe Y (2001) Fatigue science. Kodansha, Tokyo, pp 5–17
5. Mizokawa S, Tanaka M, Matumura A, Nozaki S, Watanabe Y (2003) Recovery from fatigue: changes in local brain 2- [^{18}F] fluoro-2-deoxy-D-glucose utilization measured by autoradiography and in brain monoamine levels of rat. Neuroscience Letters 353:169–172
6. Goldman-Rakic PS (1992) Working memory and the mind. Scientific Am 22:73–9
7. Pagani M, Lucini D (1999) Chronic fatigue syndrome: a hypothesis focusing on autonomic nervous system. Clin Sci 96(1):117–25
8. De Becker P, Dendale P, De Meirleir K, Campine I, Vandenborne K, Hagers Y (1998) Autonomic testing in patients with chronic fatigue syndrome. Am J Med 105(3A)22S–26S
9. Appenzeller O (1987) The autonomic nervous system and fatigue. Funct Neurol 2(4):473–85
10. Li Z, Jiao K, Chen M, Wang C (2002) Spectral analysis of heart rate variability as quantitative indicator of driver mental fatigue. SAE Tech Pap Ser: 6
11. Naschitz JE, Sabo E, Naschitz S, Rosner I, Rozenbaum M, Priselac RM, Gaitini L, Zukerman E, Yeshurun D (2002) Fractal analysis and reccuence quantification analysis of heart rate and pulse transit time for diagnosing chronic fatigue syndrome. Clin Auton Res 12:264–272
12. Yamaguchi K (2003) Evaluation of green odor as prevention from fatigue. Program No. 107.9. 2003 Abstract Viewer/Itinerary Planner. Washington, DC, Society for Neuroscience
13. Kuratsune H, Yamaguti K, Lindh G, Evengard B, Takahashi M, Machii T, Matsumura K, Takaishi J, Kawata S, Långström B, Kanakura Y, Kitani T, Watanabe Y (1998) Low levels of serum acylcarnitine in chronic fatigue syndrome and chronic hepatitis type C, but not seen in other diseases. Int J Mol Med 2(1):51–56
14. Kuratsune H, Yamaguti K, Lindh G, Evengard B, Hagberg G, Matsumura K, Iwase M, Onoe H, Takahashi M, Machii T, Kanakura Y, Kitani T, Langstrom B, Watanabe Y (2002) Brain regions involved in fatigue sensation: reduced acetylcarnitine uptake into the brain. Ann Neuroimage 17(3):1256–1265
15. Kuratsune H, Yamaguti K, Sawada M, Kodate S, Machii T, Kanakura Y, Kitani T (1998) Dehydroepiandrosterone sulfate deficiency in chronic fatigue syndrome. Int J Mol Med 1(1):143–146
16. Scott LV, Svec, F, Dinan T (2000) A preliminary study of dehydroepiandrosterone response to low-dose ACTH in chronic fatigue syndrome and in healthy subjects. Psychiatry Res 97(1):21–28
17. Tsukada H, Lindner KJ, Hartvig P, Långström B (1994) Effect of 6R-L-erythro-5,6,7,8-tetrahydrobiopterin on the extracellular levels of dopamine and serotonin in the rat striatum: a microdialysis study with tyrosine or tryptophan infusion. Brain Res 635(1–2):59–67
18. Mizuma H, Mizutani M, Nozaki S, Iizuka H, Tohyama H, Nishimura N, Watanabe Y, Kohashi R (2003) Improvement of repeated administration of 6R-tetrahydrobiopterin of 5,7-dihydroxytryptamine-induced abnormal behaviors in immature rats. Biochem Res Commun 302(1):156–161
19. Inoue M, Kuratsune H, Watanabe Y (2001) Fatigue science. Kodansha, Tokyo, pp 222–228
20. Nishino Co., Ltd. (2003) HOTLINE. July edition
21. Ministry of Health, Labour and Welfare (2003) White Paper on the Labour Economy 2003. "Gyosei": 498
22. National Institute of Industrial Health (2000) National occupational health research priorities, agenda and strategy of Japan. The press release of Ministry of Health, Labour and Welfare
23. Ministry of Health, Labour and Welfare (2003) Reports on Labour and Health 2003. Statistics and Information Department
24. Nagano Economic Research Institute (2003) Economic monthly report. March edition
25. Visser JT, De Kloet ER, Nagelkerken L (2000) Altered glucocorticoid regulation of the immune response in the chronic fatigue syndrome. Ann NY Acad Sci 917:868–875

Utility of an Advanced Trail Making Test as a Neuropsychological Tool for an Objective Evaluation of Work Efficiency During Mental Fatigue

Kei Mizuno and Yasuyoshi Watanabe

Summary

Mental fatigue caused by prolonged mental work induces not only an increase in the sensation of fatigue, but also a decrease in work efficiency. However, there have been few studies measuring the extent of the decrease in work efficiency due to mental fatigue, because previously there had been no established mental task that could measure the extent of work efficiency. In this study, we used a recently developed test to investigate changes in task performance over a 4-h period by 14 healthy volunteers. The mental tasks which the subjects performed were an advanced trail making test (ATMT) and a verbal 2-back task. The ATMT consists of selective attention and spatial working memory tests. The verbal 2-back task is a simple working memory test. The results of the ATMT showed an increase in the number of errors with time spent on the task. In contrast, the performance of the verbal 2-back test did not deteriorate with time spent on the task. These results suggest that mental fatigue induces a decrease in selective attention rather than in working memory. Therefore, the ATMT may be useful for measuring the extent of work efficiency during mental fatigue. In order to develop antifatigue medications and food supplements, the ATMT may also be useful for an objective evaluation of the extent of mental fatigue, as well as a fatigue-inducing task.

Introduction

Fatigue is an everyday experience. However, chronic or accumulated fatigue can affect a person's performance. In addition, long-term accumulated fatigue can lead to *karoshi* (death as a result of overwork). Mental fatigue is clinically defined as

Department of Physiology, Osaka City University Graduate School of Medicine, 1-4-3 Asahimachi, Abeno-ku, Osaka 545-8585, Japan

difficulty in the initiation of, or the ability to sustain, voluntary activities [1]. Mental fatigue, in contrast to neuromuscular or peripheral fatigue, represents a failure to complete mental tasks that require self-motivation and internal cues in the absence of demonstrable cognitive failure or motor weakness [2]. Therefore, mental fatigue induces not only an increase in fatigue sensation, but also a decrease in work efficiency.

When people become fatigued, they usually report difficulties in concentrating and focusing their attention on the tasks that they are required to perform. For example, Bartlett [3], in his studies in which pilots were required to fly a simulator for extended periods of time, reported that lapses in attention happened with increasing frequency, and the subjects became progressively more easily distracted. Similarly, Brown [4] noted that the main effect of mental fatigue during time spent on a driving task was a progressive withdrawal of attention from road and traffic demands, which, as expected, had adverse consequences on task performance. These results suggest that attention is affected by mental fatigue. Mental fatigue may also be linked to executive functions, which refers to the ability to regulate perceptual and motor processes for goal-directed behavior [5, 6]. van der Linden et al. [7] reported that fatigued participants showed more performance deficits than nonfatigued ones in tasks that required the flexible generation and testing of hypotheses and planning. Working memory is an important executive process used for the temporary storage, active monitoring, updating, and manipulation of information [8]. Thomas [9] reported that mental fatigue induced a decrease in the performance of a verbal working memory test in patients with sleep disorders. From these reports, it appears that decreased work efficiency due to mental fatigue may be the result of a decrease in the maintenance of attention or working memory. However, until quite recently, no mental task has been available that could objectively measure the extent of the decreased work efficiency caused by mental fatigue.

The advanced trail making test (ATMT) is a mental function test which was developed for the purpose of evaluating the level of selective attention and spatial working memory regardless of the subject's intelligence quotient or experience [10]. The ATMT consists of a visual search task in which the subject touches the figures 1 to 25 in sequential order as quickly as possible on a computer display. In patients with chronic fatigue syndrome, which is characterized by profound disabling fatigue that persists for at least 6 months without relief and is not lessened by ordinary rest, the reaction time in the ATMT was slower than that for healthy volunteers [10]. This result suggests that it is possible to use the ATMT as a neuropsychological tool to measure the extent of work efficiency during chronic fatigue. However, to date there has been no investigation into whether a decrease in task performance in the ATMT is induced by acute mental fatigue in healthy volunteers. The aim of our study was to evaluate the utility of ATMT as a neuropsychological tool for measuring the extent of decreased work efficiency due to acute mental fatigue.

Materials and Methods

Subjects

Fourteen healthy male volunteers, 22.0 ± 1.1 years of age (mean ± SD), were enrolled in the study. None of the subjects had a history of medical illness. The protocol was approved by the Ethics Committee of Osaka City University, and all subjects gave their written informed consent for the study.

Experimental Design

As their fatigue-inducing mental tasks, the subjects performed the ATMT for 30 min and the 2-back test for 30 min. Each task session was repeated four times. The mental tasks began at 1000 hours. The subjects had lunch at 1200 hours, just after the end of the second task session. The subjects started the third session after lunch at 1240 hours.

Fatigue-Inducing Tasks

For the ATMT, subjects performed visual search trials. In this test, circles numbered from 1 to 25 were randomly located on the display of a personal computer, and subjects were required to use a computer mouse to touch these circles in sequence, starting with circle number 1. When the subjects touched the 25th target, the task was finished. In task A of the ATMT, when the subjects touched a target circle it remained at the same position and its color changed from black to yellow. The positions of the other circles remained the same. In task B, when the subjects touched the first target circle it disappeared and a circle number 26 appeared on the screen. The positions of the other circles remained the same. Then touching circles 2, 3, and 4 sequentially, for example, resulted in their disappearance and the addition of circles 27, 28, and 29 to the screen. The number of circles seen on the screen always remained at 25. In task C of the test, the procedure was the same as in task B except that the positions of the other circles changed at random after each target circle had been touched. The subjects performed tasks A, B, and C consecutively in this order. They were instructed to perform them as quickly and correctly as possible.

The subjects also performed verbal 2-back tasks [11]. A series of letters was presented on successive screens, and the subject had to judge whether each letter was "different from" or "identical to" the one presented 2 screens earlier. The subjects responded by pressing the right or left button with their right middle or index finger if the target letter was identical to or different from the cue letter, respectively. The time-interval between trials was 3 s. The subjects were instructed to perform this task as quickly and correctly as possible.

Statistical Analyses

Values were presented as mean ± standard error (SE). Comparisons among four sessions of the fatigue-inducing mental tasks were performed using 1-way analysis of variance (ANOVA) for repeated measures. When statistically significant effects were found, inter-group differences among the four sessions were compared using the paired *t*-test with the Bonferroni correction. Statistical analyses were performed by using the SPSS 11.0 software package (SPSS Inc., Chicago, IL, USA).

Results

The results of the task performances in the ATMT are shown in Fig. 1. Although 1-way repeated ANOVA did not show any significant main effects of session number on the total reaction time for task A ($P = 0.406$) or task B ($P = 0.221$), it did reveal a significant main effect of session number for task C ($P = 0.043$). In

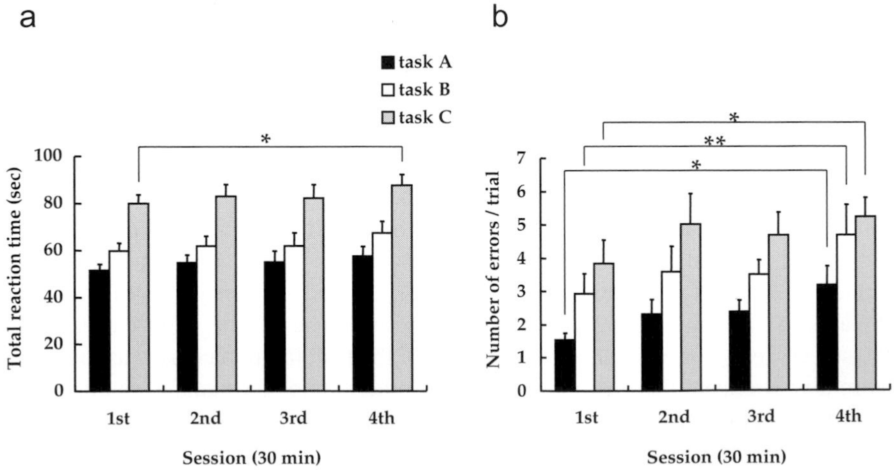

Fig. 1. Time-courses of changes in total reaction time (**a**) and number of errors per trial (**b**) in the advanced trail making test (ATMT). Subjects performed the ATMT (tasks A, B, and C) for 30 min per session per task, and each session was repeated four times. *Black columns*, task A; *white columns*, task B; *gray columns*, task C. $*P < 0.05$, $**P < 0.01$, significantly different as indicated by the brackets (one-way repeated analysis of variance followed by paired *t*-test with Bonferroni correction). Data are presented as the mean and standard error ($n = 14$)

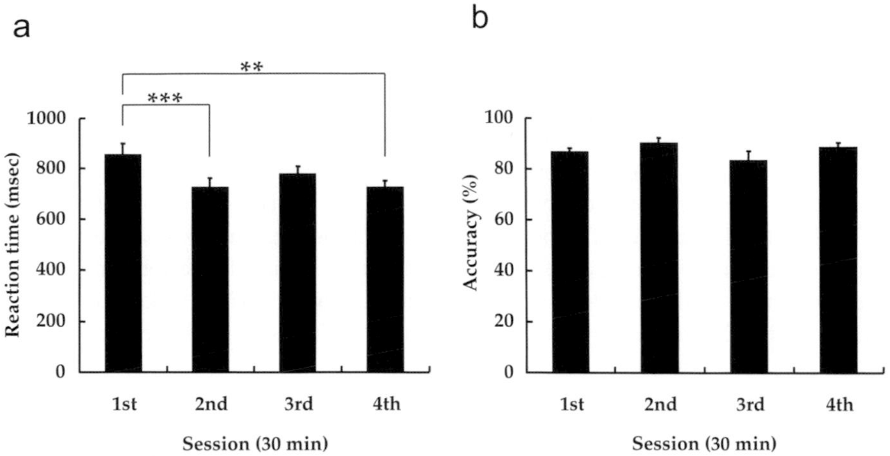

Fig. 2. Time-courses of changes in reaction time (**a**) and accuracy (**b**) of the 2-back task. Subjects performed the 2-back task for 30 min in each session, and there were four sessions. $^{**}P < 0.01$, $^{***}P < 0.001$, significantly different as indicated by the brackets (one-way repeated analysis of variance followed by paired *t*-test with Bonferroni correction). Data are presented as mean and standard error ($n = 14$)

task C, the total reaction time of the fourth session was significantly longer than that of the first session (Fig. 1a). One-way repeated ANOVA also showed significant main effects of session number on the number of errors per trial in task A ($P = 0.005$), task B ($P = 0.007$), and task C ($P = 0.025$). In all the tasks, the number of errors per trial in the fourth session was significantly greater than that in the first session (Fig. 1b).

The results of the task performances in the 2-back task are shown in Fig. 2. One-way repeated ANOVA of the reaction time showed a significant main effect of session number ($P = 0.007$). The reaction times in the second and fourth sessions were significantly shorter than that in the first session (Fig. 2a). One-way repeated ANOVA of accuracy did not show any significant main effect of session number ($P = 0.804$).

Discussion

In ATMT tasks A and B, subjects could memorize the locations of the other circles while searching for the target circle, and thus shorten their reaction time for circle touching, suggesting that the performance of these tasks required selective attention and spatial working memory. In contrast, in ATMT task C, since the locations of the circles changed every time a subject touched the target circle, and therefore every target circle had to be found within a new arrangement, this task required no memorization, suggesting that the performance of this task required only selective attention. Therefore, in tasks A and B, the reaction time for circle touching could be shortened by using the spatial working memory, whereas the spatial working memory had no effect on the performance of task C. The total reaction time in the fourth session in tasks A and B was no longer than that in the first session, but it was longer in the case of task C. The performances of the verbal 2-back test did not deteriorate with time spent on the task. These results suggest that mental fatigue induced a decrease in selective attention but not in working memory. In all the ATMT tasks, the number of errors increased with time spent on the task, suggesting that work efficiency was decreased by mental fatigue. Since the performance of the working memory did not deteriorate with time spent on ATMT tasks A and B or on the verbal 2-back task, the increased number of errors might have been caused by a decrease in the ability to maintain selective attention.

Madden et al. [12] reported that the anterior cingulate cortex was associated with selective attention, as judged from results obtained by using positron emission tomography. In addition, neuroimaging studies and event-related potentials research have established that the anterior cingulate cortex is central to performance monitoring [13–16]. The anterior cingulate cortex is thought to detect the activation of erroneous or conflicting responses and to signal the need to activate adaptive control processes, thus serving to instigate remedial performance adjustments that minimize the risk of subsequent error [17–19]. Neural activity in the anterior cingulate cortex has been found to change with time spent on a task [20, 21], suggesting that functional changes in the anterior cingulate cortex are a possible mechanism underlying mental fatigue. The monitoring function of the anterior cingulate cortex relies on the mesencephalic dopaminergic system [22, 23], which projects diffusely to the cortex and the striatum [23]. Disturbances in the striatal system have also been related to mental fatigue, supporting the theory of dopaminergic involvement in mental fatigue [2]. Therefore, the increased number of errors with time spent on the ATMTs might have resulted from the decline in function of error-monitoring and the dopaminergic system in the anterior cingulate cortex.

In the verbal 2-back task, the reaction time in the second and fourth sessions was significantly shorter than that in the first session, indicating that the improved reaction time with time spent on the task may have been an effect of learning. Thus, the verbal 2-back task is not able to measure the extent of work efficiency in mental fatigue.

We conducted this study with a limited number of subjects. In order to generalize our results, studies involving larger numbers of subjects are needed.

Conclusions

The results of a previous study showed that the ATMT is useful as a neuropsychological tool for measuring the extent of decreased work efficiency in patients with chronic fatigue syndrome [10]. However, there had been no investigation into whether a decrease in task performance in the ATMT would be induced by acute mental fatigue in healthy volunteers. In the present study, we found that the number of errors in all tasks in the ATMT increased with the time spent on the task by healthy volunteers, suggesting that this test could be useful for measuring the extent of decreased work efficiency caused by acute mental fatigue. Therefore the ATMT may be useful for an objective evaluation of the effects of antifatigue medications and food supplements during the development of these substances.

Acknowledgments. This work was supported in part by Special Coordination Funds for Promoting Science and Technology, and by the 21st Century COE Program "Base to Overcome Fatigue" from the Ministry of Education, Culture, Sports, Science and Technology, the Japanese Government. We thank Dr. Larry D. Frye for editorial help with the manuscript.

References

1. Chaudhuri A, Behan PO (2004) Fatigue in neurological disorders. Lancet 363:978–988.
2. Chaudhuri A, Behan PO (2000) Fatigue and basal ganglia. J Neurol Sci 179:34–42.
3. Bartlett FC (1943) Fatigue following highly skilled work. Proc R Soc B 131:247–257.
4. Brown LD (1994) Driver fatigue. Hum Factors 36:298–314.
5. Elliott R (2003) Executive functions and their disorders. Br Med Bull 65:49–59.
6. Fuster JM (2000) Executive frontal functions. Exp Brain Res 133:66–70.
7. van der Linden D, Frese M, Meijman TF (2003) Mental fatigue and the control of cognitive processes: effects on perseveration and planning. Acta Psychol (Amsterdam) 113:45–65.
8. Baddeley A (1992) Working memory. Science 255:556–559.
9. Thomas RJ (2005) Fatigue in the executive cortical network demonstrated in narcoleptics using functional magnetic resonance imaging: a preliminary study. Sleep Med 6:399–406.
10. Kajimoto O, Shimizu A, Takahashi T, Iwase M, Takahashi R, Kuratsune H, Watanabe Y (in press) ATMT: a computer-assisted system for assessment of fatigue. Development of advanced trail making test for evaluating mental function. J Chronic Fatigue Syndrome.
11. Braver TS, Cohen JD, Nystrom LE, Jonides J, Smith EE, Noll DC (1997) A parametric study of prefrontal cortex involvement in human working memory. Neuroimage 5:49–62.
12. Madden DJ, Turkington TG, Provanzale JM, Hawk TC, Hoffman JM, Coleman RE (1997) Selective and divided visual attention: age-related changes in regional cerebral blood flow measured by $H_2\,^{15}O$ PET. Hum Brain Map 5:389–409.
13. Carter CS, Braver TS, Barch DM, Botvinick MM, Noll D, Cohen JD (1998) Anterior cingulate cortex, error detection, and the online monitoring of performance. Science 280: 747–749.
14. Gehring WJ, Knight RT (2000) Prefrontal–cingulate interactions in action monitoring. Nat Neurosci 3:516–520.
15. Luu P, Flaisch T, Tucker DM (2000) Medial frontal cortex in action monitoring. J Neurosci 20:464–469.
16. Ullsperger M, von Cramon DY (2003) Error monitoring using external feedback: specific roles of the habenular complex, the reward system, and the cingulate motor area revealed by functional magnetic resonance imaging. J Neurosci 23:4308–4314.
17. Botvinick MM, Braver TS, Barch DM, Carter CS, Cohen JD (2001) Conflict monitoring and cognitive control. Psychol Rev 108:624–652.
18. Cohen JD, Botvinick MM, Carter CS (2000) Anterior cingulate and prefrontal cortex: who's in control? Nat Neurosci 3:421–423.
19. Kerns JG, Cohen JD, MacDonald AW, Cho RY, Stenger VA, Carter CS (2004) Anterior cingulate conflict monitoring and adjustments in control. Science 303:1023–1026.

20. Cohen RM, Semple WE, Gross M, Holcomb HH, Dowling MS, Nordahl TE (1988) Functional localization of sustained attention: comparison to sensory stimulation in the absence of instruction. Neuropsychiatr Neuropsychol Behav Neurol 1:3–20.
21. Paus T, Zatorre RJ, Hofle N, Caramanos Z, Gotman J, Petrides M, Evans AC (1997) Time-related changes in neural systems underlying attention and arousal during the performance of an auditory vigilance task. J Cogn Neurosci 9:392–408.
22. de Bruijn ER, Hulstijn W, Verkes RJ, Ruigt GS, Sabbe BG (2004) Drug-induced stimulation and suppression of action monitoring in healthy volunteers. Psychopharmacology 177:151–160.
23. Holroyd CB, Coles MG (2002) The neural basis of human error processing: reinforcement learning, dopamine, and the error-related negativity. Psychol Rev 109:679–709.

The Brief Fatigue Syndrome Scale: Validation and Utilization in Fatigue Recovery Studies

Bengt B. Arnetz[1,2,3], Lena Frenzel[3], Torbjörn Åkerstedt[4], and Jan Lisspers[5]

Summary

Medically, nonexplained fatigue is a significant clinical and public health concern. However, the construct fatigue is not easily defined, and this is reflected in the large number of different scales used to measure fatigue. In this chapter, we define fatigue using the sustained stress activation theory. It is proposed that sustained stress, with a lack of sufficient recovery periods, is characterized by a decline in the ability to concentrate, be energetic, and sleep. Based on this definition, the brief fatigue syndrome scale (BFSS) was created using visual analogue scales (VAS) to rate self-assessed energy, ability to concentrate, and quality of sleep. The BFSS consisted of one factor, with a Cronbach's α of >0.70. The validity and sensitivity of the scale was assessed by following a group of fatigued patients undergoing a 1-year lifestyle recovery program. In addition, a reference group of healthy controls was followed over the same period. Both groups responded regularly to a survey containing the BFSS. Blood samples were also collected during the first 6 months. The BFSS scores decreased significantly as the clinical conditions of the fatigued participants improved. Furthermore, self-rated mental energy, assessed by a separate and validated five-item Likert-type scale, improved with decreasing fatigue. Participants scoring above the proposed cut-off point of 8 for depression on the

[1,2]Section for Social Medicine, Department of Public Health, Uppsala University, Uppsala Science Park, SE-751 05 Uppsala, Sweden, and Division of Occupational and Environmental Health, Department of Family Medicine and Public Health Sciences, Wayne State University, 3800 Woodward Ave, Suite 808, Detroit, MI 48201, USA

[3]Center for Environmental Health and Stress Disorders (CEOS), Uppsala Academic Hospital, SE-751 85 Uppsala, Sweden

[4]Karolinska Institutet, Department of Public Health Sciences, Division of Psychosocial Factors and Health, and Institute for Psychosocial Medicine (IPM), PO Box 220, SE-171 77 Stockholm, Sweden

[5]Research Group for Behavioral Medicine and Health Psychology, Department of Social Sciences (Psychology Section), Mid-Sweden University at Östersund, SE-83125 Östersund, Sweden

hospital depression and anxiety scale had significantly higher BFSS scores. BFSS scores were also higher among subjects scoring in the burn-out range on the Shirom–Melamed scale. Decreased fatigue over time was related to improved/increased serum levels of testosterone. It is suggested that the cut-off point for fatigue vs. nonfatigue should be set at 40%. The BFSS is suggested as a valid and quick instrument to assess fatigue.

Introduction

Fatigue is a common feature of a wide range of somatic and psychiatric diseases and disorders. It is also a common problem among patients being treated for malignant conditions. The fatigue experienced is often so intense and severe that it has a major impact on the quality of life of the person affected.

An overview of studies on fatigue in primary care reported fatigue prevalence rates ranging from 7% to 45% [1]. There is a significant overlap between medically unexplained fatigue and specific medical conditions, such as depressive disorders, in which the patients commonly report fatigue, and lack of energy and motivation, both as symptoms of their disorder and as side effects of therapy [1–3].

Fatigue is also common in fibromialgic and chronic fatigue syndromes [4–6]. Furthermore, fatigue has been suggested to be one of the more characteristical aspects of syndromes such as vital exhaustion and burn-out [7,8].

Work-related fatigue is another source of concern in a growing number of industrialized countries. Excessive workload has been associated with severe forms of fatigue, including work-related death from over-work in Japan (Karoshi), burn-out, exhaustion syndrome, and "stressed-out" conditions [9–12].

Interestingly, even though it appears that chronic or severe stress is associated with increased risk of fatiguing illnesses, a study of the prevalence rates of fatiguing illnesses in the United States reported decreased rates in the aftermath of the terrorist attacks of September 11, 2001 [13].

Even though fatigue is a basic component in many clinical disorders and medically unexplained syndromes, such as chronic fatigue, and is commonly a prerequisite for the diagnosis of many psychiatric and somatic disorders, there is no universally applicable construct for fatigue. There is also no uniform theory as to the mechanisms behind fatigue [14].

Dittner et al. [15, p. 157] state that fatigue "has largely defied efforts to conceptualize or define it in a way that separates it from normal experiences such as tiredness and sleepiness." Studies from a number of settings, including primary health care settings and population-based settings, indicate that fatigue is a common and continuously distributed variable [16]. Shapiro [17] also points out the evasive and confusing art of fatigue science in an editorial entitled "Chronic fatigue—chronically confusing but growing information".

Typically, fatigue is defined as extreme and persistent tiredness, weakness or exhaustion—mental, physical, or both—in addition to decreased motivation [15].

Scales Measuring Fatigue

Many of the fatigue scales used today either focus on specific diseases, or ask the respondent to rate their fatigue in reference to work (workload) or social performance. Thus, the participant has to determine their degree of fatigue-related symptoms, and also relate them to possible causes or consequences, e.g., excessive workload or decreased motivation to participate in social activities. This increases the risk of confounding spurious associations between purported risk factors and fatigue per se.

Another common characteristic of the current scales is the view that fatigue-states are viewed as a consequence of over-exertion and a lack of sufficient periods for recovery. The term "burn-out," for example, was applied around 1940 to describe the cessation of operation of a jet or rocket engine [18]. Metaphorically, a human being suffering from a severe state of fatigue is viewed, just like a jet engine, to have been over-exerted, and lacking the necessary time for recovery and repair. This assumption is based mostly on retrospective and cross-sectional data, and is a poor definition of the possible underlying psychophysiological mechanisms contributing to the fatigue state.

The instruments available to assess fatigue in patients are either one-dimensional or multidimensional. Examples of one-dimensional scales are the visual analogue scale by Krupp et al. [19], Pearson and Byars fatigue feeling checklist [20], the Rand index of vitality [21], the tiredness scale [22], and the fatigue severity scale [23].

Multidimensional scales range from two-dimensional scales, e.g., assessing physical and mental fatigue [24], to multidimensional scales with a range of subscales, including the fatigue symptom checklist [25], the Piper fatigue self-report scale [26], and the multidimensional fatigue symptom inventory (MFSI) scale [27]. Probably one of the most commonly used fatigue instruments is the "fatigue" and "vigor" subscales of the profile of moods scale (POMS), originally developed for the assessment of psychiatric outpatients [28,29]. The checklist of individual strength (CIS) was developed for hospital use in chronic fatigue syndrome patients [30]. The CIS is a multidimensional measure of the severity and behavioral consequences of fatigue.

Theories Behind Fatigue, and Relevance to Scale Development and Validation

As discussed earlier in this chapter, the construct of medically nonexplained fatigue is not very well delineated, and neither is the theoretical and psychophysiological underpinning which attempts to explain the root causes of fatigue. Dittner et al. [15, p. 166] point this out in their review article of instruments used to assess fatigue. They write "Fatigue assessment depends on a clear understanding of the phenomenology and aetiology of fatigue within a condition. In developing fatigue scales, there is a "catch-22" situation: before a concept can be measured, it must be defined, and before a definition can be agreed, there must exist an instrument for assessing phenomenology." However, even before trying to define what constitutes fatigue, we need to identify the key components of fatigue that we believe reflect the current view of central nervous systems changes that contribute to fatigue.

The current criteria of chronic fatigue syndrome, for example, require severe disabling fatigue symptoms *and* a combination of symptoms including impairment of concentration and short-term memory, sleep disturbance, and musculoskeletal pain [31]. Clearly, the requirement is that the fatigue experienced in chronic fatigue syndrome should be disabling. However, this is not only a function of the fatigue experienced, but is also influenced by factors such as motivation and underlying drive or energy, which are also important aspects in diagnosing depressive disorders [1]. An alternative would be to apply the hypothesis that fatigue is the end result of: (1) sustained activation or over-exertion/over-reach, and (2) lack of recovery. That approach would guide us in the direction of psychophysiological stress research. Naturally, it might also be that the influence on human performance from factors such as diseases and/or drugs might lower the threshold at which exertion elicits persistent fatigue.

In this chapter, it is postulated that the sustained activation of psychophysiological systems and over-reach will result in changes in the central nervous system which are similar to those found in depressive disorders. The changes will be characterized by a hyperactive hypothalamic–pituitary axis at the same time as the peripheral stress–response system is attenuated, which is predominantly measured as decreased stress-related cortisol secretion from the adrenal cortex [32]. Moreover, many of the more depression-like states, such as those found in severe fatigue, are also linked to changes in the serotonin system and in 5-hydroxytryptamine receptors [33]. Long-term stress has also been linked to sleeping disorders, memory impairment, inability to concentrate, and lowered serum testosterone levels [12,16].

Based on the stress-related theory described above, it is hypothesized that the fatigue construct should include at least the following three dimensions: lack of energy, inability to concentrate, and sleep disturbance. Based on this theory and concept, we have developed and validated a very brief scale, called the brief fatigue syndrome scale (BFSS). This scale is the sum of the aggregate scores for three separate items which give a self-rated assessment of:

1. energy;
2. ability to concentrate;
3. sleep.

In what follows, we will demonstrate the psychometric properties of the BFSS, the means used to validate the scale, and the effects, as measured by the BFSS, from a prospective, controlled intervention program aimed at counteracting fatigue and enhancing the participants' energy and level of function.

Participants

The reliability and validity of the fatigue syndrome scale was tested using the study population described below. The participants consisted of three groups.

1. Group A consisted of 24 people, 18 men and 6 women, who were participating in a rehabilitation program offered at the Föllinge Rehabilitation Clinic, Sweden. Typically, this group was already suffering from lifestyle-related diseases such as cardiovascular disorders.
2. Group B consisted of 17 people, 9 men and 8 women, at the Föllinge Rehabilitation Clinic who took part in a primary prevention lifestyle modification program. The aim was not only to prevent a further deterioration of their health, but also to encourage positive behavioral changes.
3. Group C consisted of a reference group of healthy subjects ($n = 21$, 13 men and 8 women) living in the local area where the clinic was situated. They were part of the voluntary first-responder organization of the area, in addition to having regular jobs.

There were no statistically significant differences between groups A and B at baseline with regard to ratings on the BFSS (Group A, mean 60.5 percentage points, SD 20.8, SEM 4.4 vs. 51.5 percentage points, SD 21.4, SEM 5.5 for Group B). Both groups scored significantly higher on the BFSS than did Group C, the reference group (33.4 percentage points, SD 13.8, SEM 3.0), using Tukey's post-hoc tests, following a significant one-way ANOVA (F_2 24.11, $P < 0.01$). Groups A and B were therefore combined into one group and termed the *recovery/treatment* group. In what follows, the *recovery* group is compared with the *reference* group, i.e., group C above.

In addition to the reference group described above, and in preparation for this chapter, the BFSS's reliability and validity was assessed in three other study groups.

1. Subjects rating their own health using a public web-based system with many thousands of responders.
2. Participants who were part of a prospective web-based intervention study ($n >$ 300 respondents, [34,35]).
3. Subjects attending an academic stress clinic (>200 respondents).

Data from these three additional study groups are not used in this report, but they did support the recommended cut-off points for defining healthy vs. fatigued subjects as well as the reliability of the proposed BFSS (data available from the senior author, BBA, upon request).

The Fatigue Syndrome Scale

Based on prior research and current theory of stress-related fatigue, we identified three basic components of medically unexplained fatigue that we wanted to evaluate in our assessment of fatigue. As described above, the three areas were: self-rated sleep, ability to concentrate, and energy.

In order to decrease, as far as possible, confounding or spill-over effects from previous experiences of the symptoms we wanted to assess, i.e., sleep, ability to concentrate, and energy, we asked each participant to assess their *current* status. We did this by defining the time period we were interested in assessing and asking the respondents to rate their feelings "right now." With regard to quality of sleep, we asked them to rate how they slept the previous night.

Responses were given on a visual analogue scale (VAS), which was 100 mm in length with anchoring statements in both ends. For ability to concentrate and ability to sleep, the anchoring statements were "very poor" and "very good," respectively. For energy, the anchoring statements were "no energy" and "full of energy."

In previous work we used validated scales, based on the aggregate scores on scales made up of Likert-type items, to assess the validity of single-item VAS-based scales to measure the concept energy and work-related fatigue. We also used the same methods to assess the validity of single-item VAS scales to assess quality of sleep. We found a substantial and significant correlation between single-item VAS and the more extensive and validated Likert-type scales [34,35]. Therefore, we believe it is valid to use these single-item VAS scales in this development and assessment of a brief fatigue syndrome scale.

Some earlier work also used a prospective controlled stress-intervention program to assess the impact on self-rated health and energy and its relationship to biological measures of the stress response [36]. In this study, we used a more elaborate scale for measuring self-rated mental energy. The mental energy scale consists of five Likert-type items that are summarized to an overall score and converted into a percentage scale, ranging from a low of 0% to a high of 100% [12]. The mental energy scale was also used in this study in validation of the BFSS.

Intervention

The purpose of this study was to assess whether the fatigue syndrome scale was sensitive enough to detect clinically relevant improvements from this validated and proven intervention program.

The intervention programs offered to groups A and B are described in detail elsewhere, and they have been found to decrease risk factors for, and recurrence of, cardiovascular disease [37,38]. Briefly, group A participated in a 1-year program focusing on return to work and secondary prevention of cardiovascular disease. The program consists of an initial intensive phase of 3 weeks duration during which the person lives at the Föllinge Rehabilitation Clinic in the north of Sweden. Following these 3 weeks, the person goes home and continues with a structured program. Later they return to the clinic for an additional week of behavioral and lifestyle changes. Following that there is a 10-month sustainability phase while the person is living at home. The intervention program consists of a multitude of interventions, including a review of exercise and nutritional habits, stress management training, return-to-work strategies, and, when warranted, smoking cessation training. The long-term goal of the program is the secondary prevention of cardiovascular disease, or any other form of chronic disease. The other goal is to optimize the person's return to work.

Group B is exposed to a prevention program focusing on stress and lifestyle factors. The main purpose is the primary prevention of cardiovascular disease among high-risk people. Typically, these people are still working but they are tired and stressed, and perceive that they never have enough time. In addition, they commonly smoke, are obese, have unhealthy diets, and lack sleep. The intervention program runs over a 9-month period and consists of 10 days of on-site, intensive lifestyle and stress management interventions at the Föllinge Rehabilitation Clinic. The participants continue with their lifestyle modification training back home for an additional 2 months, during which time they are part of a sustainability effort to ensure that they keep up the beneficial changes achieved during the initial intensive part of the program. They then return for 3 days of training at the clinic. Finally, there is an additional 4 months of domestic training and sustainability training, concluding with a final 2 days at the clinic. After these steps, there is a 3-month follow-up period while the person is back at home in order to ensure, as far as possible, that positive lifestyle changes are retained. Both programs combine group-based interventions with individual coaching sessions.

The Human Investigative Committees of Uppsala and Umeå Universities, respectively, approved the study.

Brief Fatigue Scale Validation: Results

Factor analysis, using principal components analysis and varimax rotation, confirmed that the three VAS items, measuring ability to concentrate, energy, and sleep, formed a single component/factor. This factor was termed the brief fatigue syndrome scale (BFSS). Cronbach's α on the scale was 0.70 or higher. The single component solution and the internal consistency were confirmed in three subsequent measurements of the participants over a 1-year period. Figure 1 shows a histogram of the distribution of the scores on the BFSS at the initial ratings by all participants.

The changes in ratings on the BFSS of the recovery and reference groups are shown in Fig. 2. There was a significant group × time interaction (Greenhouse–Geisser, $F_{2.44}$ 4.37, $P = 0.01$). Thus, while changes in self-rated fatigue in the reference group were modest over the 1-year study period, the recovery group exhibited

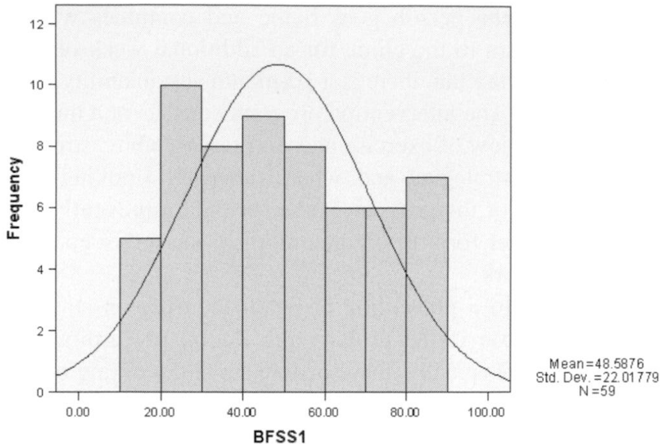

Fig. 1. Histogram showing a normal curve of the score distribution on the brief fatigue syndrome scale (BFSS1) at the first assessment, including all respondents

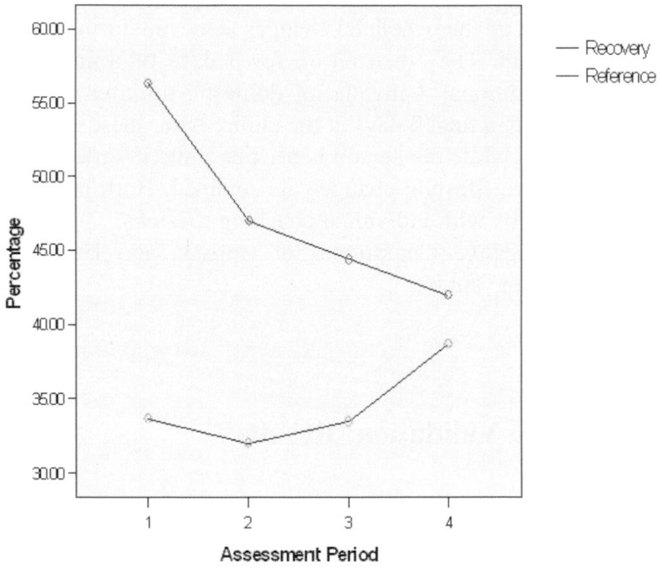

Fig. 2. Changes in brief fatigue syndrome scores in subjects recovering from fatigue as part of a rehabilitation program and healthy controls. The ratings were done at the start of the project, and after 3, 6, and 12 months

a significant decrease over time in self-rated fatigue as their intervention program progressed.

In Fig. 3, a box plot chart shows mean and dispersion measures on the BFSS for participants scoring less than 8 points vs. 8 points and above on the depression subscale of the hospital anxiety and depression (HAD) scale [39]. Subjects rating

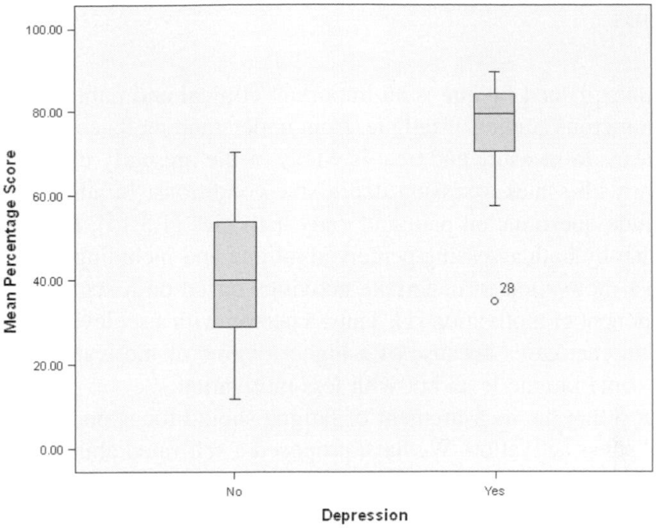

Fig. 3. A box plot depicting the mean and dispersion measures on the BFSS of participants scoring below 8 points, which is suggested to be indicative of nondepression, and 8 points and above (which is indicative of depression) on the hospital depression and anxiety scale, the depression subscale

above the cut-off point of 8 have been suggested by the developers of the scale to be more likely to suffer from depression. The mean (SD, SEM) BFSS score for participants scoring less than 8 points on the HAD was 40.23% (16.67, 2.44) vs. 75.42% (14.29, 3.81) for those scoring 8 points or above ($t_{57} = 7.11$, $P < 0.001$).

Mean BFSS scores for participants scoring less than 2.75 on the Shirom–Melamed burnout scale were 31.68 (14.86, 3.16), for those scoring between 2.75 and 4.75 they were 49.71 (17.38, 3.62), and for those scoring above 4.75 they were 73.30 (12.27, 3.27). The differences between groups were significant: one-way ANOVA F_2 2 = 31.44, $P < 0.001$. Tukey post-hoc tests were also significant for any contrasting groups. The cut-off point on the Shirom–Melamed scale is based on clinical impressions from the stress rehabilitation center affiliated with the Karolinska Institutet, Stockholm, Sweden.

Since the construct and theory behind the BFSS were based on the sustained stress activation theory, we also studied the possible relationship between changes in serum testosterone during the first 6 months of the intervention and changes in BFSS scores during the same period. The rationale for doing this is that testosterone is supposed to increase as sustained stress activation is decreased. We hypothesized that decreasing fatigue scores would be associated with increasing levels of serum testosterone over time [12]. Our findings revealed that decreased fatigue scores were modestly related to increased serum testosterone levels ($r = 0.2$, $P = 0.01$).

We also observed that with decreasing BFSS scores, self-rated energy, using the five-item Likert-based mental energy scale, improved, thus adding further statistical support that BFSS is a valid and sensitive measure of fatigue.

Discussions

Medically unexplained fatigue is an important clinical and public health concern. There are numerous studies of fatigue, from understanding its conceptualization to finding a means to measure and treat it. Many of the presently used scales overlap substantially with scales assessing depressive conditions. In addition, scales also tend to include questions on pain and daily activities [1,3,15]. However, it could be argued that by both assessing perceived fatigue and including questions related to a person's motivation to undertake activities based on a set fatigue level, one adds a component of motivation [1]. Thus, a person with a set level of fatigue might be undertaking activities because of a higher degree of motivation than a person scoring the same fatigue level but with less motivation.

We suggest that the measurement of fatigue should focus on symptoms related to sustained stress activation. We have proposed a self-rated ability to concentrate, a self-rated assessment of energy, and a self-rated quality of sleep as being relevant indicators of sustained stress activation without sufficient recovery. Scores on a fatigue scale based on this concept could then be related to activities of daily life, motivation, sick leave, biological markers, overall health, and related issues of interest. However, we do not believe such subsequent and consequential questions should be part of a fatigue scale.

We propose a cut-off level on the brief fatigue syndrome scale (BFSS) for medically unexplained fatigue of 40%t or higher on a 100% scale. This proposed level for diagnosing medically unexplained fatigue needs to be further refined in future studies. However, by proposing a cut-off point, it will be easier to use the scale in comparative studies as well as examine its feasibility in daily clinical practice.

The BFSS is a very brief, three-item scale. Its briefness makes it easy to use in studies involving a range of other scales and outcome measures. It might also be helpful to clinicians and patients interesting in following fatigue development over time, and in assessing the effects of various interventions.

The BFSS needs to be studied further with regard to its reliability and validity, as well as its feasibility in daily medical practice. However, this initial study suggests acceptable psychometric properties and predictive validity. The scores on the BFSS also relate to weekly changes in serum testosterone. This suggests that there are biologically relevant and measurable processes related to fatigue development as measured using the BFSS.

Acknowledgments. This study was supported by grants from Folksam Insurance Research Fund and the Swedish council for Working Life and Social Research (FAS). Bengt Arnetz proposed the items on the brief fatigue syndrome scale. All authors took an active part in the design, execution, and analyses of the study. Bengt Arnetz was the chief writer of the manuscript, with significant input from the other authors.

References

1. Fehnel SE, Bann CM, Hogue SL, Kwong WJ, Mahajan SS (2004) The development and psychometric evaluation of the motivation and energy inventory (MEI). Qual Life Res 13:1321–1336
2. Masand PS, Gupta S (1999) Selective serotonin reuptake inhibitors: an update. Harvard Rev Psychiatr 7:69–84
3. Stein KD, Martin SC, Hann DM, Jacobsen PB (1998) A multi-dimensional measure of fatigue for use with cancer patients. Cancer Pract 6:143–152
4. Kent-Braun JA, Sharma KR, Weiner MW, Massie B, Miller RG (1993) Central basis of muscle fatigue in chronic fatigue syndrome. Neurology 43:125–131
5. Kroenke K, Wood DR, Mangelsdorff DA, Meirer NJ, Powell JB (1988) Chronic fatigue in primary care: prevalence, patient characteristics, and outcome. J Am Med Assoc 260:929–934
6. Melillo N, Corrado A, Quarta L, D'Onofrio F, Trotta A, Cantatore FP (2005) Fibromialgic syndrome: new perspectives in rehabilitation and management. A review. Minerva Med 96:417–423
7. Appels A, de Vos Y, van Diest R, Höppner P, Mulder P, de Groen J (1987) Are sleep complaints predictive of future myocardial infarction? Activitas Nervosa Superior 29:147–151
8. Melamed S, Ugarten U, Shirom A, Kahana L, Lerman Y, Froom P (1999) Chronic burnout, somatic arousal and elevated salivary cortisol levels. J Psychosom Res 46:591–598
9. Kalia M (2002) Assessing the economic impact of stress. The modern-day hidden epidemic. Metabolism 51 Suppl 1:49–53
10. Uehata T (1991) Karoshi due to occupational stress-related cardiovascular injuries among middle-aged workers in Japan. J Sci Labour 67:20–28
11. Winwood PC, Winefield AH, Dawson D, Lushington K (2005) Development and validation of a scale to measure work-related fatigue and recovery: the occupational fatigue/recovery scale (OFER). J Occup Environ Med 47:594–606
12. Anderzén I, Arnetz BB (2005) The impact of a prospective survey-based workplace intervention program on employee health, biological stress markers, and organizational productivity. J Occup Environ Med 47:671–682
13. Heim C, Bierl C, Nisenbaum R, Waginer D, Reeves WC (2004) Regional prevalence of fatiguing illnesses in the United States before and after the terrorist attacks of September 11, 2001. Psychosom Med 66:672–678
14. Lewis G, Wessely S (1992) The epidemiology of fatigue: more questions than answers. J Epid Com Health 46:92–97
15. Dittner AJ, Wessely SC, Brown RG (2004) The assessment of fatigue. A practical guide for clinicians and researchers. J Psychosom Res 56:157–170
16. Arnetz BB, Ekman R (2006) Fatigue and recovery. In: Arnetz B, Ekman R (eds) Wiley–VCH, New York, pp 298–309
17. Shapiro CM (2004) Chronic fatigue: chronically confusing but growing information. Editorial. J Psychosom Res 56:153–155
18. Felton JS (1998) Burnout as a clinical entity: its importance in health care workers. Occup Med 48:237–250
19. Krupp LB, Alvarez LA, LaRocca NG, Scheinberg LC (1988) Fatigue in multiple sclerosis. Arch Neurol 45:435–437
20. Pearson PG, Byars GE (1956) The development and validation of a checklist measuring subjective fatigue. Report no. 56-115, School of Aviation, USAF, Randolf AFB, Texas
21. Brook RH, Ware JE, Davies-Avery A, Stewart AL, Donald CA, Rogers WH, Williams KN, Johnston SA (1979) Overview of adult health status measures fielded in Rand's health insurance study. Med Care 17 (Suppl):1–55
22. Montgomery GK (1983) Uncommon tiredness among college undergraduates. J Con Clin Psychol 51:517–525

23. Krupp B, LaRocca NG, Muir-Nash J, Steinberg AD (1989) The fatigue severity scale. Application to patients with multiple sclerosis and systematic lupus erythematosus. Arch Neurol 46:1121–1123
24. Wessely S, Powell R (1989) Fatigue syndromes: a comparison of chronic postviral fatigue with neuromuscular and affective disorders. J Neurol Neurosurg Psychol 52:940–948
25. Haylock PJ, Kart LK (1979) Fatigue in patients receiving localized radiation. Cancer Nursing 2:461–467
26. Piper BF, Lindsey AM, Dodd MJ, Ferketich S, Paul SM, Weller S (1989) The development of an instrument to measure the subjective dimension of fatigue. In: Funk SG, Tornquist EM, Campagene MT, Archer Gropp LM, Wiese RA (eds) Key aspects of comfort: management of pain, fatigue and nausea. Springer, New York, pp 199–208
27. Stein KD, Martin Sc, Hann DM, Jacobsen PA (1998) A multidimensional measure of fatigue for use with cancer patients. Cancer Pract 6:143–152
28. Fawzy FI, Cousin N, Fawzy NW, Kemeny ME, Elashoff R, Morton D (1990) a structured psychiatric intervention for cancer patients. Arch Gen Psychiatr 18:35–59
29. Salinsky MC, Storzbach D, Dodrill CB, Binder LM (2001) Test–retest bias, reliability, and regression equations for neuropsychological measures repeated over a 12–16-week period. J Int Neuropsychol Soc 7:597–605
30. Vercoulen JHMM, Swanink CMA, Fennis JFM, Galama JMD, van der Meer JWM, Bleijenberg G (1994) Dimensional assessment of chronic fatigue syndrome. J Psychosom Res 38:383–392
31. Fukuda K, Straus SE, Hickie I, Sharpe MC, Dobbins JG, Komaroff A (1994) The chronic fatigue syndrome. A comprehensive approach to its definition and study. Ann Intern Med 121:953–959
32. Raison CL, Miller AH (2003) When not enough is too much: the role of insufficient glucocorticoid signaling in the pathophysiology of stress-related disorders. Am J Psychiatr 160: 1554–1565
33. Svenningsson P, Chergui K, Rachleff I, Flajolet M, Zhang X, El Yacoubi M, Vaugeois J-M, Nomikos GG, Greengard P (2006) Alterations in 5-HT_{1b} receptor function by p11 depression-like states. Science 311:77–80
34. Hasson D, Anderberg UM, Theorell T, Arnetz BB (2005) Psychophysiological effects of a web-based stress management system. A prospective, randomized controlled intervention study of IT and media workers. BMC Public Health 5:78 (hccp;//www.biomedcentral.com/1471-2458/5/78)
35. Hasson D, Arnetz BB (2005) Validation and findings comparing VAS vs. Likert scales for psychosocial measurements. Int Electron J Health Educ 8:178–192
36. Arnetz BB (1996) Techno-stress. A prospective psychophysiological study of the impact of a controlled stress-reduction program in advanced telecommunication systems design work. JOEM 38:53–65
37. Lisspers J, Sundin Ö, Öhman A, Hofman-Bang C, Rydén L, Nygren Å (2005) Long-term effects of lifestyle behavior change in coronary artery disease: effects on recurrent coronary events after percutaneous coronary intervention. Health Psychol 24:41–48
38. Lisspers J, Hofman-Bang C, Nordlander R, Rydén L, Sundin Ö, Öhman A, Nygren Å (1999) Multifactorial evaluation of a program for lifestyle behavior change in rehabilitation and secondary prevention of coronary artery disease. Scand Cardiovasc J 33:9–16
39. Zigmond AS, Snaith RP (1983) The hospital anxiety and depression scale. Acta Psychiatr Scand 67:361–370

Chronic Fatigue Syndrome

Hirohiko Kuratsune[1] and Yasuyoshi Watanabe[2]

Summary

Chronic fatigue syndrome (CFS) is an operational concept for clarifying the unknown etiology of the syndrome characterized by the sensation of abnormally prolonged fatigue. The vast majority of patients with CFS are interrupted in their daily or social lives by prolonged fatigue, headache, myalgia, arthralgia, sleep disturbance, or brain dysfunctions. However, the pathogenesis of CFS remains unclear, and so there are still many medical doctors around the world who are skeptical about the disease.

Recently, we organized a study group of Japanese investigators from various fields, such as virology, immunology, endocrinology, physiology, biochemistry, psychiatry, and neuroscience, and as a result of the efforts of this group the mechanism underlying CFS is now becoming a little clearer. We are now able to suggest that CFS can be understood to be a special condition based on an abnormality of the psycho-neuro-endocrino-immunological system caused by psycho-social stress, and which has some genetic components. A reactivation of various types of herpes virus infections and/or chronic mycoplasma infection might occur as a result of immune dysfunction, causing the abnormal production of several cytokines. A distinctive feature of CFS is thought to be a secondary brain dysfunction caused by the abnormal production of such cytokines.

In this chapter, we would like to introduce not only the recent findings on the pathogenesis of CFS, but also the prevalence, diagnosis, therapy, and prognosis of CFS in Japan.

---

[1]Department of Health Science, Faculty of Health Science for Welfare, Kansai University of Welfare Sciences, 3-11-1 Asahigaoka, Kasiwara, Osaka 582-0026, Japan

[2]Department of Physiology, Osaka City University Graduate School of Medicine, 1-4-3 Asahimachi, Abeno-ku, Osaka 545-8585, Japan

Introduction

In 1999, a Japanese study group supported by the Ministry of Health and Welfare of Japan (group leader Teruo Kitani) investigated the incidence of fatigue in 4000 Japanese residents (Nagoya area) based on their response to a questionnaire, and 3015 of these responses (75.4%) were analyzed. From this study, it became clear that 59.1% of Japanese people have felt fatigue, and that 35.8% of Japanese people had chronic fatigue (lasting more than 6 months). Surprisingly, 5.1% of these felt a deterioration in their ability to perform personal daily tasks, and 1.8% of them had a loss of daily work-related activity because of chronic fatigue of unknown cause. Only 8 of the 3015 (0.26%) fulfilled the chronic fatigue syndrome (CFS) criteria proposed by the CDC [1].

In 2004, a Japanese study group supported by the Japanese Ministry of Education, Culture, Sports, Science, and Technology (group leader Yasuyoshi Watanabe) again studied the incidence of fatigue by using the same questionnaire in the Osaka area, and 2742 questionnaires were analyzed. This survey suggested that the incidence and clinical features of fatigue in Osaka were very similar to those in Nagoya. That is, 56.0% of these respondents have felt fatigue and 39.0% had chronic fatigue. Of the patients with chronic fatigue, 45% had loss of daily activity, but the cause of fatigue was found in only 19.0%.

When we investigated the annual economic impact of fatigue in Japan by using the above survey data, we estimated a total loss of $4.0 billion due to CFS and $6.0 billion due to idiopathic chronic fatigue (ICF). Therefore, chronic fatigue is becoming not only an important medical problem, but also a serious social problem because of its large economic impact. Our survey also revealed that even medical doctors found the cause of fatigue in only 40% of patients with chronic fatigue, and so ICF has become a major problem in clinical practice.

Concerning the pathogenesis of CFS, a variety of theories have been proposed, such as virus infections, hypothalamo–pituitary–adrenal (HPA) axis abnormality, immune dysfunction, metabolic abnormalities, autonomous nerve unbalance, or brain dysfunction, based on each researcher's own viewpoint. It is true that these theories might reflect some of the features of CFS, but it would seem that they do not grasp the whole picture, which is reminiscent of the story of "the blind men and the elephant."

In view of this situation, our proposal for studying the neuronal and molecular mechanisms of the sensation of fatigue was adopted in 1999 by the Japanese Ministry of Education, Culture, Sports, Science, and Technology (MEXT) as pioneering research in the 21st century. More recently, it was also adopted by MEXT as the 21st century Center of Excellent (COE) Program "Formation of a Scientific and International Base to Overcome Fatigue" in Osaka City University. The pathogenesis of CFS has been investigated by workers from various fields such as virology, immunology, endocrinology, physiology, biochemistry, psychiatry, and neuroscience, and its mechanism is now becoming a little clearer.

In this chapter, we introduce our recent results and put forward a hypothesis for the neuronal and molecular mechanisms resulting in chronic fatigue which account for the relationships among each of the abnormalities found in CFS. We also introduce the Japanese Diagnostic Criteria for CFS, which is a self-check list for evaluating the levels of fatigue, the treatments, and the prognosis of patients with CFS in Japan.

Social Stress Events

It is well known that stressful social events frequently become the trigger for acute mental fatigue, and occasionally cause chronic fatigue. There are some reports indicating that stressful events are associated with the onset of CFS, but there are others giving data showing the opposite. Thus, the role of stress in CFS has been unclear.

Therefore, our co-worker, Tomoko Ueda, studied the social-stress events of 71 Japanese patients with CFS and 223 aged-matched healthy controls by using a questionnaire. Social stress was investigated by counting the events described in the Social Readjustment Rating Scale proposed by Holmes and Rahe [2]. In the CFS group, the social-stress events were studied at the time of onset of CFS and during medical treatment. Most of the CFS patients in this study denied any association between social stress and their complaints. However, the average count of stressful life events per year in the CFS group was 8.3 at the time of onset and 6.0 at the time of medical treatment. These values were significantly higher than the values for the healthy control group (4.4, $P < 0.01$, Mann–Whitney U-test). Furthermore, the relative impact of a variety of stressful events in the CFS group was 223.0 at the time of onset, which was significantly higher than the value for the healthy control group (112.3, $P < 0.01$, Mann–Whitney U-test).

The stressful events that had a significantly higher frequency in patients with CFS than in the controls were: personal injury or illness; marital reconciliation; a change in the health of a family member; foreclosure of a mortgage or loan; trouble with in-laws; a change in living conditions; a change in residence/school/recreation; a change in sleeping/eating habits.

It therefore became clear that most of the Japanese CFS patients were under considerable social stress, with or without being aware of it. However, we should emphasize that this result does not mean that CFS is a psychological illness. As described later, stressful social events are related to an abnormality of the psycho-neuro-endocrino-immunological system, and a secondary brain dysfunction caused by the abnormal production of several cytokines and/or autoantibodies which might be a key feature of CFS.

Genetic Background

When evaluating a stress-related disease, we should pay attention not only to the absolute magnitude or frequency of stressful events, but also to the patient's susceptibility to, and resistance against, stress, since these factors are thought to be related to personal character or disposition. Indeed, when we studied the personality of the patients with CFS, most of them had a predisposition toward perfectionism and/or over-adaptation, and these tendencies were not related to the existence or not of mental illness. We suspect that such a predisposition might be related to the genetic polymorphism of transporters and/or receptors of various neurotransmitters.

Recently, we examined the polymorphism of the promoter region of the serotonin transporter (5-HTT) gene in 78 CFS patients by performing polymerase chain reaction (PCR) amplification of their blood genomic DNA [3]. This promoter region affects the transcriptional efficiency of the 5-HTT gene. A significant increase in the frequency of longer (L and XL) allelic variants was found in the CFS patients compared with that in the controls by both genotype-wise and allele-wise analyses ($P < 0.05$). Efficiency in the transportation of 5-HTT is known to be higher with the L allele than with the S allele. There was no significant difference in two other 5-HT-related polymorphisms, i.e., the 5-HT 2A receptor promoter polymorphism and the 5-HTT intron 2 VNTR polymorphism, between the CFS patient group and the control group. Therefore, we speculate that a polymorphism within the 5′ upstream region of the 5-HTT gene is closely linked to CFS, and may be a risk factor for this disorder. There is also a possibility of the existence of polymorphisms of genes for transporters and/or receptors of other neurotransmitters, and such studies are currently on-going in our laboratory.

Immunological Abnormalities

It is known that the prevalence of a past history of allergy is high in patients with CFS. Furthermore, CFS patients were reported to have many immunological abnormalities of various types, such as low natural killer cell function, an abnormality of the T cell population, elevated levels of several types of cytokines, the presence of antinuclear antibody, an increased level of immune complexes, and an abnormality of the RNase-L pathway [4–9]. Therefore, there is no doubt that immunological abnormalities are another of the factors involved in the pathogenesis of CFS.

It is also well known that flu-like symptoms are a common side-effect of interferon (IFN) therapy, and an elevated activity of 2′,5′-oligoadenylate synthetase, an enzyme involved in antiviral infection, is frequently found in peripheral blood mononuclear cells from CFS patients [7,8]. Therefore, much attention has been paid to the relationship between IFN and the pathogenesis of CFS. The abnormality of the RNase-L pathway is located in the downstream part of the IFN pathway.

Recently Katafuchi et al. [10], who are members of our fatigue project, found a close association between the changes in the IFN-α mRNA content in the brain and immunologically induced fatigue. An intraperitoneal injection of a synthetic double-stranded RNA, poly I : C 3 mg/kg, was given to rats to produce immunologically induced fatigue. The daily amounts of spontaneous running-wheel activity decreased to about 40%–60% of the preinjection level until day 9, with a normal circadian rhythm being maintained. A quantitative analysis of mRNA levels, conducted by using the real-time capillary reverse transcriptase–polymerase chain reaction (RT–PCR) method, revealed that IFN-α mRNA contents in the cortex, hippocampus, hypothalamic medial preoptic, paraventricular, and ventromedial nuclei were higher in the poly I : C group than in the saline or heat-exposed groups on day 7. These results suggest that brain IFN-α may play a role in the animal model for immunologically induced fatigue mimicking that induced by a viral infection.

Katafuchi et al. [10] also found that the expression of 5-HTT mRNA in the brain was increased in this model, and that treatment with a selective serotonin re-uptake inhibitor (SSRI) was effective at blocking the decrease in the daily amount of spontaneous running-wheel activity and the loss of appetite. These results suggest that our fatigue sensation during a common cold might be related to serotonergic dysfunction, and that SSRI might be an effective protection against some of the symptoms of the common cold.

Moreover, there is a possibility that abnormalities of transforming growth factor-β (TGF-β) are also strongly involved in the sensation of fatigue. For example, Inoue et al. [11] found that intracranial administration of cerebrospinal fluid (CSF) from exercise-exhausted rats to naïve mice produced a decrease in spontaneous motor activity, whereas CSF from sedentary rats had no such effect. This finding suggests the presence of a substance which suppresses the urge for motion as a response to fatigue. Using a bioassay system, they found that the level of TGF-β in the CSF from exercise-fatigued rats had increased, but there was no such increase in the CSF from the sedentary rats. Furthermore, the injection of recombinant TGF-β into the brains of sedentary mice elicited a similar dose-dependent decrease in spontaneous motor activity. These results suggest that TGF-β might be involved in the fatigue developed after exercise and thus suppress spontaneous motor activity.

An elevated serum level of bioactive TGF-β was also frequently found in patients with CFS [5], and we also confirmed such an increase in the majority of our CFS patients. TGF-β was reported to inhibit the production of dehydroepiandrosterone sulfate (DHEA-S) [12], which is known to regulate positively the activity of carnitine acetyltransferase [13], the enzyme that catalyzes the transfer of free carnitine to acylcarnitine, and especially to acetylcarnitine. We found that most Japanese CFS patients had a deficiency in DHEA-S [14] as well as in acetylcarnitine [15], and so the increase in TGF-β would appear to be related to these abnormalities.

In addition, the presence of autoantibodies, including antinuclear antibody, is also thought to be an important key immunological abnormality involved in the pathogenesis of CFS. It is known that antinuclear antibody is frequently found in fatigued patients throughout the world who have various indefinable complaints. However, the role of these autoantibodies in such patients is unclear.

Recently, using a sensitive radio-ligand assay, we examined the sera of CFS patients ($n = 60$), patients with autoimmune disease ($n = 33$), and healthy controls ($n = 30$) for autoantibodies against various neurotransmitter receptors, i.e., recombinant human muscarinic cholinergic receptor 1 (CHRM1), μ-opioid receptor

(OPRM1), 5-hydroxytryptamine receptor 1A (HTR1A), and dopamine receptor D2 (DRD2) [16]. The mean anti-CHRM1 antibody index was significantly higher in patients with CFS ($P < 0.0001$) and autoimmune disease ($P < 0.05$) than in healthy controls, and over a half of the patients with CFS (53.3%, 32/60) had anti-CHRM1 antibody. Antinuclear antibodies were also found in 56.7% (34/60) of the CFS patients, but their titers did not correlate with the activities of the four autoantibodies listed above.

The CFS patients who were positive for autoantibodies against CHRM1 had a significantly higher mean score (1.81) of "feeling of muscle weakness" than those who were negative for these autoantibodies (1.18, $P < 0.01$). Higher scores on "painful lymph nodes," "forgetfulness," and "difficulty in thinking" were also found in CFS patients with anti-CHRM1 antibodies than in those without them, but no statistical significance was reached. Anti-OPRM1 antibodies, anti-HTR1A antibodies, and anti-DRD2 antibodies were also found in 15.2, 1.7, and 5.0%, respectively, of patients with CFS, but no significant relationship was found between the symptoms and the existence of these antibodies. Since anti-CHRM1 antibody is also frequently found in patients with schizophrenic disorders, mood disorders, and other psychiatric disorders, it is clearly not specific to CFS, but autoimmune-induced abnormalities in neurotransmitter receptors might cause secondary brain dysfunction, including CFS.

Infections

At the onset of CFS, patients frequently complain of flu-like symptoms such as headache, sore throat, fever, painful lymph nodes, myalgia, and arthralgia. Mass outbreaks of CFS have also been reported to occur sometimes throughout the world. Therefore, many investigators have tried to find pathogens or pathogenic organisms which might be suspect candidates for causing CFS, and many viruses and microorganisms have been reported to be involved in the pathogenesis of CFS. Examples include various herpes viruses (Epstein–Barr (EB) virus, human herpes virus-6, *Herpes simplex* virus, *Varicella zoster* virus, and cytomegalovirus), influenza virus, retroviruses, coxsackie B virus, Borna disease virus, hepatitis C virus, parvovirus, mycoplasma infection, and chronic rickettsial infections. Indeed, we have found that some patients acquire CFS after developing an acute infection such as mononucleosis caused by EB virus infection.

However, the vast majority of pathogens or pathogenic organisms found in patients with CFS do not represent an initial acute infection, but rather a reactivation of various kinds of herpes viruses and/or chronic mycoplasma infections [17–19]. These infections might be related to a deterioration of immune function, but the infections themselves seem not to be a serious danger to health. The important point is that most complaints reported by these patients stem from cytokines produced by the immune response to these pathogens or pathogenic organisms, and these cytokines cause secondary brain dysfunction.

Regarding a specific viral infection related to CFS, we should consider a Borna disease virus (BDV) infection. Recently, Ikuta et al. [20] reported that antibodies against BDV in plasma and BDV RNA in peripheral blood mononuclear cells (PBMCs) were found in several patients with CFS. They also reported that anti-BDV antibodies and BDV transcripts in PBMCs were found in Japanese family clusters of patients with CFS [21]. After their reports, they followed-up these family clusters and found that most of these antibodies and transcripts disappeared after the patient had recovered from CFS. There is one report indicating that there is no relationship between CFS and BDV infection [22], but we think that at least some cases of CFS are closely associated with BDV infection.

Hypothalamo–Pituitary–Adrenal (HPA) Dysfunction

In 1991, Demitrack et al. [23] reported the impaired activation of the HPA axis in patients with CFS, and thereafter several investigators addressed HPA dysfunction in patients with CFS, including lower basal plasma cortisol levels, reduced salivary cortisol levels, lower adrenocorticotropic hormone (ACTH) response in an insulin-tolerance test and a psycho-social stress test, reduced ACTH responses to corticotropin-releasing hormone (CRH) and prolonged suppression of salivary free cortisol in the low-dose dexamethasone suppression test [24–26]. We also found that the majority of Japanese patients with CFS had a deficiency in serum DHEA-S [14]. Serum DHEA-S is one of the most abundantly produced hormones secreted from the adrenal glands, and its physiological role is thought to be that of a precursor of sex steroids. However, DHEA-S itself was recently shown to have physiological properties, such as acting as a neurosteroid associated with such psychophysiological phenomena as memory, stress, anxiety, sleep, and depression. Therefore, the deficiency in DHEA-S might be related to the neuropsychiatric symptoms in patients with CFS. As described above, there is also a possibility that the DHEA-S deficiency is associated with the increased serum level of TGF-β.

Acylcarnitine Metabolism

Carnitine has important roles not only in the transport of long-chain fatty acids into the mitochondria as the long-chain fatty acid carnitine, but also in the modulation of the intramitochondrial CoA/acyl-CoA ratio [27]. A deficiency in carnitine results in abnormal energy metabolism and/or the accumulation of toxic acyl-CoA compounds in the mitochondria. Therefore, we investigated whether CSF patients had carnitine abnormalities or not, and found an acylcarnitine deficiency in serum from these patients [15].

Since the physiological and biological roles of serum acylcarnitine were unclear at that time, we also studied the dynamics of acylcarnitine in several tissues in the

Rhesus monkey and in humans by using positron emission tomography (PET), and found an important feedback system in the acylcarnitine metabolism [28]. This is that the mammalian liver can supply a large amount of acylcarnitine for energy metabolism at a time of danger, and immediately salvage and conserve the unused acylcarnitine to provide for subsequent energy crises when the state of the energy metabolism has improved. A high brain uptake of [2–^{11}C]acetyl-L-carnitine was also found. These results suggest that endogenous serum acylcarnitine might be an important substance in mammals, and that it has some role in conveying an acetyl moiety into the brain, especially in an energy crisis.

It was also found that the acetyl moiety taken up into the brain through acetylcarnitine is mainly utilized for the biosynthesis of glutamate, and that this uptake was significantly lower in patients with CFS than that in controls in several brain regions, namely, in the prefrontal (Brodmann's area 9/46d) and temporal (BA21 and 41) cortices, anterior cingulum (BA24 and 33), and cerebellum [29]. Thus, the levels of biosynthesis of neurotransmitters through acetylcarnitine might be reduced in some brain regions of chronic fatigue patients, and this abnormality might be one of the keys to unveiling the mechanisms of the chronic fatigue sensation.

However, there have been some conflicting reports of the levels of serum carnitine and acylcarnitine in patients with CFS. After our first report, Plioplys and Plioplys [30] also found lower than normal levels of acylcarnitine in their patients with CFS in the USA, but their CFS patients also had low levels of free carnitine. Conversely, Soetekouw et al. [31] reported no significant difference in the levels of carnitine and acylcarnitine in patients in The Netherlands with or without CFS, and Jones et al. [32] also reported no difference in carnitine and acylcarnitine levels between British patients with CFS and controls.

There are several explanations for this discrepancy. The first is the possibility that there was a difference in the time of the blood samples. As mentioned above, we found that the level of acylcarnitine quickly drops after eating [28]. Therefore, if there is any difference in the time at which the blood samples were taken, the levels of acylcarnitine would obviously be expected to vary. For this reason, we collected all blood samples from CFS patients and controls in the morning after an overnight fast. The second reason is the possibility that there are different subsets of patients with CFS. Recently, Ruud et al. [33] reported that the levels of plasma acetylcarnitine in 58 CFS patients who had a good response to azithromycin were lower than those in their patients with CFS who had no response to this drug. The last possibility is that there are species differences. The levels of free carnitine and acylcarnitine are well known to vary among different species due to differences in food habits and/or constitutional size.

Recently, Vermeulen et al. [34] reported that acetylcarnitine had a beneficial effect on fatigue and attention (mental concentration) in an open-label, randomized study on CFS patients. We also found beneficial effects in several Japanese patients with CFS [35], and so acylcarnitine dysmetabolism is thought to be another component involved in the pathogenesis of CFS.

Brain Dysfunction

Regarding the brain dysfunction in patients with CFS, the details are described in chapter by K. Mizuno of this book. However, we now provide some brief abstracts.

Brain Magnetic Resonance Imaging (MRI)

In 1993, Natelson et al. [36] reported that patients with CFS had significantly more abnormal MRI scans than controls. The abnormalities seen were foci of increased white-matter T2 signals. However, in 1997 Costa et al. [37] gave an opposing opinion. They reported that patients with CFS had several punctate hyperintense foci in the brain, but these abnormalities were reported not to be specific to CFS. In response to this finding, Natelson et al. [38] again reported that CFS patients without a psychiatric diagnosis showed a significantly larger number of brain abnormalities on T2-weighted images than CFS patients with a psychiatric diagnosis or than healthy control (HC) groups, and that no significant difference was found when both CFS groups were combined and compared with the HC group. Moreover, they also reported in 2001 [39] that the presence of brain abnormalities in CFS was significantly related to subjective reports of physical function, and that CFS subjects with MRI brain abnormalities were more physically impaired than those patients without brain abnormalities.

We also found that patients with CFS had a significant reduction in gray-matter volume in their bilateral prefrontal areas, and that there was a significant negative correlation between the gray-matter volume of the right prefrontal cortex and the performance status of the CFS group [40]. de Lange et al. [41] also reported a significant reduction in global gray-matter volume in CFS patients as compared with the volume for controls, and showed that the decline in gray-matter volume was linked to the reduction in physical activity. Therefore, these data suggest that CFS is not only a functional disorder, but also an organic disorder in an advanced phase.

Single-Photon Emission Computed Tomography (SPECT)

Recent single-photon emission computed tomography (SPECT) studies using 99mTc-hexamethyl–propylene–amine oxime revealed that most CFS patients showed cerebral hypoperfusion in a variety of brain regions such as the frontal, temporal, parietal, and occipital cortices, and the anterior cingulum, basal ganglia, and brainstem, and suggested that the central nerve system (CNS) dysfunction might be related to the neuropsychiatric symptoms of CFS patients [42–44].

Positron Emission Tomography (PET)

Regional cerebral blood flow (rCBF) using ^{15}O-labeled water ($H_2{}^{15}O$)

Recently, we showed that rCBF was lower in the CFS patient group than in the control group in several brain regions, including the frontal, temporal, and occipital cortices, anterior cingulum, basal ganglia, and brainstem [29]. Our results from the first quantitative rCBF study on CFS patients done with PET are in good agreement with the data from the above-mentioned SPECT studies [42–44]. Brain regions showing the decrease in rCBF in CFS patients correspond to those involved in various neuropsychiatric complaints, including autonomic imbalance, sleep disturbance, many types of pain, and the loss of concentration, thinking, motivation, and short-term memory. Therefore, various neuropsychiatric complaints in CFS patients might be related to dysfunction in these regions of the CNS.

[^{18}F]fluorine-Deoxyglucose (^{18}FDG) Study

Regional cerebral glucose metabolism (rCMRglu) measured with 2-[^{18}F]fluoro-2-deoxyglucose (FDG) and PET somehow reflects neural activity. Using [^{18}F]FDG and PET, Tirelli et al. [45] reported that their CFS patient group had a significant hypometabolism in the right mediofrontal cortex and brainstem in comparison with the healthy controls, and that the brainstem hypometabolism seemed to be a marker for the in vivo diagnosis of CFS. However, Siessmeier et al. [46] reported that abnormalities in FDG–PET were only detectable in approximately half the CFS patients examined, and that no specific pattern for CFS could be identified. In these two reports, most of the CFS patients had an abnormality of neural activity, but the discrepancy between them might have come from the different subsets of CFS patients studied by the two groups. As in the case of the MRI studies, stratified analysis will be needed to clarify brain dysfunction in CFS.

Acetyl-L-Carnitine Uptake

As mentioned in the section on acylcarnitine metabolism, when we studied the uptake in eight CFS patients and eight age- and sex-matched normal controls by using PET [29], a significant decrease was found in the cerebral uptake of [2-^{11}C]acetyl-L-carnitine in several brain regions of the CFS patient group, namely, the prefrontal (Brodmann's area 9/46d) and temporal (BA21 and 41) cortices, anterior cingulum (BA24 and 33), and cerebellum.

The subdivision of BA9, BA9/46d, is responsible for executive function, such as motivation and planning for new things, and BA24 is strongly related to concentration, attention, and some autonomic functions. BA21 is a part of the TE area, which is responsible for the integration of visual information, visual attention/memory, and the association of stimulus and reward, and the dentate nucleus area of the cerebellum is related to the vestibular function. Thus, the dysfunction of these regions may explain some of the characteristics of the fatigue state.

5-HT Transporter (5-HTT)

When we studied 5-HT transporter (5-HTT) density in 10 patients with CFS and 10 age-matched normal controls by using PET with the radiotracer [^{11}C](+)McN5652, the density of 5-HTT in the rostral subdivision of the anterior cingulum was significantly reduced in the CFS patients [47]. In addition, the density of 5-HTT in the dorsal anterior cingulum was negatively correlated with the pain score. These loci are spatially different from the locus of the rostral subdivision of the anterior cingulum. Therefore, the reduction in the density of serotonin transporters in the rostral subdivision of the anterior cingulum might be related to the chronic fatigue itself, and not to the nonspecific symptom of pain. Thus, an alteration in the serotoninergic neurons in the anterior cingulum may play a key role in the pathophysiology of CFS.

Hypothesis: Neuronal and Molecular Mechanisms Leading to Chronic Fatigue

It is becoming clear that various abnormalities found in CFS patients might not exist independently, but might be related to each other. That is, CFS can be understood to be a special condition based on the abnormality of the psycho-neuro-endocrino- immunological system caused by psycho-social stress together with some genetic components (Fig. 1). Under these conditions, a reactivation of various types of herpes virus infections and/or chronic mycoplasma infection might occur as a result of immune dysfunction, causing the abnormal production of several cytokines. A distinctive feature of CFS is thought to be the secondary brain dysfunction caused by the abnormal production of such cytokines.

As described above, the increase in TGF-β might inhibit the production of DHEA-S, which in turn might be related to the dysmetabolism of acetyl-L-carnitine through the modulation of carnitine acetyltransferase activity. Indeed, when we administered DHEA-S to CFS patients in a double-blind study, an apparent increase in serum acetylcarnitine was found in the patients treated with DHEA-S. Therefore, one of the pathways leading to CFS may be described as follows: "increase in TGF-β" $\rightarrow$ "decrease in DHEA-S" $\rightarrow$ "acetylcarnitine dysmetabolism" $\rightarrow$ "deterioration of biosynthesis of glutamate in the anterior cingulum" $\rightarrow$ "autonomic imbalance and prolonged fatigue."

As mentioned in the section on immunological abnormalities, the abnormal production of IFN is another important pathway whose activation results in CFS. That is, "reactivation of various types of herpes virus infections or chronic mycoplasma infection" $\rightarrow$ "abnormal production of IFN in the brain" $\rightarrow$ "elevation of

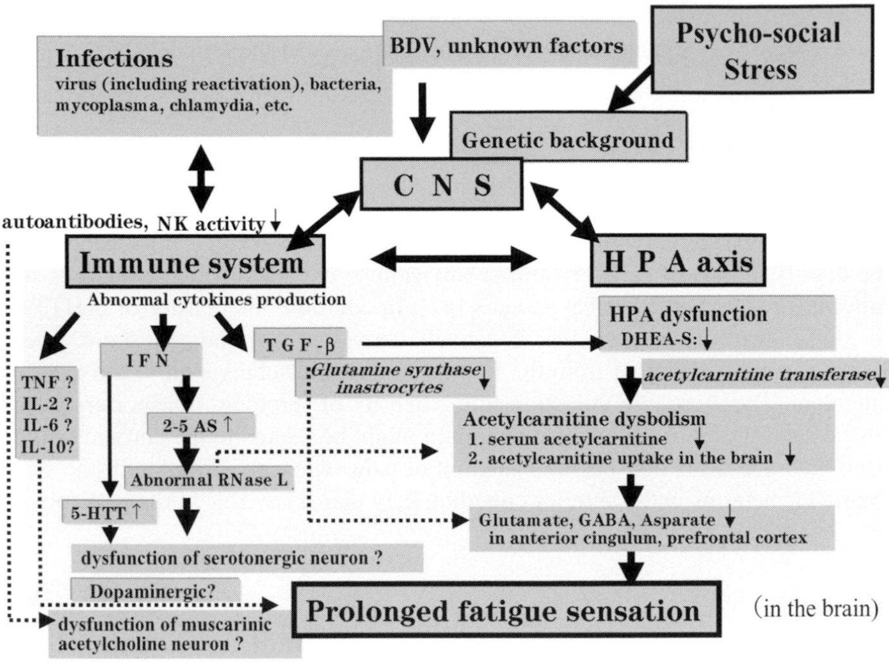

Fig. 1. Hypothesis: neuronal and molecular mechanisms leading to chronic fatigue

5-HTT mRNA content in the brain" → "5-HT deficiency in the synapse" → "depression, chronic pain disorder, and prolonged fatigue." The abnormal production of IFN is thought to trigger yet another pathway leading to CFS, that is, "abnormal production of IFN" → "elevation of 2′,5′-oligoadenylate synthetase activity" → "abnormality of RNase-L pathway" → "CNS dysfunction" →" various neuropsychiatric complaints." Recently, an abnormal RNase-L pathway has been considered to be a good candidate biomarker of CFS [48], and we also found an abnormality of the RNase-L pathway in several Japanese CFS patients.

In this review, we have focused on TGF-β and IFN, but tumor necrosis factor (TNF) might also be involved in fatigue sensation, since it is known that TNF is associated with the symptoms found in cachexic patients with advanced cancer [49]. Also, an increased TNF-α level has been reported in CFS patients [6]. There is a possibility that other types of cytokines, such as IL-2, IL-4, IL-6, and IL-10, might also be involved in the secondary brain dysfunction in CFS. Furthermore, recent PET studies by our group have revealed that the brain dysfunction found in CFS involves not only abnormal serotonergic and glutaminergic metabolism, but also abnormal dopaminergic metabolism. There is a possibility that the muscarinic–cholinergic system might also be defective in patients with CFS. Therefore, even if a distinctive feature of CFS is summarized as secondary brain dysfunction caused by abnormal production of cytokines, its pathogenesis would obviously be heterogeneous. In addition, autoantibodies against neurotransmitter receptors might also be involved in the pathogenesis of CFS in some cases.

Japanese Diagnostic Criteria for CFS

In 1990, we reported the first patients with CFS in Japan to the Japanese Society of Internal Medicine (Kinki Branch), and this event prompted the Japanese Ministry of Health and Welfare to establish a Japanese study group for CFS (group leader Teruo Kitani, Osaka University). In 1991, this study group agreed on the Japanese Diagnostic Criteria for CFS based on the Holmes Center for Disease Control (CDC) criteria [1] with two modifications. The first was that CFS should be classified into two groups, one being the "definitive CFS," which meets the Holmes CDC criteria, and the other, "suspected CFS," which meets the major but not the minor criteria of the Holmes CDC criteria. At that time, we thought that Holmes CDC criteria were suitable only for searching for the pathogenesis of CFS, and so we introduced the concept of "suspected CFS" for practical use in the clinic. This concept is reflected in the Fukuda CDC criteria (1994) as idiopathic chronic fatigue [50].

The second modification was that the Japanese criteria should adopt an objective measure as the performance status for evaluating the fatigue state. In the Holmes CDC criteria, the level of fatigue in CFS must be severe enough to reduce or impair the average daily activity below 50% of the patient's premorbid activity level for a period of at least 6 months. However, when Japanese medical doctors used this criterion to evaluate patients with chronic fatigue, we found that the levels of fatigue for diagnosing CFS varied considerably from doctor to doctor. Therefore, we adopted the concept of performance status (PS) for evaluating the fatigue state (Table 1). In CFS, PS is classified from PS 0 to PS 9 (on a 0–9 scale), and the level of fatigue for a diagnosis of CFS must be PS level 3 or above. Except for these two modifications, the remainder of the Japanese CFS criteria are identical to the Holmes CDC criteria, and so we will not give any further details here.

Recently, the committee for revision of the CFS diagnostic criteria in Japanese Association of Fatigue Science (President; H. Kuratsune) made a new guideline for diagnosis of CFS, and reported it at the conference of Japanese Association of Fatigue Science (June 30–July 1, 2007). Its detail will be published in the Journal of Japanese Association of Fatigue Science in 2008.

Self-Checking List for Evaluating the Level of Fatigue

In the Holmes CDC criteria [1], several somatic and neuropsychiatric symptoms are thought to be features of CFS. Therefore, many patients with chronic fatigue are coming to our hospital with a self-diagnosis check list obtained from the media of mass communication. They usually judge their symptoms by noughts-and-crosses, and when they find 8 or more of the 11 symptoms of the minor criteria, they self-diagnose themselves as having CFS. However, there have never been any

Table 1. Performance status in CFS for evaluating the severity of the disease

PS 0:	Able to carry on normal activity without fatigue
PS 1:	Able to carry on normal activity, but sometimes feels fatigue
PS 2:	Able to carry on normal activity or to do active work with effort; requires occasional rest
PS 3:	Several days a month, unable to carry on normal activity or to do active work; requires rest at home without work
PS 4:	Several days a week, unable to carry on normal activity or to do active work; requires rest at home without work
PS 5:	Unable to carry on normal activity or to do active work at all, but able to do light tasks; requires rest at home without work several days a week
PS 6:	Requires rest without work at home over half a week; able to do light tasks in good health
PS 7:	Unable to carry on normal activity or to do light tasks at all; able to care for self without assistance
PS 8:	Stays in bed over half a day; able to care for self to some extent, but requires frequent assistance
PS 9:	Unable to care for oneself; stays in bed with all-day assistance.

Japanese CFS criteria

previous studies evaluating the levels and incidence of these symptoms in Japanese CFS patients and in healthy controls. Therefore, we studied them in 127 patients with CFS (35.8 ± 8.6 years old) and 104 healthy controls (39.3 ± 11.0 years old). Ninety-seven patients with CFS were in the aggressive phase (above PS level 3), and the other 30 were in the recovery phase (below PS level 2). We studied the levels and incidence of the following 20 symptoms, divided into two categories.

1. Fatigue symptoms from physical diseases (10 symptoms): 1, feeling of exhaustion; 2, mild fever; 3, sore throat; 4, painful lymph nodes; 5, unexplained generalized muscle weakness; 6, myalgia; 7, prolonged generalized fatigue after levels of exercise that would have easily been tolerated in the patient's premorbid state; 8, generalized headaches; 9, migratory arthralgia without joint swelling; 10, debilitating fatigue that does not resolve with bed-rest.
2. Fatigue symptoms from mental diseases (10 symptoms): 1, depression; 2, anxiety; 3, flagging interest; 4, forgetfulness; 5, photophobia; 6, confusion; 7, difficulty in thinking; 8, hypersomnia; 9, insomnia; 10, inability to concentrate.

All of the above symptoms were evaluated on an ascending risk scale of 0–4 (5-level rating system). Symptoms (1) and (2) were both judged from 0 to 40, and the total fatigue score (1 + 2) was thus judged from 0 to 80.

Judging from the scores of the healthy controls, there was no difference in either physical or mental fatigue scores between males and females (Table 2). There was also no difference by age bracket (data not shown). On the contrary, both the physical and mental fatigue scores of CFS patients in the recovery phase (PS < 3) were significantly higher than those of healthy controls ($P < 0.001$). Moreover, both physical and mental fatigue scores of patients with CFS in the aggressive phase (PS = 3) were significantly higher than those of healthy controls or of patients with

CFS in the recovery phase (PS < 3) ($P < 0.001$). Therefore this scoring system seems to be useful for evaluating the fatigue state.

In Japan, there are many "workaholics," i.e., people who work more than 260 h per month, and it has been suggested that these people fall into a high-risk group for sudden death or "Karoushi," due to overwork. Unfortunately, most of them do not appear to notice the abnormality of their health by themselves. Therefore, we are now studying their mental and physical fatigue state using several different methods, such as heart rate variability, long-term body motion (assessed by use of an actigraph), and brain function. Our preliminary study suggests that this self-check list for evaluating the levels of fatigue is an easy-to-use approach for picking up heath problems of which the sufferer is not aware.

Treatment and Prognosis

The pathogenesis of CFS has not yet been entirely clarified, and there is currently no "magic bullet" for the treatment of CFS. However, as mentioned above, its mechanism is now becoming a little clearer, and some treatments have been reported to be effective for the signs and symptoms of patients with CFS. We now turn to some of the treatments which are often used for CFS patients in Japanese fatigue clinics.

Herbal Medicine

Some classic Chinese herbal medicines are reported to be effective for the signs and symptoms of CFS, i.e., low-grade fever, general fatigue, and depression. We therefore studied the effects of one herbal medicine (TJ-41, Tsumura, Hochu-ekki-to, 7.5 g/day) on 29 patients with CFS for 8 or 12 weeks. Judging by the change in their performance status (Table 2), an apparent improvement was found in 10 of these patients (34.5%). Two showed a slight improvement, and 15 showed no change. The remaining 2 showed a slight worsening of their symptoms. The numbers (percentages) of patients with symptoms before and after treatment, respectively, were as follows: severe fatigue, 16 (55.2%) and 10 (34.5%); moderate

Table 2. Fatigue check-list score of healthy controls and CFS patients

	A symptoms	B symptoms	Total fatigue score
Healthy controls			
Males ($n = 50$)	4.2 +/− 3.4	6.0 +/− 3.5	10.1 +/− 6.4
Females ($n = 54$)	4.5 +/− 4.5	6.6 +/− 4.4	11.0 +/− 8.6
Total ($n = 104$)	4.3 +/− 4.0	6.3 +/− 4.0	10.5 +/− 7.5
CFS patients			
Recovery phase (PS < 3, $n = 30$)	14.2 +/− 6.0*	15.0 +/− 7.0*	29.2 +/− 11.6*
Aggressive phase (PS ≥ 3, $n = 97$)	22.0 +/− 7.6**	20.4 +/− 8.1**	42.4 +/− 14.3**

* $P < 0.001$ vs. healthy controls; ** $P < 0.001$ vs. both healthy controls and recovery phase

fatigue, 12 (41.4%) and 8 (27.6%); mild fatigue, 1 (3.4%) and 11 (37.9%). Unfortunately, none were totally cured of their fatigue symptoms after treatment, but Hochu-ekki-to seemed to be an effective drug for treatment of their fatigue state.

Symptoms such as difficulty in thinking and the inability to concentrate are known to be the main factors involved in the loss of social activity. The percentage of patients who were frequently unable to concentrate was dramatically reduced from 12 (41.4%) to 2 (6.9%). Therefore, Hochu-ekki-to appeared to improve their quality of life.

Moreover, 10 of 17 patients studied had low natural killer (NK) activity before treatment, but all except one of these 10 patients showed an increase in their NK activity after treatment. Low NK activity is frequently found in CFS, and so the enhancement of NK activity was one of the important effects of this herbal medicine.

High-Dose Administration of Vitamin C

It is well known that vitamin C provides protection against oxidation, and that it is beneficial for a suppressed immune system. Recently, Watanabe and co-workers used mice which had been deprived of sufficient sleep as a mouse model for fatigue. When they studied the animals' fatigue state before and after loading them into a weight-loaded forced swimming test, they found that the swimming time was significantly reduced after loading compared with that before loading. Next, the effect of vitamin C on this fatigue model was examined, and the results showed that a high-dose administration of vitamin C improved the swimming time after loading. A daily vitamin C dose of 50–100 mg (one or two oranges are included) is adequate to protect against vitamin C deficiency in human beings, but the dose needed for protection against oxidation is many times higher than this daily dose. Therefore, we usually administer 3000–4000 mg vitamin C per day to patients with CFS. One-third of our CFS patients who took this high dose of vitamin C reported an improvement in several CFS symptoms, such as low-grade fever, fatigue, and myalgia.

Vitamin B Complex

It has been reported that vitamin B1 plays an important role in glucose metabolism, in particular since it is involved in the change from pyruvic acid to acetyl-CoA. When we studied the effect of vitamin B1 on fatigue-model mice using the same weight-loaded forced swimming test as in the vitamin C study, we found that vitamin B1 administration also improved the swimming time. Vitamin B1 is also reported to have an important role in neural function, and so we usually give CFS patients 30–100 mg vitamin B1 per day.

Vitamin B12 also has an important role in neural function. When we administered a high dose of vitamin B12 (3000 μg/day) to patients with CFS, some of them showed an objective improvement in their sleep disturbance. As there are few adverse effects of vitamins B1 and B12, we routinely prescribe both for patients with CFS.

Selective Serotonin Re-uptake Inhibitor (SSRI) and Serotonin Noradrenaline Re-uptake Inhibitor (SNRI)

As mentioned when considering the pathogenesis of CFS, we speculate that a polymorphism within the 5′ upstream region of the 5-HTT gene is closely linked to CFS and may be a risk factor for this disorder. When we used fluvoxamine maleate, an SSRI, to treat 39 Japanese patients with CFS, 11 of them withdrew from the treatment within 2 weeks because of side-effects such as nausea, increased fatigue, and loss of the ability to think. However, the remaining 28 patients were given the inhibitor for more than 2 months. As a result, 2 of these patients were cured of CFS after the treatment, and 8 of them recovered enough to return to work. Therefore, we consider that serotonergic hypofunction is one of the aspects of the pathogenesis of CFS.

Paroxetine is also classified as an SSRI, and we found that it was equally as efficacious as fluvoxamine maleate for the treatment of patients with CFS. However, its drug formula is quite different from that of fluvoxamine maleate. It is interesting that patients who have an adverse reaction to fluvoxamine maleate tolerate paroxetine well, and vice versa. Recently, milnacipran hydrochloride (an SNRI) was also found to have a beneficial effect similar to that of SSRIs on CFS patients, and so we usually use these agents creatively.

We would like to stress that these SSRI and SNRI drugs are not only used for the treatment of patients in a depressive state. We found that some CFS patients without depression did have serotonergic hypofunction, and that an SSRI or SNRI was frequently effective against the fatigue or the pain itself. Furthermore, some CFS patients feel a sense of rejection when told that they are being treated with an antidepressant. Consequently, we usually take the time to explain the reason for the use of these drugs, and this time is well spent if it establishes a good rapport with the patient.

Acetylcarnitine

As mentioned in the section on acylcarnitine metabolism, acylcarnitine dysmetabolism is thought to be a part of the pathogenesis of CFS. When we administered acetylcarnitine to several CFS patients who had acetylcarnitine deficiency, some of them showed a marked improvement in their daily activities and a reduction in their symptoms [35]. However, when the effectiveness of a therapy is estimated by the treatment of a disease, the placebo effect should also be considered. Recently, Vermeulen et al. [34] confirmed that acetylcarnitine had a beneficial effect on fatigue and attention in an open-label, randomized study on CFS. Since few side-effects are caused by acetyl-L-carnitine, supplementation with acetyl-L-carnitine might possibly become a useful new treatment for CFS patients, or at least those with an acylcarnitine deficiency.

Amantadine

Amantadine is well known to be effective for the treatment of Parkinsonism. This effect is believed to release brain dopamine from nerve endings, thus making it more available to activate dopaminergic receptors. It is also known that amantadine has antiviral activity toward influenza type A.

Recently, Bode et al. [51] reported the successful inhibition of BDV by amantadine in cultured cells and in an infected human individual. At that time, we had two family clusters of patients with CFS. One family consisted of a father, mother, two sons, and one daughter, and all members except the elder son had been diagnosed with CFS. All members with CFS had antibodies against BDV in their plasma and BDV RNA in their peripheral blood mononuclear cells. [21] This father is a medical doctor, and when he learned about the report by Bode et al., he decided to use amantadine to treat his affected family members. After 12 weeks administration of amantadine (200 mg per day), all of them showed a good response, which included a marked improvement in their daily activities and a reduction in the degree of their symptoms. When we tested for BDV RNA in their peripheral blood mononuclear cells after a 1-year administration of the drug, we could not detect BDV RNA in any of them.

Therefore, we administered amantadine (200 mg per day) to 22 patients with CFS. Three of them withdrew from the study because of side-effects such as increased fatigue, loss of concentration, and staggering. The other 19 were able to take amantadine (200 mg per day) for 8 weeks, and our therapeutic rating revealed the following results: 1 patient showed an excellent response, 8 showed a good response, 6 showed a poor response, and 4, showed no response. When we evaluated the effect of amantadine on patients with and without antibodies against BDV in their plasma, 6 of 11 patients with antibodies against BDV showed a good response, whereas only 2 of 6 patients without antibodies showed a good response. Therefore, there is a possibility that the effect of amantadine might be different depending on the presence or absence of antibodies against BDV. Since the report from Bode et al., there have been many conflicting reports indicating that amantadine does not have any antiviral activity against BDV. Therefore, the mechanism of the effect of amantadine is now unclear, but we consider amantadine to be one of a range of valuable therapies for patients with CFS in the absence of a "magic bullet."

Supportive Care

Patients with CFS are frequently plagued by a broad range of symptoms such as myalgia, arthralgia, sleep disturbance, digestive symptoms, and vegetative symptoms. Therefore, we frequently use various kinds of traditional medicine, such as acupuncture, massage, aroma therapy, laughter therapy, etc., depending on the symptoms.

Prognosis and the Relationship to Psychiatry

When we studied the prognosis of our CFS patients who had been treated by Oriental medicine (a herbal medicine plus a high-dose administration of vitamin C) in Osaka University Hospital, none of them died due to the CFS itself. However, only 9 of 74 patients (12.2%) were cured after 2 years of treatment; and 13 of 46 patients (28.3%) were cured after 5 years of treatment. Therefore, CFS does not have a good prognosis.

All of these patients had selected the Oriental medicine of their own accord. However, half of them had psychiatric symptoms. Therefore, we classified these patients into 3 groups by using the *Diagnostic and Statistical Manual of Mental Disorders,* 4th ed. (DSM-IV). One group comprised patients without mental disorders (Group I), the second group comprised those who had developed mental disorders after the onset of CFS (Group II), and the last group comprised those who had met the diagnostic criteria for mental disorder at the onset of CFS (Group III). This classification was recommended by the psychiatric group in Osaka University (Okajima and Shimizu). The improvement after 5 years of treatment was 8/20 for Group I, 3/8 for Group II, and 2/18 for Group III. When the patients who did not have a concurrent mental disorder at the onset of CFS (Groups I + II) were compared with those who did (Group III), the recovery rates were significantly higher in Group I + II ($P < 0.05$) than in Group III (Okajima et al., submitted for publication). Therefore, the presence or absence of a concurrent mental disorder at the onset of CFS plays a greater role in the outcome of the disease than a mental disorder which develops after the onset of CFS. For this reason, we make a point of letting our CFS patients meet a psychiatrist before making a differential diagnosis.

Acknowledgments. Most of the studies presented here were performed with the support of the Special Coordination Funds for Promoting Science and Technology from the Ministry of Education, Culture, Sports, Science, and Technology of the Japanese Government (MEXT), and by a grant (JSPS-RFTF 98L00201) from the Research for the Future (RFTF) program of the Japan Society for the Promotion of Science (JSPS), awarded to Y.W. The details of the studies performed in our Japanese fatigue project will be presented at the 2nd International Conference on Fatigue Science on February 9–11, 2005, in Karuizawa, Japan.

References

1. Holmes GP, Kaplan JE, Gantz NM, Komaroff AL, Schonberger LB, Strauss SE, Jones JF, Dubois RE, Cunningham-Rundles C, Pahwa S, Tosato G, Zegans LS, Purtilo DT, Browh N, Schooles RT, Brus I (1988) Chronic fatigue syndrome: a working case definition. Ann Intern Med 108:387–389
2. Holmes TH, Rahe RH (1967) The social readjustment rating scale. J Psychosom Res 11:213–218
3. Narita M, Nishigami N, Narita N, Yamaguti K, Okado N, Watanabe Y, Kuratsune H (2003) Association between serotonin transporter gene polymorphism and chronic fatigue syndrome. Biochem Biophys Res Commun 311(2):264–266
4. Klimas NG, Salvato FR, Morgan R, Fletcher MA (1990) Immunologic abnormalities in chronic fatigue syndrome. J Clin Microbiol 28(6):1403–1410
5. Bennett AL, Chao CC, Hu S, Buchwald D, Fagioli LR, Schur PH, Peterson PK, Komaroff AL (1997) Elevation of bioactive transforming growth factor-beta in serum from patients with chronic fatigue syndrome. J Clin Immunol 17(2):160–166
6. Moss RB, Mercandetti A, Vojdani A (1999) TNF-alpha and chronic fatigue syndrome. J Clin Immunol 19(5):314–316
7. Suhadolnik RJ, Reichenbach NL, Hitzges P, Sobol RW, Peterson DL, Henry B, Ablashi DV, Müller WE, Schröder HC, Carter WA, Strayer DR (1994) Upregulation of the 2–5A synthetase/RNase L antiviral pathway associated with chronic fatigue syndrome. Clin Infect Dis 18(Suppl 1):S96–104
8. Ikuta I, Yamada T, Shimomura T, Kuratsune H, Kawahara R, Ikawa S, Ohnishi E, Sokawa Y, Fukushi H, Hirai K, Watanabe Y, Kurata T, Kitani T, Sairenji T (2003) Diagnostic evaluation for 2′,5′-oligoadenylate synthetase activities and antibodies against Epstein–Barr virus and *Coxiella burnetii* in patients with chronic fatigue syndrome in Japan. Microbes Infect 5(12):1096–1102
9. Demettre E, Bastide L, D'Haese A, De Smet K, De Meirleir K, Tiev KP, Englebienne P, Lebleu B (2002) Ribonuclease L proteolysis in peripheral blood mononuclear cells of chronic fatigue syndrome patients. J Biol Chem 277(38):35746–35751
10. Katafuchi T, Kondo T, Yasaka T, Kubo K, Take S, Yoshimura M (2003) Prolonged effects of polyriboinosinic:polyribocytidylic acid on spontaneous running-wheel activity and brain interferon-alpha mRNA in rats: a model for immunologically induced fatigue. Neuroscience 120(3):837–845
11. Inoue K, Yamazaki H, Manabe Y, Fukuda C, Hanai K, Fushiki T (1999) Transforming growth factor-beta activated during exercise in brain depresses spontaneous motor activity of animals. Relevance to central fatigue. Brain Res 846(2):145–153
12. Stankovic AK, Dion LD, Parker CR Jr. (1994) Effects of transforming growth factor-beta on human fetal adrenal steroid production. Mol Cell Endocrinol 99(2):145–151
13. Chiu KM, Schmidt MJ, Shug AL, Binkley N, Gravenstein S (1997) Effect of dehydroepiandrosterone sulfate on carnitine acetyl transferase activity and L-carnitine levels in oophorectomized rats. Biochim Biophys Acta 1344(3):201–209
14. Kuratsune H, Yamaguti K, Sawada M, Kodate S, Machii T, Kanakura Y, Kitani T (1998) Dehydroepiandrosterone sulfate deficiency in chronic fatigue syndrome. Int J Mol Med 1:143–146
15. Kuratsune H, Yamaguti K, Takahashi M, Misaki H, Tagawa S, Kitani T (1994) Acylcarnitine deficiency in chronic fatigue syndrome. Clin Infect Dis 18(Suppl 1):S62–S67
16. Tanaka S, Kuratsune H, Hidaka Y, Hakariya Y, Tatsumi KI, Takano T, Kanakura Y, Amino N (2003) Autoantibodies against muscarinic cholinergic receptor in chronic fatigue syndrome. Int J Mol Med 12:225–230
17. Levy JA (1994) Viral studies of chronic fatigue syndrome. Clin Infect Dis 18(Suppl 1): S117–120

18. Ablashi DV, Eastman HB, Owen CB, Roman MM, Friedman J, Zabriskie JB, Peterson DL, Pearson GR, Whitman JE (2000) Frequent HHV-6 reactivation in multiple sclerosis (MS) and chronic fatigue syndrome (CFS) patients. J Clin Virol 16(3):179–191
19. Vojdani A, Choppa PC, Tagle C, Andrin R, Samimi B, Lapp CW (1998) Detection of Mycoplasma genus and *Mycoplasma fermentans* by PCR in patients with chronic fatigue syndrome. FEMS Immunol Med Microbiol 22(4):355–365
20. Nakaya T, Takahashi H, Nakamura Y, Asahi S, Tobiume M, Kuratsune H, Kitani T, Yamanishi K, Ikuta K (1996) Demonstration of Borna disease virus RNA in peripheral blood mononuclear cells derived from Japanese patients with chronic fatigue syndrome. FEBS Lett 378:145–149
21. Nakaya T, Takahashi H, Nakamur Y, Kuratsune H, Kitani T, Machii T, Yamanishi K, Ikuta K (1999) Borna disease virus infection in two family clusters of patients with chronic fatigue syndrome. Microbiol Immunol 43(7):679–689
22. Evengård B, Briese T, Lindh G, Lee S, Lipkin WI (1999) Absence of evidence of Borna disease virus infection in Swedish patients with chronic fatigue syndrome. J Neurovirol 5(5):495–499
23. Demitrack MA, Dale JK, Straus SE, Laue L, Listwak SJ, Kruesi MJ, Chrousos GP, Gold PW (1991) Evidence for impaired activation of the hypothalamic-pituitary-adrenal axis in patients with chronic fatigue syndrome. J Clin Endocrinol Metab 73(6):1224–1234
24. Roberts AD, Wessely S, Chalder T, Papadopoulos A, Cleare AJ (2004) Salivary cortisol response to awakening in chronic fatigue syndrome. Br J Psychiatr 184:136–131
25. Gaab J, Engert V, Heitz V, Schad T, Schürmeyer TH, Ehlert U (2004) Associations between neuroendocrine responses to the insulin tolerance test and patient characteristics in chronic fatigue syndrome. J Psychosom Res 56(4):419–424
26. Gaab J, Hüster D, Peisen R, Engert V, Schad T, Schürmeyer TH, Ehlert U (2002) Low-dose dexamethasone suppression test in chronic fatigue syndrome and health. Psychosom Med 64(2):311–318
27. Rebouche CJ (1988) Carnitine metabolism and human nutrition. J Appl Nutr 40:99–111
28. Yamaguti K, Kuratsune H, Watanabe Y, Takahashi M, Nakamoto I, Machii T, Jacobsson G, Onoe H, Matsumura K, Valind S, Langstrom B, Kitani T (1996) Acylcarnitine metabolism during fasting and after refeeding. Biochem Biophys Res Commun 225:740–746
29. Kuratsune H, Yamaguti K, Lindh G, Evengård B, Hagberg G, Matsumura K, Iwase M, Onoe H, Takahashi M, Machii T, Kanakura Y, Kitani T, Långström B, Watanabe Y (2002) Brain regions involved in fatigue sensation: reduced acetylcarnitine uptake into the brain. Neuroimage 17(3):1256–1265
30. Plioplys AV, Plioplys S (1995) Serum levels of carnitine in chronic fatigue syndrome: clinical correlates. Biol Psychiatr 32:132–138
31. Soetekouw PM, Wevers RA, Vreken P, Elving LD, Janssen AJ, van der Veen Y, Bleijenberg G, van der Meer JW (2000) Normal carnitine levels in patients with chronic fatigue syndrome. Neth J Med 57(1):20–24
32. Jones MG, Goodwin CS, Amjad S, Chalmers RA (2005) Plasma and urinary carnitine and acylcarnitines in chronic fatigue syndrome. Clin Chim Acta 360(1–2):173–177
33. Vermeulen RC, Scholte HR (2006) Azithromycin in chronic fatigue syndrome (CFS): an analysis of clinical data. J Trans Med 4:34
34. Vermeulen RC, Scholte HR (2004) Exploratory open label, randomized study of acetyl- and propionylcarnitine in chronic fatigue syndrome. Psychosom Med 66(2):276–282
35. Kuratsune H, Yamaguti K, Watanabe Y, Takahashi M, Nakamoto I, Machii T, Jacobson GB, Onoe H, Matsumura T, Valind S, Langstrom B, Kitani T (1997) Acylcarnitine and chronic fatigue syndrome. In: DeSimone C, Famularo G (eds) Carnitine today. Molecular Biology Intelligence Unit, Landes Bioscience, pp 195–213
36. Natelson BH, Cohen JM, Brassloff I, Lee HJ (1993) A controlled study of brain magnetic resonance imaging in patients with the chronic fatigue syndrome. J Neurol Sci 120(2):213–217

37. Greco A, Tannock C, Brostoff J, Costa DC (1997) Brain MR in chronic fatigue syndrome. Am J Neuroradiol 18(7):1265–1269
38. Lange G, DeLuca J, Maldjian JA, Lee H, Tiersky LA, Natelson BH (1999) Brain MRI abnormalities exist in a subset of patients with chronic fatigue syndrome. J Neurol Sci 171(1):1–2
39. Cook DB, Lange G, DeLuca J, Natelson BH (2001) Relationship of brain MRI abnormalities and physical functional status in chronic fatigue syndrome. Int J Neurosci 107(1–2):1–6
40. Okada T, Tanaka M, Kuratsune H, Watanabe Y, Sadato N (2004) Mechanisms underlying fatigue: a voxel-based morphometric study of chronic fatigue syndrome. BMC Neurol 4(1):14
41. de Lange FP, Kalkman JS, Bleijenberg G, Hagoort P, van der Meer JW, Toni I (2005) Gray matter volume reduction in chronic fatigue syndrome. Neuroimage 26(3):777–781
42. Ichise M, Salit IE, Abbey SE, Chung DG, Gray B, Kirsh JC, Freedman M (1992) Assessment of regional cerebral perfusion by 99Tcm-HMPAO SPECT in chronic fatigue syndrome. Nucl Med Commun 13:767–772
43. Costa DC, Tannock C, Brostoff J (1995) Brainstem perfusion is impaired in chronic fatigue syndrome. QJM 88:767–773
44. Fischler B, D'Haenen H, Cluydts R, Michiels V, Demets K, Bossuyt A, Kaufman L, De Meirleir K (1996) Comparison of 99m Tc HMPAO SPECT scan between chronic fatigue syndrome, major depression and healthy controls: an exploratory study of clinical correlates of regional cerebral blood flow. Neuropsychobiology 34:175–183
45. Tirelli U, Chierichetti F, Tavio M, Simonelli C, Bianchin G, Zanco P, Ferlin G (1998) Brain positron emission tomography (PET) in chronic fatigue syndrome: preliminary data. Am J Med 105(3A):54S–58S
46. Siessmeier T, Nix WA, Hardt J, Schreckenberger M, Egle UT, Bartenstein P (2003) Observer-independent analysis of cerebral glucose metabolism in patients with chronic fatigue syndrome. J Neurol Neurosurg Psychiatry 74(7):922–928
47. Yamamoto S, Ouchi Y, Onoe H, Yoshikawa E, Tsukada H, Takahashi H, Iwase M, Yamaguti K, Kuratsune H, Watanabe Y (2004) Reduction of serotonin transporters in patients with chronic fatigue syndrome. Neuroreport 15:2571–2574
48. Demettre E, Bastide L, D'Haese A, De Smet K, De Meirleir K, Tiev KP, Englebienne P, Lebleu B (2002) Ribonuclease L proteolysis in peripheral blood mononuclear cells of chronic fatigue syndrome patients. J Biol Chem 277(38):35746–35751
49. Oliff A, Defeo-Jones D, Boyer M, Martinez D, Kiefer D, Vuocolo G, Wolfe A, Socher SH (1987) Tumors secreting human TNF/cachectin induce cachexia in mice. Cell 50(4):555–563
50. Fukuda K, Straus SE, Hickie I, Sharpe MC, Dobbins JG, Komaroff A (1994) The chronic fatigue syndrome: a comprehensive approach to its definition and study. International Chronic Fatigue Syndrome Study Group. Ann Intern Med 121(12):953–959
51. Bode L, Dietrich DE, Stoyloff R, Emrich HM, Ludwig H (1997) Amantadine and human Borna disease virus in vitro and in vivo in an infected patient with bipolar depression. Lancet 349(9046):178–179

Development and Validation of a New Fatigue Scale for Fatigued Subjects With and Without Chronic Fatigue Syndrome

Sanae Fukuda[1], Shoko Takashima[3], Masao Iwase[2], Kouzi Yamaguti[1,3], Hirohiko Kuratsune[3,4], and Yasuyoshi Watanabe[1]

Summary

The objective of our study was to develop a new fatigue scale for the assessment of patients with chronic fatigue syndrome (CFS) as well as people who feel they are chronically fatigued but do not meet the diagnostic criteria for CFS. A new fatigue scale was developed by one psychiatrist and two physicians who specialize in CFS. This scale consists of various psychosomatic symptoms, psychiatric symptoms, and diagnostic criteria for CFS. It was completed by 325 patients with CFS, 311 fatigue patients who did not fulfill the diagnostic criteria for CFS, 92 healthy workers, and 80 university students. The Chalder fatigue scale, the profile of mood states (POMS), the performance status (PS), which is included in the Japanese diagnostic criteria for CFS, and the visual analogue scale (VAS) for fatigue were also assessed with the agreement of patients who consulted our center from December 2004 to April 2006. Seventy-two university students also completed the questionnaire, including this new scale, the Chalder fatigue scale, and other lifestyle factors, and we reconfirmed the effectiveness of the new scale among fatigue patients with and without CFS and normal controls. There was a high degree of internal consistency in the results, and principal components analysis supported the notion of an 8-factor solution (42 items covering fatigue, anxiety and depression, loss of attention and memory, pain, overwork, autonomic imbalance, sleep problems, and infection). Only "anxiety and depression," "pain," and "infection" factors were able to distinguish CFS from not CFS. The sensitivity and specificity of CFS were 67.7 and 64.4, respectively, using

[1]Department of Physiology, Osaka City University Graduate School of Medicine, 1-4-3 Asahimachi Abeno-ku, Osaka 545-8585, Japan

[2]Department of Psychiatry, Osaka University Graduate School of Medicine, Osaka, Japan

[3]Department of Internal Medicine, Osaka City University Graduate School of Medicine, Osaka, Japan

[4]Department of Health Science, Faculty of Health Sciences for Welfare, Kansai University of Welfare Sciences, Kansai, Japan

a cut-off score of 25 points for this subscore. We concluded that the new fatigue scale used in this study was useful for differentiating CFS patients from not CFS patients and fatigued people from a healthy sample.

Introduction

According to the US Centers for Disease Control and Prevention (CDC), chronic fatigue syndrome (CFS) is defined as a sensation of abnormal and unexplained mental and physical fatigue of at least 6 months' duration [1].

The cause of CFS and chronic continuous fatigue is poorly understood, and few pharmacological or somatic treatments have been shown to be effective. It is important to develop a clear clinical picture, as well as a simple screening questionnaire that distinguishes CFS from fatigue symptoms that do not fulfill the diagnostic criteria of CFS (hereafter referred to as "not CFS"). A few studies have used depression rating scales or fatigue rating scales to distinguish CFS [2,3] from "not CFS," but these scales have not been shown to be adequate at distinguishing between CFS and "not CFS" at our clinical fatigue center, where many people consult us complaining of fatigue. We need to understand not only fatigue itself, but also its related symptoms, in order to clarify the clinical picture of CFS.

About 60% of people in Japan report that they feel fatigue [4]. About 40% of these complain of continuous fatigue for more than 6 months. In other countries, the prevalence of fatigue ranges from 14.3% to 38.0% (United States, 14.3% and 20.4%; Norway, 22%; Australia, 25.0%; the United Kingdom, 38.0%) [5–8]. In a cross-cultural epidemiological study, the prevalence of unexplained fatigue of 1-month duration ranged from 2.7% to 15.1% [9]. It is important to detect and cope with the general symptoms of fatigue as soon as possible after the symptoms appear, as fatigue might be related to the presence of various diseases, including cancer [10–13], or might induce Karoshi [14] and a decrease in the amount and inventiveness of work. In addition, fatigue may be associated with economic losses.

The aim of our study was to examine the reliability and validity of a new scale for both healthy, pathologically fatigued people (i.e., not CFS) and those with CFS.

Methods

A new fatigue scale which included the symptoms of CFS, i.e., sleep difficulties, depression, attention problems, somatic symptoms, loss of motivation, delayed recovery from diseases, and overload, was developed by one psychiatrist (M.I.) and two physicians (H.K. and K.Y). The questionnaire associated with this scale consisted of 64 questions (see Appendix). All 64 questions were scored using a Likert scale (0–4). The questionnaire was completed by 325 patients with CFS (mean age

(±SD) 36.9 (±10.0) years, 65.8% of whom were female) and 311 people who consulted the clinical fatigue center but did not fulfill the CFS criteria, that is "not CFS" (mean age (±SD) 42.9 (±15.3) years, 53.1% of whom were female). It was also completed by two groups of subjects with no symptoms of fatigue, including 92 healthy workers in A company (mean age (±SD) 39.3 (±10.9) years, 48.9% of whom were female) and 80 Osaka City University medical students (group 1) (mean age (±SD) 20.9 (±2.0) years, 32.5% of whom were female). For test–retest reliability, we asked 56 CFS patients (who were not included in the CFS patients group above) who consulted our center from September 2006 to February 2007 (mean age (±SD) 36.6 (±10.4) years, 58.9% of whom were female) to complete the new questionnaire twice at an interval of between 14 and 50 days, and we used only the results from subjects who completed the questionnaire twice within less than 30 days.

The Chalder fatigue scale, the profile of mood states (POMS), and the performance status (PS), which is now included in the diagnostic criteria for CFS in Japan (Table 1), as well as a visual analogue scale (VAS) for fatigue [13], were completed by people who consulted the center from December 2004 to April 2006. In addition, the university students in group 1 also completed the PS, the Chalder fatigue scale, and the VAS.

Another 72 university students (group 2) also completed the new questionnaire, and we reconfirmed the effectiveness of the scale with this group.

A translation of the draft scales into English was performed by two different editorial companies using an interactive forward–backward translation.

Table 1. Performance status scores for evaluating the daily activity, working status, and severity of fatigue in chronic fatigue syndrome (CFS) patients

Scores	Content
0	Able to carry on normal daily social activity without fatigue
1	Able to carry on normal daily social activity and work, but often feels fatigue
2	Able to carry on normal daily social activity and work, but often needs a rest because of fatigue
3	Several days a month, unable to carry on normal daily social activity and works with generalized fatigability
4	Several days a week, unable to carry on normal daily social activity and works with generalized fatigability
5	Unable to carry on normal daily social activity and work. Able to work on light duties, but several days a week needs a rest at home
6	Able to work at light duties only on good days, but after more than half a week needs a rest at home
7	Able to take care of oneself without assistance, but unable to carry on normal daily social activities or light work duties
8	Able to take care of oneself with assistance, but must be in bed more than half a day
9	Unable to take care of oneself, needs daily assistance, and must be in bed all day

The Chalder Fatigue Scale

This scale was developed by Chalder et al. [15] to measure the severity of fatigue. It consists of 14 questions, and has been found to be both reliable and valid, with a high degree of internal consistency. The principal components of this scale are physical and mental fatigue.

Performance Status (PS)

This proprietary scale was described in the Japanese CFS diagnostic criteria to evaluate daily activity, working status, and the severity of fatigue (Table 1).

VAS for Rating Fatigue

We asked patients, students, and workers to express the intensity of the fatigue they were experiencing at that time on a 100-mm VAS, ranging from not fatigued at all to extremely fatigued [13].

Other Psychological Parameters

We also asked the 72 university students (group 2) the following questions in order to determine the effectiveness of the scale for mental problems.

"Did you experience not feeling well, or were you unable to go to school without any reason and had to stay at home to rest?"

"Did you notice that you were tired or lacking in energy for more than 30 days, did not feel better after getting plenty of rest, and missed school because of tiredness or weakness?"

"Do you feel stress?"

"Do you continue to get tired easily, and not feel much better after having a rest?"

Statistical Analysis

All data were statistically analyzed using SPSS version 13.0J (SPSS Inc., Tokyo, Japan). The statistical methods for evaluating the new fatigue scale are shown in detail in the results. This scale was developed by factor analysis (principal factor method) of the draft items followed by Promax rotation. We used only data from

CFS patients for this analysis. Interscale correlations were evaluated by calculating Pearson's correlations among the Chalder fatigue scale, PS, VAS, and POMS. Reliability was evaluated by examining Cronbach's α coefficient. The mean differences of the new fatigue scale and its subscales were tested by one-way analysis of variance among CFS, not CFS, and healthy people [workers and students (group 1)]. Test–retest reliability was assessed by Pearson's correlations comparing scores reported on two separate occasions, and we used only samples with an interval of less than 30 days. We examined the relationships between fatigue or mental health factors and the new fatigue scale by the Mann–Whitney nonparametric test or the Kruskal–Wallis test, and calculated their sensitivity and specificity, respectively.

Results

The characteristics of all participants are shown in Table 2. Promax rotation analysis of the principal component method was performed to confirm the principal axes of the questionnaire. Although 12 factors were selected at the first step, we could conceptualize only the first 8 factors (Table 3). These 8 factors accounted for 52.5% of the total variance. We used 42 questions that did not overlap with these 8 factors (load > 0.4) (Table 4). Cronbach's α for each factor was 0.96, 0.94, 0.92, 0.87, 0.80, 0.71, 0.79, and 0.69, respectively, and its total score was 0.96. Because each factor has a different number of questions, we re-calculated each score to go up to 20 points, and assigned those scores to subscales (factors 1 through 8, where factor 1 = fatigue, factor 2 = anxiety and depression, factor 3 = loss of attention and memory, factor 4 = pain, factor 5 = overwork, factor 6 = autonomic imbalance, factor 7 = sleep problems, and factor 8 = infection) of the new fatigue scale (Table 4).

Table 5 shows the results of the correlation coefficients between the new scale and other scales. The short version of the new fatigue scale was highly correlated with the Chalder fatigue scale, PS, and VAS ($r > 0.4$). Factors 1 and 4 were positively associated with the Chalder fatigue scale, PS, and VAS ($r > 0.4$). Factor 2 was highly correlated with the Chalder fatigue scale and POMS (tension–anxiety and depression–dejection) ($r > 0.4$). Factor 3 was correlated with the Chalder

Table 2. Characteristics of the participants

Sample	n	Age (years) Mean	SD	Sex (% female)
Workers	92	39.3	10.9	48.9
University students 1 (2006)	80	20.9	2.03	32.5
Fatigued people but not CFS	311	42.9	15.3	53.1
CFS (20042006)	325	36.9	10.0	65.8
CFS (test-retest)	56	36.6	10.4	58.9
University students 2 (2007)	69	20.6	0.94	39.1

Table 3. Factor analysis (principal factor method by Promax rotation) of the new fatigue scale

Factor	Eigen value	Percent of variance	Cumulative percent
1	18.96	29.63	29.63
2	3.70	5.78	35.40
3	2.60	4.06	39.46
4	2.46	3.84	43.29
5	2.17	3.40	46.69
6	1.34	2.09	48.78
7	1.28	1.99	50.77
8	0.95	1.48	52.25
9	0.87	1.35	53.60
10	0.69	1.08	54.68
11	0.63	0.98	55.66
12	0.57	0.89	56.55

Table 4. Principal factor analysis with Promax rotation of items in a new fatigue scale

Factor number	Factor name	Item number
Factor 1	Fatigue	9, 10, 15, 18, 31, 43, 50, 51
Factor 2	Anxiety and depression	2, 11, 20, 21, 26, 27, 29, 33, 34, 38, 52
Factor 3	Loss of attention and memory	6, 17, 30, 47, 53
Factor 4	Pain	7, 22, 23, 58, 62
Factor 5	Overwork	24, 32, 44, 49, 61
Factor 6	Autonomic imbalance	36, 39, 63, 64
Factor 7	Sleep problems	4, 54, 59
Factor 8	Infection	35, 57

fatigue scale, the POMS confusion scale, and PS ($r > 0.4$). Factors 6 and 7 were correlated with the Chalder fatigue scale ($r > 0.4$).

Table 6 shows the differences in the means of each factors' score and total score. The scores of all factors except factor 5 and the total score showed significant differences between "CFS and workers," "CFS and students," "not CFS and workers," and "not CFS and students." Only factors 2, 4, and 8 showed a significant difference between CFS and not CFS ($P < 0.0001$).

Thereafter, we added factor 4, factor 8, and the reciprocal of factor 2, and assigned this score into a new category (factor 248). We used the mean area under the receiver operating characteristic curves (ROC) of factor 248 to determine the cut-off point from the ROC curve to distinguish CFS from controls or "not CFS." The ROC was 0.77, and we set the cut-off points from 22 to 26 for every 1 point (Table 7). The most suitable cut-off point for distinguishing CFS from not CFS was 25 points, and from healthy controls it was 23 points.

The test–retest correlation coefficients of each factor and the total score between the first and second sessions were all above 0.56 ($P < 0.001$) (Table 8).

Table 5. Correlation coefficients between each factor of a 64-item developmental fatigue scale and other fatigue scales

	Chalder fatigue scale	POMS (n = 607)						PS	VAS
		Tension-anxiety	Depression-dejection	Anger-hostility	Vigor	Fatigue	Confusion		
Factor 1	0.68*** (n = 676)	0.20*** (n = 605)	0.21*** (n = 602)	0.17*** (n = 602)	–0.21*** (n = 605)	0.38*** (n = 604)	0.28*** (n = 604)	0.67*** (n = 607)	0.61*** (n = 70)
Factor 2	0.66*** (n = 677)	0.41*** (n = 604)	0.42*** (n = 601)	0.32*** (n = 601)	–0.30*** (n = 604)	0.34*** (n = 603)	0.38*** (n = 603)	0.36*** (n = 607)	0.36*** (n = 672)
Factor 3	0.73*** (n = 677)	0.23*** (n = 606)	0.20*** (n = 603)	0.17*** (n = 603)	–0.16*** (n = 606)	0.26*** (n = 605)	0.41*** (n = 605)	0.43*** (n = 607)	0.36*** (n = 672)
Factor 4	0.53*** (n = 676)	0.13*** (n = 603)	0.10*** (n = 600)	0.09* (n = 600)	–0.03 (n = 603)	0.18*** (n = 602)	0.18*** (n = 602)	0.44*** (n = 607)	0.40*** (n = 671)
Factor 5	0.22*** (n = 676)	0.19*** (n = 603)	0.11** (n = 600)	0.09* (n = 600)	–0.13** (n = 604)	0.16*** (n = 602)	0.13** (n = 602)	–0.11** (n = 607)	0.11** (n = 672)
Factor 6	0.44*** (n = 677)	0.15*** (n = 605)	0.09* (n = 602)	0.12** (n = 602)	–0.07 (n = 605)	0.16*** (n = 604)	0.17 (n = 604)	0.33*** (n = 607)	0.24*** (n = 672)
Factor 7	0.46*** (n = 678)	0.16*** (n = 606)	0.11** (n = 603)	0.16** (n = 603)	–0.06 (n = 606)	0.22*** (n = 605)	0.23 (n = 605)	0.25*** (n = 607)	0.21*** (n = 673)
Factor 8	0.31*** (n = 678)	0.04 (n = 607)	–0.05 (n = 604)	–0.05 (n = 604)	0.07 (n = 607)	0.02 (n = 606)	0.04 (n = 606)	0.34*** (n = 607)	0.18*** (n = 647)
Total	0.75*** (n = 652)	0.27*** (n = 583)	0.22*** (n = 580)	0.20*** (n = 580)	–0.16*** (n = 584)	0.32*** (n = 582)	0.35*** (n = 582)	0.52*** (n = 607)	0.46*** (n = 647)

*** $P < 0.001$; ** $P < 0.01$; * $P < 0.05$

The values in the table are correlation coefficients

Table 6. Comparison of the mean scores in a 42-item fatigue scale among CFS, not CFS, and healthy people (university students and workers)

	CFS $n = 324$	Not CFS $n = 300$	Students $n = 78$	Workers $n = 92$	F	P	
Factor 1	14.47 ± 4.87	14.73 ± 4.71	4.19 ± 3.71	3.15 ± 2.95	260.52	<0.0001	a,b,e,f
Factor 2	6.86 ± 4.77	9.41 ± 5.46	4.25 ± 3.46	2.73 ± 2.14	59.67	<0.0001	a,b,c,e,f
Factor 3	11.15 ± 5.43	10.29 ± 5.81	5.27 ± 3.67	4.48 ± 2.99	58.35	<0.0001	a,b,e,f
Factor 4	9.68 ± 5.42	8.35 ± 5.44	2.71 ± 3.01	1.71 ± 2.34	86.64	<0.0001	a,b,c,e,f
Factor 5	4.46 ± 4.54	5.27 ± 4.85	5.73 ± 4.54	4.92 ± 4.00	2.44	0.06	
Factor 6	4.29 ± 4.03	4.25 ± 4.21	1.83 ± 2.57	0.99 ± 1.89	26.54	<0.0001	a,b,e,f
Factor 7	9.06 ± 5.79	8.49 ± 5.93	6.32 ± 4.23	3.59 ± 3.25	27.13	<0.0001	a,b,e,f
Factor 8	6.80 ± 5.31	3.94 ± 4.69	0.94 ± 2.11	0.84 ± 2.04	64.26	<0.0001	a,b,c,e,f
42-item	66.56 ± 26.0	64.32 ± 27.3	17.61 ± 2.05	15.58 ± 15.6	113.31	<0.0001	a,b,e,f
(20-Factor 2) + Factor 4 + Factor 8	29.57 ± 8.56	22.97 ± 8.47	19.42 ± 4.58	19.42 ± 4.58	70.88	<0.0001	a,b,c,e,f

A, CFS vs workers; b, CFS vs students; c, CFS vs not CFS; d, students vs workers; e, students vs not CFS; f, not CFS vs workers

Missing values: factor 1, two CFS, 2 not CFS, and 2 students; factor 2, five not CFS; factor 3, one CFS, 2 not CFS, and one student; factor 4, one CFS and 5 not CFS; factor 5, two CFS and 4 not CFS; factor 6, 1 CFS and 3 not CFS; factor 7, 2 CFS and not CFS; factor 8, 2 CFS and one student; total, 9 CFS, 8 not CFS, and 4 students

All statistics used one-way analysis of variance

Table 7. Screening characteristics between CFS and not CFS or healthy controls from a new fatigue scale (factors 2, 4, and 8) for different cut-off scores

	Not CFS		Healthy	
Threshold score	Sensitivity (%)	Specificity (%)	Sensitivity (%)	Specificity (%)
22	78.8	51.9	78.8	83.4
23	87.0	55.6	**87.0**	**87.0**
24	71.4	62.0	71.4	90.5
25	**67.7**	**64.4**	67.7	93.5
26	61.8	69.2	61.8	95.3

"not CFS" indicates patients who visited the clinical fatigue center in Osaka City University Hospital with complaints of fatigue but who were not diagnosed with chronic fatigue syndrome. Bold type fonts mean the most suitable cut-off point, respectively

Table 8. Test-retest reliability of the total scale and each subscale

Test-retest reliability (correlation coefficient) (n = 56)	
Factor 1	0.77***
Factor 2	0.78***
Factor 3	0.81***
Factor 4	0.78***
Factor 5	0.82***
Factor 6	0.72***
Factor 7	0.81***
Factor 8	0.56***
Total	0.81***

*** $P < 0.001$
The values in the table are correlation coefficients

We reconfirmed the effectiveness of the scale in the other university students, because we developed this questionnaire to apply not only to CFS, but also to "not CFS." Only the mean score of factor 2 showed significant differences between subjects who did not feel well and those who felt well ($Z = -2.25$, $P = 0.03$) (Table 9). The total score and subscores, except for factor 5, showed significant differences between subjects who were tired for more than 30 days and those who were not tired for more than 30 days (factor 1, $Z = -3.02$, $P = 0.003$; factor 2, $Z = -3.69$, $P < 0.0001$; factor 3, $Z = -3.00$, $P = 0.003$; factor 4, $Z = -2.74$, $P = 0.006$; factor 6, $Z = -3.19$, $P = 0.001$; factor 7, $Z = -2.24$, $P = 0.03$; factor 8, $Z = -2.03$, $P = 0.04$; total, $Z = -3.30$, $P = 0.001$). The total score and subscores, except for factors 5, 7, and 8, showed significant differences between subjects who tired easily and those who did not tire easily (factor 1, $\chi^2 = 6.53$, $P = 0.04$; factor 2, $\chi^2 = 12.99$, $P = 0.002$; factor 3, $\chi^2 = 12.25$, $P = 0.002$; factor 4, $\chi^2 = 11.49$, $P = 0.003$; factor 6, $\chi^2 = 11.26$, $P = 0.004$; total, $\chi^2 = 9.50$, $P = 0.009$). The total score and subscores,

Table 9. The relationship between mental problems and the new fatigue scale (mean ± SD)

Factor	1	2	3	4	5	6	7	8	Total
A Not well ($n = 15$)	5.88 ± 5.32	5.80 ± 4.42	4.87 ± 4.55	2.40 ± 3.29	4.80 ± 5.24	1.33 ± 2.52	8.00 ± 4.64	1.33 ± 3.39	34.4 ± 25.3
Well ($n = 54$)	3.28 ± 3.42	3.45 ± 4.08	3.35 ± 4.20	2.09 ± 3.43	4.94 ± 4.78	0.53 ± 1.37	6.91 ± 5.45	0.47 ± 1.55	24.9 ± 21.3
		*							
B Tired ($n = 10$)	8.75 ± 6.08	8.85 ± 4.74	7.50 ± 4.97	5.20 ± 5.29	5.20 ± 5.29	3.00 ± 3.40	10.5 ± 5.45	2.25 ± 4.16	52.9 ± 31.8
Not tired ($n = 59$)	3.01 ± 2.88	3.14 ± 3.58	3.03 ± 3.85	1.64 ± 2.68	1.64 ± 2.68	0.32 ± 0.72	6.58 ± 5.07	0.39 ± 1.39	22.6 ± 17.2
	**	***	**	**		**	*	*	**
C Much ($n = 13$)	7.31 ± 6.05	9.73 ± 5.09	7.85 ± 5.16	4.38 ± 4.84	8.23 ± 5.96	2.21 ± 3.15	8.08 ± 6.76	1.35 ± 3.63	49.1 ± 32.4
Moderate ($n = 37$)	3.56 ± 3.12	3.30 ± 2.91	2.89 ± 3.76	1.81 ± 3.20	4.41 ± 4.21	0.47 ± 0.95	7.70 ± 5.52	0.69 ± 1.85	24.7 ± 17.5
Little ($n = 19$)	2.01 ± 2.15	1.32 ± 1.19	2.37 ± 2.79	1.32 ± 1.60	3.63 ± 4.39	0.13 ± 0.57	5.44 ± 3.03	0.13 ± 0.57	16.3 ± 9.54
	*	***	**	*		**			**
D No symptom ($n = 58$)	3.15 ± 3.14	3.06 ± 3.32	2.84 ± 3.62	1.55 ± 2.60	4.57 ± 4.73	0.36 ± 0.84	6.49 ± 4.92	0.48 ± 1.53	22.4 ± 16.7
>1 month ($n = 6$)	5.00 ± 2.82	8.08 ± 4.84	7.17 ± 4.62	3.17 ± 3.82	4.17 ± 3.60	1.25 ± 2.50	8.89 ± 5.02	2.08 ± 5.10	39.8 ± 21.6
>6 months ($n = 5$)	10.5 ± 7.72	9.50 ± 6.60	9.20 ± 5.72	8.00 ± 5.48	9.80 ± 5.54	4.00 ± 3.89	12.7 ± 6.83	1.00 ± 2.24	64.7 ± 40.4
	*	**	**	**		**			**

A; a subject who does not feel well, or cannot go to school but has no reason, or has to go home to rest

B: a subject who was tired or lacking in energy for more than 30 days, does not feel much better after getting plenty of rest, and was absent from school because of tiredness or weakness

C: a subject who feels stress

D: a subject who continues to get tired easily, and does not feel much better after having a rest

*** $P < 0.001$; ** $P < 0.01$; * $P < 0.05$

A and B were tested by the Mann-Whitney test, and C and D were examined by the Kruskal-Wallis test except for factors 5, 7, and 8, showed significant differences between subjects who felt stress and those who did not feel stress (factor 1, $\chi^2 = 8.66$, $P = 0.01$; factor 2, $\chi^2 = 25.67$, $P < 0.0001$; factor 3, $\chi^2 = 11.47$, $P = 0.003$; factor 4, $\chi^2 = 8.48$, $P = 0.01$; factor 6, $\chi^2 = 10.22$, $P = 0.006$; total, $\chi^2 = 11.40$, $P = 0.003$).

Discussion

In this study, we explored a new fatigue scale to see if it could be used to discriminate between CFS and "not CFS." The new fatigue scale was conceptualized into eight main factors by factor analysis: 1, fatigue; 2, anxiety and depression; 3, loss of attention and memory; 4, pain; 5, overwork; 6, autonomic imbalance; 7, sleep problems; 8, infection. We reconstructed a new 42-item fatigue scale that showed good reliability. This new scale and its subscales were significantly correlated with other psychiatric scales. The mean scores of the new scale and its subscales showed differences between healthy people and people with CFS. Only three factors showed differences between CFS and not CFS. Therefore, we categorized a new subscale that included these three factors, and examined the specificity and sensitivity of screening for CFS in a mixed group of not CFS and healthy people. The most suitable cut-off point for discriminating between CFS and not CFS was 25 points (sensitivity, 65.3; specificity, 64.1), and between CFS and healthy people it was 23 points (sensitivity, 81.5; specificity, 83.4). These values are considered to be high bearing in mind the complexity of the clinical picture.

De Vries et al. [16] examined six fatigue questionnaires completed by a working population and reported that the fatigue assessment scale [17] represented the most promising fatigue measure for the working population [16]. Our new scale has the advantage that it can be used for both patients and healthy people.

The limitations of this study include a small sample size (patients and controls) and the fact that we did not examine the validity of the scale in different populations. Further surveys are clearly needed, but this new scale might be useful in clinical practice for discriminating between CFS and not CFS. Because 42 questions are too many for fatigued patients as well as for epidemiological studies, we need to develop a shorter version of the scale.

There were relationships between some mental problems and the new fatigue scale. In addition, the sensitivity and specificity of this scale for fatigued students within a group of university students (group 2) were 60.0 and 74.1, respectively, using a cut-off score of 33 points. However, the fitness of this cut-off score was not good, and further research is needed to clarify this point (data not shown).

Each psychosocial variable of depression, anxiety, optimism, internal health, locus of control, amount of social support, satisfaction with social support, and sleep quality is partially mediated by emotional intelligence and fatigue [18–20]. Siegrist [21] presented an effort and reward imbalance model in the working population. Some studies show that higher levels of exposure for the effort and reward imbalance component over-commitment are associated with an increasing prevalence of sleep disturbance and fatigue [22,23]. Kato et al. [24] reported that elevated premorbid stress is a significant risk factor for chronic fatigue-like illness. In order to develop a higher-accuracy scale for various populations, we need to include fatigue variables from multiple dimensions, including the recovery phase from fatigue, motivation, personality, social support, environment, and lifestyle.

In conclusion, the new fatigue scale used in this study was useful for differentiating CFS patients from "not CFS" patients, and fatigued people from healthy controls.

Acknowledgments. This research was conducted with support from the 21st Century COE Program "Base to Overcome Fatigue" from the Ministry of Education, Culture, Sports, Science and Technology, the Japanese Government, and RISTEX of JST (Japan Science and Technology Agency). We thank Masaaki Tanaka, Kei Mizuno, Emi Yamano, Kaoru Yoshida, Asami Eguchi, and Kanako Tajima for their support.

References

1. Fukuda K, Straus SE, Hickie I, Sharpe MS, Dobbins JG, Komaroff A (1994) The chronic fatigue syndrome: a comprehensive approach to its definition and study. International Chronic Fatigue Syndrome Study Group. Ann Intern Med 121:953–959
2. Morris RK, Wearden AJ, Mullis R (1998) Exploring the validity of the Chalder fatigue scale in chronic fatigue syndrome. J Psychosom Res 45:411–417
3. Henderson M, Tannock C (2005) Use of depression rating scales in chronic fatigue syndrome. J Psychosom Res 59:181–184
4. Survey from 2004 by the Research Group "Revealing Fatigue and its Neuro/Molecular Mechanism and Overcoming Fatigue" (in Japanese). Supported by the Ministry of Education, Culture, Sports, Science and Technology Foundation
5. Chen MK (1986) The epidemiology of self-perceived fatigue among adults. Prev Med 15:74–81
6. Kage JH, Ekeberg O, Kaasa S (1998) Fatigue in the general Norwegian population: normative data and associations. J Psychosom Res 45:53–65
7. Hickie IB, Hooker AW, Hadzi-Pavlovic D, Bennett BK, Wilson AJ, Lloyd AR (1996) Fatigue in selected primary care settings: sociodemographic and psychiatric correlates. Med J Aust 164:585–588
8. Pawlikowska T, Chalder T, Hirsch SR, Wallace P, Wright DJ, Wessely SC (1994) Population-based study of fatigue and psychological distress. Br Med J 308:763–766
9. Skapinakis P, Lewis G, Mavreas V (2003) Cross-cultural differences in the epidemiology of unexplained fatigue syndrome in primary care. Br J Psychiatr 182:205–209
10. Bjornsson E, Simren M, Olsson R, Chapman RW (2004) Fatigue in patients with primary sclerosing cholangitis. Scand J Gastroenterol 39:961–968
11. Bower JE, Ganz PA, Desmond KA, Rowland JH, Meyerowitz BE, Belin TR (2000) Fatigue in breast cancer survivors: occurrence, correlates, and impact on quality of life. J Clin Oncol 18:743–753
12. Wilbur J, Shaver J, Kogan J, Buntin M, Wang E (2006) Menopausal transition symptoms in midlife women living with fibromyalgia and chronic fatigue. Health Care Women Int 27:600–614
13. Okuyama Toru, Akechi T, Kugaya A, Okamura H, Shima Y, Maruguchi M, Hosaka T, Uchitomi Y (2000) Development and validation of the cancer fatigue scale: a brief, three-

dimensional, self-rating scale for assessment of fatigue in cancer patients. J Pain Symptom Manage 19:5–14
14. Uehata T (2005) Karoushi: death by overwork (in Japanese). Nippon Rinsho 63:1249–1253
15. Chalder T, Berelowitz G, Pawlikowska T, Watts L, Wessely S, Wright D, Wallace EP (1993) Development of a fatigue scale. J Psychosom Res 37:147–153
16. De Vries J, Michielsen HJ, Van Heck GL (2003) Assessment of fatigue among working people: a comparison of six questionnaires. Occup Environ Med 60 (Suppl 1):i10–i15
17. Michielson HJ, De Vries J, Van Heck GL (2002) Psychometric qualities of a brief self-rated fatigue measure: the Fatigue Assessment Scale (FAS). J Psychosom Res 54:345–352
18. Godin I, Kittel F, Coppieters Y, Siegrist J (2005) A prospective study of cumulative job stress in relation to mental health. BMC Public Health 5:67
19. Watt T, Groenvold M, Bjorner JB, Noerholm V, Rasmussen N-A, Bech P (2000) Fatigue in the Danish general population. Influence of sociodemographic factors and disease. J Epidemiol Community Health 54:827–833
20. Beckers DGJ, van der Linden D, Smulders PGW, Kompier MAJ, van Veldhoven MJPM, van Yperen NW (2004) Working overtime hours: relations with fatigue, work motivation, and the quality of work. J Occup Environ Med 46:1282–1289
21. Siegrist J (1996) Adverse health effects of high-effort/low-reward conditions. J Occup Health Psychol 1:27–41
22. Fahlen G, Knutsson A, Peter R, Akerstedt T, Nordin M, Alfredsson L, Westerholm P (2006) Effort–reward imbalance, sleep disturbances and fatigue. Int Arch Occup Environ Health 79:371–378
23. Takaki J, Nakao M, Karita K, Nisikitani M, Yano E (2006) Relationships between effort–reward imbalance, over-commitment, and fatigue in Japanese information technology workers. J Occup Health 48:62–64
24. Kato K, Sullivan PF, Evengard B, Pedersem NL (2006) Premorbid predictors of chronic fatigue. Arch Gen Psychiatr 63:1267–1272

Appendix

1	Feeling shaky on my feet
2	Feeling restless due to anxiety
3	Getting a low backache
4	Dozing off frequently
5	Having a mild fever
6	Feeling less able to think
7	My legs feel heavy lately
8	Having difficulty breathing
9	Feeling so tired that I want to lie down at times
10	Feeling tired and without energy
11	Being reluctant to socialize with people
12	Being unable to sleep well
13	My eyes easily become tired
14	Not feeling energetic lately
15	Becoming very tired with just a small amount of exercise or work
16	Catching a cold often, and it is difficult to get better
17	Forgetting things at times
18	Feeling sluggish lately
19	My eyelids and muscles twitch
20	Cannot help feeling disgusted with myself

(continued)

21	Feeling depressed
22	Feeling muscle pain recently
23	My arms feel heavy lately
24	Having no time to rest and relax
25	A hoarse voice
26	Unable to get enthusiastic about things
27	Unable to have fun no matter what I do
28	Feeling anxious about the condition of my own body
29	Having no desire to work
30	Unable to remember small things
31	A recent lack of physical energy
32	Being busy and unable to get enough sleep
33	Having thoughts of being better off dead
34	Not wanting to read or write anything
35	Getting swollen lymph nodes
36	A portion of what is in front of my eyes disappears at times
37	Thinking about leaving my current job at times
38	Becoming irritated and touchy
39	Becoming dizzy when there is bright light
40	Feeling sluggish
41	Getting headaches and feeling heavy-headed
42	Having an upset stomach
43	Thinking that the way I get tired recently is abnormal
44	Having work and things to do until late at night
45	Getting caught in a daze
46	Getting stiff shoulders easily
47	Making many careless mistakes
48	Feeling nauseous and sick to my stomach
49	Having a heavy workload and it is burdensome
50	Feeling sluggish all over lately
51	Even after a night's sleep, do not feel refreshed
52	Not having self-confidence in the things I do
53	A decline in my ability to concentrate
54	Cannot help but feel sleepy lately
55	Going to work every day is very difficult
56	Having no desire to eat lately
57	Getting a sore throat
58	My back feels heavy lately
59	No matter what, I sleep too much
60	Dropping things I am holding in my hand
61	Even after returning home, being unable to get work off my mind
62	Having sore joints
63	Breaking out into a cold sweat at times
64	Getting shaky hands and/or legs

Psychiatric Assessment and Treatment for Chronic Fatigue Syndrome in Japan

Masao Iwase[1], Shoji Okajima[1], Rei Takahashi[1], Tamiko Mogami[2], Nahoko Kusaka[3], Hirohiko Kuratsune[2], Masatoshi Takeda[1], and Akira Shimizu[2]

Summary

Chronic fatigue syndrome (CFS) is an intractable pathological state characterized by chronic fatigue for 6 months or more with unknown cause. For its diagnosis, it is necessary to exclude any physical or psychiatric conditions which could cause chronic fatigue. Psychiatric co-morbidity is commonly observed in cases diagnosed as CFS, and we propose a classification of the therapeutic role of physicians and psychiatrists according to the psychiatric classification of the chronic fatigue episode. Recently, a series of studies proved the effectiveness of cognitive behavioral therapy (CBT) for CFS. In CBT for CFS, it is considered to be important not to seek physical causes, to accept the pathological state as it is, to monitor and record the patient's daily activity and recognize the cognitive and behavioral patterns which might prolong fatigue, to maintain a constant activity level, and to make planned increases in daily activity. In CFS, our data showed that the rate of complete recovery was about 20% at the 2-year follow-up, and 40% at the 5-year follow-up, and that the prognosis of patients with psychiatric co-morbidity from the onset of a fatigue episode was far poorer than that of patients with no psychiatric co-morbidity or with psychiatric co-morbidity subsequent to a fatigue episode. We conclude that the psychiatric classification of the course of chronic fatigue is important for planning a therapeutic strategy and predicting the outcome of this state.

History and Background of the Disease Entity Called "Chronic Fatigue Syndrome"

The disease that has come to be called "chronic fatigue syndrome" (CFS) was first noted in 1984 in Nevada in the United States, after a massive outbreak of flu-like symptoms (fatigue, pharyngalgia, myalgia, arthralgia, low-grade fever, etc.). The

[1]Psychiatry and Behavioral Science, Osaka University Graduate School of Medicine, 2-2 D3 Yamadaoka, Suita, Osaka 565-0871, Japan

[2]Kansai University of Welfare Sciences, 3-11-1 Asahigaoka, Kashihara, Osaka 582-0026, Japan

[3]Doshisha Women's College of Liberal Arts, Kodo, Kyotanabe, Kyoto 610-0395, Japan

American Center for Disease Control (CDC) prepared a case definition for a diagnosis of CFS in 1988, among its steps to identify the cause of this condition [1]. Initially, the involvement of viruses was suspected on the basis of the clinical symptoms. To date, however, no particular virus has proved to be a causal agent in this condition. Typical patients with CFS suddenly develop flu-like symptoms after leading healthy lives. Unexplained fatigue is accompanied by a variety of persistent physical symptoms (low-grade fever, among others) and neuropsychiatric symptoms. Since this disease exhibits diverse neuropsychiatric symptoms, it tends to be confused with mental illness. In fact, CFS is often complicated by mental problems. The case definition of CFS resembles that of neurasthenia proposed in 1869 by Beard, a name which continues to be used in the ICD-10. It is plausible to suppose that patients with CFS symptoms have been observable in the population throughout history. In recent years, the association and similarities of neurasthenia with panic disorder and depression have been reported [2]. Patients with CFS are often depressed or suffer from panic disorder. Furthermore, it is known that both neurasthenia and CFS sometimes develop shortly after an infection. We therefore consider that the terms neurasthenia and CFS have been used historically to refer to the same condition, although in different eras. Because CFS was initially viewed as a physical disease, it did not attract close attention in psychiatric practice. However, like the concept of "neurasthenia," which spread explosively after it began to be used, the concept of CFS is now spreading, primarily among lay people, and this condition is gradually becoming one that psychiatric practice cannot ignore. It is in these circumstances that this chapter will discuss how the relationship between CFS and mental illness should be considered during the diagnosis and treatment of patients with CFS. We will describe how cognitive behavioral therapy (the only valid means of treatment available for CFS at present) should be performed. This material is based primarily on our experience at the Outpatient Fatigue Clinic of the Department of Internal Medicine and at the Department of Psychiatry, Osaka University Hospital.

Criteria for the Diagnosis of Chronic Fatigue Syndrome

In Japan, the criteria for a diagnosis of CFS were made public by the Ministry of Health and Welfare (later renamed the Ministry of Health, Labour and Welfare), and were partially amended in March 1995. The criteria are divided into major and minor items. Among the major criteria, fatigue intense enough to markedly interfere with daily living is seen as a major symptom. This symptom needs to continue for 6 months or longer, or to show repeated cycles of remission and relapse (covering 50% or more of a given period) in order to fulfill the criteria for a diagnosis of CFS. The intensity of fatigue needed to support a diagnosis of CFS is equivalent to Performance Status 3 (the state in which general malaise makes it impossible for the patient to work or conduct other social activities, and obliges them to rest at home for several days each month) or higher [3]. The overall effects of fatigue on daily life are evaluated case by case when evaluating whether or not each case satisfies the major criteria. The minor criteria are divided among symptom criteria and physical criteria. There are 11 symptoms, i.e., low-grade fever or chill, pharyngalgia, swollen lymph nodes, muscular weakness, myalgia, fatigue after exertion, headache, migrating arthralgia, neuropsychiatric symptoms (one or more from among: photophobia, temporary scotoma, amnesia, irritability, confusion, reduced ability to think, reduced concentration, and depression), sleep disorders (both sleeplessness and drowsiness), and the sudden onset of illness. The physical criteria include the requirement that low-grade fever, nonexudative pharyngitis, and swollen lymph nodes must be noted twice or more frequently within 1 month. A diagnosis of CFS is made in cases where unexplained chronic fatigue satisfying the major criteria is present, with either at least 6 items from among the symptom criteria and 2 items among the physical criteria, or at least 8 items among the symptom criteria alone, and none of the exclusion criteria listed below are present. The prevalence of CFS is estimated to be about 0.3% [4].

The medical and psychiatric exclusion criteria are included in the diagnostic criteria for CFS. Psychiatric illnesses which serve as exclusion criteria are schizophrenia, drug addiction, manic-depressive psychosis, psychotic depression, and organic mental diseases. Cases where depression or neurosis developed before any episodes of fatigue are excluded from a diagnosis of CFS, while cases where depression or neurosis developed simultaneously with fatigue episodes are not excluded. The following medical screening tests are recommended to identify cases of somatic diseases which can cause fatigue, and fatigue experienced by patients with such diseases is not viewed as being caused by CFS: hematological tests (blood appearance, erythrocyte sedimentation rate, C-reactive protein (CRP), glycoprotein, cholesterol, creatinine, blood urea nitrogen (BUN), Na, K, Ca, aspartate aminotransferase (AST), alanine aminotransferase (ALT), lactic dehydrogenase (LDH), alkaline leukocyte phosphatase (ALP), total bilirubin, creatine phosphokinase (CPK), aldorase, uric acid, thyroid-stimulating hormone (TSH) as an indicator of thyroid function, T3, T4, antinuclear antibody), tests of urine and feces (urinary protein, urinary glucose, urobilinogen, urinary sediment, occult fecal blood), simple chest X-ray, and ECG.

Psychiatric Classification of the Course of Chronic Fatigue Episodes

We classify episodes of chronic fatigue (CF) which satisfy the major criteria of CFS into four groups on the basis of the relationship between the time of the first onset of a CF episode and the time when the diagnostic criteria for mental illness were satisfied (Fig. 1) [3]. Group I contains cases where the diagnostic criteria for mental illness have not been satisfied to date since the first onset of the CF episode. Group II contains cases where the diagnostic criteria for mental illness were not satisfied at the first onset of a CF episode but were satisfied later. Group III contains

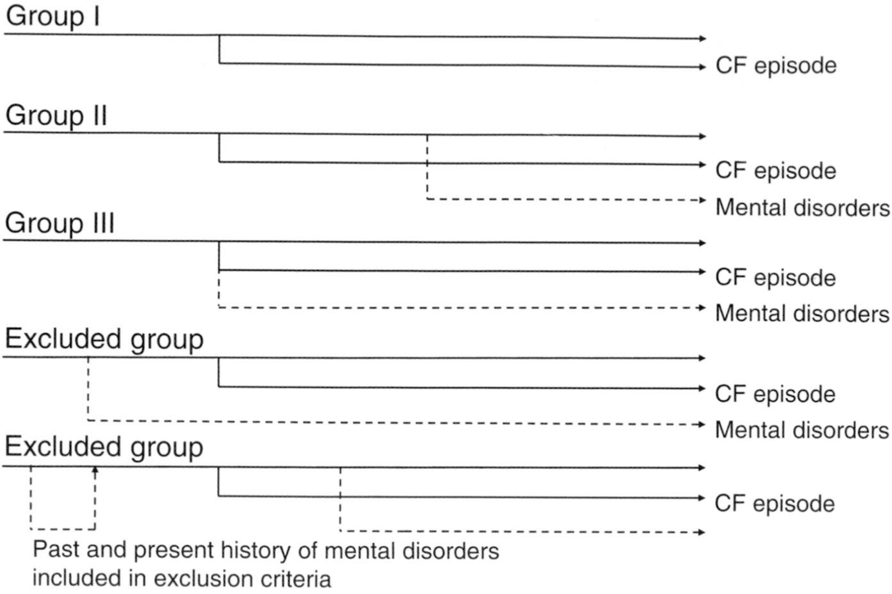

Fig. 1. Psychiatric classification of the course of a chronic fatigue episode

cases where the criteria were satisfied at the first onset of a CF episode. The excluded group, which contains cases where the CF episodes developed before complete remission of the preceding mental illness, or where mental illness which falls under the exclusion criteria for the diagnosis of CFS is the case at present or was the case in the past. Because the psychiatric classification of the course of chronic fatigue episodes is made at the time of the patient's first visit to the psychiatric clinic, it is possible for group I cases (cases later complicated by mental illness) to fall into the group II category. Group III may be interpreted not only as cases where both CFS and mental illness have developed at the same time, but also as cases where the symptoms of the mental illness accidentally satisfy the diagnostic criteria for CFS as well. The latter interpretation is probably more rational, according to common sense. The "excluded group" may include cases where CF episodes seem to be the remaining symptoms of mental illness, and cases where CF episodes have developed independently of mental illness. None of these cases is rated as being CFS. When diagnosing and treating CFS, we attach greater importance to the psychiatric classification of the course of the CF episodes than to the diagnosis of the condition made by the psychiatrist. This is because the classification of CF episodes is related to the therapeutic strategy used and the prognosis for the patient. Previously after the introduction of the case definition for CFS, the distribution of cases did not differ markedly between groups I, II, and III, and the number of cases in the excluded group was very small. However, as CFS was identified more extensively, the number of group III cases and of excluded-group cases increased, accounting for more than 50% of all cases.

Psychiatric Screening to Identify Chronic Fatigue Episodes

At the Osaka University Hospital, patients with a chief complaint of chronic fatigue who were suspected of having CFS were first examined in the Outpatient Fatigue Clinic of the Department of Hematology and Oncology. These patients then received psychiatric screening in the Department of Psychiatry. Later, they visited the Outpatient Fatigue Clinic again, where a therapeutic strategy was worked out on the basis of a general assessment of the medical screening results and the psychiatric findings.

At the beginning of the screening, the patient answers questions contained in several different questionnaires. The questionnaires used in the Department of Psychiatrics, Osaka University, include the draft Japanese version of Chalder's fatigue assessment scale [5], SDS, which is the Japanese version of SSAS (the somatosensory amplification scale) [6], JIBT-20 (the Japanese version, called the irrational belief test) [7], MOS-SF36 (the medical outcome study/short form 36) [8], and the Japanese version of the PDQ-R (personality diagnostic questionnaire, revised version) [9]. The Jikaku Sho Shirabe and Chalder's fatigue assessment scale are useful for evaluating the degree of fatigue. The SDS is useful as a means of simplifying the evaluation of the degree of depressive symptoms. The SSAS is a test designed to evaluate the patient's sensitivity to physical symptoms. The JIBT-20 is useful for checking for cognitive biases. The MOS-SF36 is suitable for evaluating the effects of fatigue on daily life, and has frequently been used in studies of CFS in many countries. The PDQ-R is a test for screening for personality disorders, but care must be taken because there is a high false-positive rate with this test.

During a face-to-face interview, the patient is asked about their developmental, educational, and occupational history and pre-onset adaptation. The patient is then asked about how the CF episode developed, in order to determine whether or not the CF episode can be viewed as representing a mental illness. The patient's history after the onset of the CF episode is analyzed to check for any psychiatric episodes occurring after the onset. Finally, the patient's current condition is judged psychiatrically. Through these steps, a psychiatric classification of the course of the illness is made, as well as a psychiatric diagnosis of the patient's condition. For group II, group III, and the excluded-group cases, the psychiatric findings and the necessity for treatment are explained to the patient. In cases where a great deal of time has elapsed since the onset of the CF episode, the diagnosis tends to be less accurate, due to the paucity of information and the ambiguities of the condition. However, we think it is important from a therapeutic point of view that the psychiatrist dealing with such cases reaches a decision about the patient's condition while taking these limitations into account.

Chronic Fatigue Syndrome Complicated by Mental Illness

The percentage of patients with CFS complicated by mental illness is as high as 60%–70% [10]. The mental illness which most frequently complicates CFS is a major depressive disorder. According to many reports, major depressive disorder accompanies CFS in 15%–44% of all patients, and about 60%–70% of CFS patients had experience of suffering from a major depressive disorder in their past history [11–16]. CFS was accompanied by anxiety disorders in about 20% of patients, and this had also been the case in the past in about 30% of patients according to many reports [11–16]. Among somatoform disorders, somatization disorder is estimated to be present in 5%–15% of all patients with CFS [11–16].

Co-morbidity with Major Depressive Disorder

Major depressive disorder is a mental illness which has many similarities to CFS. Symptoms common to CFS and major depressive disorder are depressive mood, sleep disorder, a tendency to fatigue or loss of vigor, reduced thinking ability or concentration, myalgia, headache, and so on. Patients with CFS are more likely to show loss of interest and joy, changes in body weight, inappropriate self-reproachful mood, and suicidal ideation. They tend to attribute their illness to physical factors. Since most patients with CFS satisfy the diagnostic criteria for dysthymic disorder, our screening does not regard compliance with the criteria for dysthymic disorder as indicating a complication by mental disease.

Co-morbidity with Anxiety Disorders

Panic disorder and generalized anxiety disorder are frequent types of anxiety disorder seen in patients with CFS. Co-morbidity with panic disorder is often seen after the onset of CFS, and close attention to this problem is needed during the management of CFS. Generalized anxiety disorder is occasionally seen in patients with CFS. Although patients with CFS often show a tendency toward an obsessive personality, it is rare that a diagnosis of obsessive–compulsive disorder can be made. In cases where co-morbidity with anxiety disorder has been detected, it is necessary to judge whether the anxiety disorder developed secondarily to the onset of the CF episode, or simultaneously with or before the onset of the CFS (group III or the excluded group).

Co-morbidity with Somatoform Disorders

Somatoform disorders have many similarities to CFS. If the diagnostic criteria are applied directly, all cases of CFS may be diagnosed as having undifferentiated somatoform disorder. For this reason, we refrain from making a diagnosis of co-morbidity with mental illness even if the patient was diagnosed as having undifferentiated somatoform disorder during screening. When we encounter a symptom which is included among the case definitions during screening, it is almost impossible to determine whether the symptom is an organic physical symptom or a somatized mental symptom. We make it a rule to avoid making a diagnosis of pain disorder or conversion disorder unless the association between a given symptom and psychological factors is evident. We make a diagnosis of hypochondriasis only if the patient complains of symptoms other than those listed as physical symptoms in the case-definition for CFS, and we take care to avoid making a hasty diagnosis of somatoform disorder.

Co-morbidity with Adjustment Disorders

We make a diagnosis of adjustment disorder if the fatigue can be attributed to some particular stress factors. We often encounter cases where we notice adjustment disorders only after the fatigue was alleviated in response to the elimination of stress factors. The diagnosis of adjustment disorder seems to be rational in many cases of CF episodes caused by overwork. However, it is not uncommon that we encounter cases where CF episodes caused by overwork do not subside despite more than 6 months of rest. In such cases, no appropriate diagnosis other than dysthymic disorder is available in the DSM-IV. According to the ICD-10, "prolonged depressive reaction" corresponds to such cases, but the duration of this condition is usually considered to be 2 years or less. In practice, it is not rare that CF episodes caused by overwork last for 2 years or longer.

Co-morbidity with Personality Disorders

It is said that patients with CFS often show a tendency to obsessive–compulsive personality, or a tendency to avoidant personality characterized by fear of aggravated fatigue. Few patients with CFS satisfy the diagnostic criteria for personality disorders according to DSM-IV, and acting out "difficult to control" is also rare among patients with CFS. According to one report, patients with CFS have high scores on histrionic, avoidant, obsessive–compulsive, and borderline personality disorders when rated using the PDQ-R [17], suggesting a relationship of fatigue to some particular personality tendencies.

Treatment

Therapeutic Strategy on the Basis of the Psychiatric Classification of the Course of the Disease

We treat cases of CFS using the following strategies, depending on the classification of the CF episodes. Group I is primarily treated medically. Medical treatments for this type include Kampo (traditional Chinese) therapy using herbal preparations such as Hochu-Ekki-To, as well as vitamin B12 and C therapy. For group II, we administer psychiatric therapy in parallel with the medical therapy. For group II cases, if the mental illness is in remission, we sometimes forgo the immediate application of psychiatric therapy. For group III and the excluded group, psychiatric therapy is emphasized. Patients complaining of chronic fatigue tend to attribute their sickness to physical factors and are reluctant to receive psychiatric therapy. Psychiatric therapy is sometimes difficult to administer in this situation. When dealing with cases of CFS, we think it necessary that the roles of physicians and psychiatrists be clearly distinguished, i.e., physicians assume the duties of diagnosing CFS and managing the physical problems of the patients, while psychiatrics conduct cognitive behavioral therapy or drug therapy to deal with the psychological symptoms.

Drug Therapy

Herbal preparations and vitamin preparations are prescribed, irrespective of the psychiatric classification of the disease course. Psychotropic agents such as selective serotonin re-uptake inhibitors (SSRIs), anxiolytics, hypnotics, etc., are used as needed. According to a randomized study involving patients with CFS, SSRI was effective against the accompanying depression, but was ineffective against fatigue [18]. We have the impression that SSRI is effective in some cases, and needs to be discontinued earlier than the usual complete course owing to adverse reactions in other cases. No clinical study results about the effects of central nervous system (CNS) stimulants such as methylphenidate upon cases of CFS have been reported, and unpublished data from small-scale studies do not suggest that they are effective in cases of CFS. Because drug therapy for CFS tends to be applied for long periods of time, we think it advisable to avoid the use of CNS stimulants, since this group of drugs is likely to cause addiction. Furthermore, CNS stimulants may induce the following adverse reactions: aggravation of insomnia (a symptom of CFS), hypertension (due to methylphenidate), and drug-induced hepatitis (due to pemoline) [19]. Because CFS patients often drop out of treatment owing to an intolerance of the drugs, it is advisable to adopt one of the following two strategies. One strategy is to start psychotropic drug therapy at low dose levels and increase the dose carefully. The other strategy is to start at effective dose levels, but to review the dose levels immediately if adverse reactions appear. In any event, we respect the patient's discretion to some degree when selecting drug therapy. For groups II and III, drug therapy is tailored to the mental illness.

Our Stance on Alternative Therapies

Alternative therapies of massage, relaxation, acupuncture and moxibustion, bathing, food supplement therapy, aroma-therapy, forest therapy, humor–laughter therapy, etc., have been proposed, but none of them has been adequately documented as being effective. We do not actively recommend these therapies, but if a patient consults us about such therapies, we support them if the patient can continue the chosen therapy for a long period of time without sustaining a large economic burden. This is because, when dealing with CFS, which has a main symptom of long-term loss of vigor, it is desirable for patients to have some activities that they can engage in and take satisfaction from.

Cognitive Behavioral Therapy

In recent years, reports of randomized studies demonstrating the effectiveness of cognitive behavioral therapy (CBT) and graded exercise (GE) have been published [20]. In earlier reports, CBT was shown to be ineffective. Later reports, however, showed that the response rate to CBT or GE was 35%–75%, and that the daily activity level of patients and their recovery from fatigue were significantly better after CBT or GE than among patients who had relaxation therapy [21–27]. Basically, CBT seems to be indicated for all cases of CFS. However, in cases where the fatigue is too severe to allow the smooth performance of graded exercise, particular care will be needed when using a behavioral therapy approach.

The following important information needs to be conveyed by the therapist to the patient when CBT is used for the treatment of CFS. CFS is an unexplained condition and no radical means of treatment is available. Unfortunately, it is unlikely that the CFS will subside immediately. The percentage of patients who completely recover from CFS is 20% within 2 years and about 40% within 5 years. However, some degree of alleviation can be expected for most patients with CFS. It is useless and inadvisable to make excessive efforts to identify the cause of the fatigue. CBT is not intended to cure fatigue, but is designed to help the patient coexist better with the fatigue. They are simply told not to overstrain themselves or overindulge themselves.

At first glance the reader may think that it would be difficult to give this information to a patient during their first visit to the clinic. However, most patients will accept these warnings relatively calmly. This is because patients visiting the clinic with a suspicion of CFS have often heard these pieces of information already. The validity of these precautions is evident from overseas studies as well as our studies. It is necessary and important to give accurate precautions and information to each patient at the beginning of treatment. If this information is shared by the therapist and the patient, it will be possible for the therapist to avoid becoming excessively impatient or feeling a sense of blame even if the patient does not respond to the therapy immediately after the start of treatment. It is often difficult for patients to keep appointments because of their physical discomfort. It seems better for the therapist to accept these irregularities on the part of the patient, unless the irregularities are unacceptably marked.

The next step is to inquire into the conduct of the patient's daily life. To this end, the practice of taking activity records is useful. When you read the term "CBT," you may call to mind columns of dysfunctional thought records. However, we believe that behavioral techniques are more effective than cognitive techniques in the early stages of CBT for CFS. This is because the fatigue is not directly linked to some particular negative and automatic thinking habits (thoughts or images that appear unintentionally and habitually when triggered by some events), as is the case with depression. Rather, activities during a single day or over several days will affect the person's activity for several subsequent days. Even when the patients record their thoughts while experiencing strong fatigue, they often cannot understand why they are so tired. Although automatic negative thoughts can appear secondarily to fatigue or physical symptoms, how to deal with these thoughts is a task we have to resolve after the patient's fatigue has come under some degree of control. The daily activity record is designed to allow the entry of daily activities for every hour. Each activity, and the degree of fatigue caused by it, is scored on a 10-point scale, and a slash is drawn through the hours of sleep. Using this record, the basic activity level, patterns of fatigue aggravation, and sleep–awake rhythms can be checked. Disturbed sleep–awake rhythms are seen relatively frequently. Some degree of symptom alleviation can be expected just by correcting these rhythms.

Next, the patterns of fatigue aggravation are checked. Two patterns are often noted: (1) a pattern characterized by the repetition of cycles of good and poor general conditions, and (2) a pattern characterized by there always being a strong complaint of fatigue accompanied by a low overall activity level. As a behavioral characteristic of patients with CFS, it has been reported that they can be roughly divided into the relatively active group and the relatively passive group [28]. Relatively active patients place heavy demands on themselves; they want to do many things and cannot accept their present situation. Passive patients think that physical activity can aggravate their symptoms, and their activity level is often low. The former group can be characterized by obsessive and excessively adaptive tendencies, while the latter group can be characterized by a tendency to anxiety and avoidance. If individual patients with CFS are roughly divided into these two groups, it will be easier to devise a CBT strategy tailored for each case. Relatively active patients often overstrain themselves when their general condition is relatively good, resulting in a repetition of cycles of aggravation and remission of fatigue. When dealing with such patients, it is advisable for the therapist to guide and support the patient to become aware of their excessive adaptation and the disadvantages of that behavior, and to help the person to modify their behavior voluntarily. This group of patients often has the belief that they should quickly resume the activity level prevailing before the onset of disease. When patients have this attitude, the therapist should advise them to accept their current situation. For passive patients, the therapist should explain the disadvantages of excessive rest and advise a gradual increase in activity level. During this discussion, it is a good idea for the therapist to propose a schedule that the patient can actively commit to. Through a collaborative therapeutic relationship, the therapist should guide the patient to confirm that a gradual increase in activity level does not always aggravate fatigue.

We have proposed nine cognitive and behavioral characteristics of patients with CFS. These are: (1) a tendency to excessive adaptation, (2) excessive consideration of human relationships, (3) perfectionism, (4) lack of appropriate rest, (5) a tendency to avoid activity, (6) excessive rest, (7) physical attribution of symptoms, (8) fear of relapse, and (9) a sense of alienation (the feeling that: "No one understands me"). The first four characteristics are often seen in relatively active patients, the fifth and sixth are often seen in passive patients, and the last three are common to all patients with CFS.

Table 1 lists examples of valid means of coping with chronic fatigue, tailored to the cognitive and behavioral characteristics of CFS. Because of the great impact of fatigue on the daily life of patients with CFS, it is desirable: (1) to guide the patient toward understanding that their daily life can be enriched by adopting an

Table 1. Effective coping for chronic fatigue

1. Work and activity
   - Divide a given task into several stages, to make it easier to suspend and resume
   - Use memoranda and plan the schedule to compensate for reduced memory
   - Prevent overwork:
     - (a) Be resistant to the insufficient activity level
     - (b) Abandon self-esteem based on accomplishment
     - (c) Notice the disadvantage of overwork
     - (d) Check your activity level with a pedometer, etc., to prevent overwork
   - Increase activity level gradually. Cope with transient aggravation of fatigue composedly
2. Rest
   - Rest according to a plan. Sleep in a regular pattern
   - List recreational activities that you can enjoy without special effort, and pursue these activities
   - Master relaxation techniques
3. Physical symptoms
   - Understand that excessive focus on physical symptoms aggravates your prognosis
   - Promote awareness of the relationship between stress and physical symptoms
4. Others
   - Deal with emotions such as anger, discouragement, self-reproach in a constructive manner
   - Develop the ability to explain your disease to health-care workers, family, friends, colleagues, etc.

energy-saving style of behavior throughout the day, and that excessive rest can delay recovery from fatigue, and (2) to support the patient in devising a step-wise recovery plan which can be implemented without too much effort.

Prognosis of Chronic Fatigue Syndrome

Table 2 summarizes data about the prognosis of CFS [24, 29–33]. Many published reports deal with the short-term prognosis for CFS, and few pertain to the long-term prognosis (5 years or longer). Because the criteria for a decision about recovery varied slightly among different reports, it was not possible to compare these data precisely. However, if the data in these reports are summarized, the CFS recovery rate is found to be 3%–37%, indicating that the functional prognosis for CFS is not good. However, the investigators had the impression that some alleviation was observed in most cases. In these reports, alleviation close to complete recovery was needed for a judgment of recovery to be made. As a result, the recovery rate tended to be underestimated. It is known that advanced age, longer duration of illness, co-morbidity with mental disease, and adherence of patients to physical symptoms are associated with a poor prognosis for CFS [34].

Also according to our data, the percentage of groups I + II cases showing alleviation after 2 years of medical treatment was 23%, while the percentage for group III cases was significantly lower (4%) [33]. These results clearly indicate that the psychiatric classification of the course of CF episodes is important when devising a strategy of treatment for CFS. Prior to the present study, the relatively recent study conducted by Tiersky et al. [35] was the only study involving the classification of CFS patients by the timing of the onset of mental disease. In that study, patients with CFS were divided into three groups (a group free of psychiatric co-morbidity at present, a group currently co-morbid with mental disease which had developed before the diagnosis of CFS, and a group complicated by mental disease after the diagnosis of CFS). They analyzed the roles played by their psychiatric

Table 2. Reports on the prognosis of CFS

Ref.	Follow-up (years)	*n*	Measurements	Recovery rate (%)
29	1	78	4-point self-rate	8
30	9	341	VAS	12
31	13	46 (child)	4-point self-rate	37
24	5	25 (CBT)	MOS-SF36 etc.	24
		28 (relaxation)		4
32	5	33	Multiple measures	3
33	2	48 (groups I + II)	PS	23
		26 (group III)		4

VAS, visual analogue scale; CBT, cognitive behavioral therapy; MOS-SF36, medical outcome study short form 36; PS, performance status; groups I, II, III, psychiatric classification of course of chronic fatigue episode (see text)

condition on the health-related quality of life (QOL) of these patients in comparison to healthy controls. Their study revealed that physical function did not differ between patients with CFS co-morbid with mental disease and patients with CFS without mental disease, but that emotional health was lower in the former patients, with the decrease in emotional health being most marked in patients where mental disease had developed before the diagnosis of CFS. Ciccone et al. [36] also reported that CFS was often co-morbid with mental disease or personality disorder, although this co-morbidity did not markedly affect the physical function or defects of the patients. These earlier reports indicate that when seen in cross section, co-morbidity with mental disease or personality disorder does not markedly affect the physical function of patients with CFS. However, when our data were analyzed longitudinally from the viewpoint of prognosis, it was evident that a psychiatric evaluation of patients with CFS is important when predicting the long-term prognosis or devising a therapeutic strategy. At the same time, the data suggest that psychiatric treatment is valid and necessary for group-III CFS cases. It is suggested that psychiatric treatment is highly likely to provide a valid and indispensable means of dealing with group-III CFS cases. An important theme related to the management of patients with CFS will be the grouping of patients and establishing a therapeutic strategy tailored to individual groups.

Acknowledgments. This work was supported in part by the Special Coordination Funds for Promoting Science and Technology, and in part by a Grant-in-Aid for Science Research to M.I. (17591211) from the Ministry of Education, Culture, Sports, Science and Technology of the Japanese Government.

References

1. Holmes GP, Kaplan JE, Gantz NM, Komaroff AL, Schonberger LB, Straus SE, Jones JF, Dubois RE, Cunningham-Rundles C, Pahwa S, et al. (1988) Chronic fatigue syndrome: a working case definition. Ann Intern Med 108:387–389
2. Kato S (2004) Panic disorder and depression in contemporary Japan: current neurasthenia (in Japanese). Jpn J Psychiatr Treat 19:955–961
3. Kitani T, Kuratsune H (1992) Chronic fatigue syndrome (in Japanese). J Jpn Soc Intern Med 81:573–582
4. Kuratsune H (2003) Pathogenesis and diagnosis of chronic fatigue syndrome (in Japanese). J Clin Exp Med (Igaku No Ayumi) 204:381–386
5. Chalder T, Berelowitz G, Pawlikowska T, Watts L, Wessely S, Wright D, Wallace EP (1993) Development of a fatigue scale. J Psychosom Res 37:147–153
6. Barsky AJ, Wyshak G (1990) The somatosensory amplification scale and its relationship to hypochondriasis. J Psychiatr Res 24:323–334
7. Cash TF (1984) The irrational beliefs test: its relationship with cognitive–behavioral traits and depression. J Clin Psychol 40:1399–1405
8. Ware JE, Snow K, Kosinski M, Gandek B (1993) SF-36 health survey manual and interpretation guide. Health Institute, New England Medical Center
9. Hyler SE, Skodol AE, Kellman HD, Oldham JM, Rosnic L (1990) Validity of the personality diagnostic questionnaire revised: comparison with two structured interviews. Am J Psychiatry 174:1043–1048

10. Shimizu A, Okajima S, Takahashi R, Takaishi J (1994) Psychiatric evaluation of chronic fatigue syndrome (in Japanese). In: Kitani T (ed) 1993 annual report of domestic survey and research on pathogenesis of chronic fatigue syndrome. Osaka, pp 62–66
11. Wessely S, Powell R (1989) Fatigue syndromes: a comparison of chronic "postviral" fatigue with neuromuscular and affective disorders. J Neurol Neurosurg Psychiatry 52:940–948
12. Hickie I, Lloyd A, Wakefield D, Parker G (1990) The psychiatric status of patients with chronic fatigue syndrome. Br J Psychiatry 156:534–540
13. Lane TJ, Manu P, Matthews DA (1991) Depression and somatization in chronic fatigue syndrome. Am J Med 91:335–344
14. Farmer A, Jones I, Hillier J, Llewelyn M, Borysiewicz L, Smith A (1995) Neuraesthenia revisited: ICD-10 and DSM-III-R psychiatric syndromes in chronic fatigue patients and comparison subjects. Br J Psychiatry 167:503–506
15. Buchwald D, Pearlman T, Kith P, Katon W, Schmaling K (1997) Screening for psychiatric disorders in chronic fatigue and chronic fatigue syndrome. J Psychosom Res 42:87–94
16. Wilson A, Hickie I, Hadzi-Pavlovic D, Wakefield D, Parker G, Straus SE, Dale J, McCluskey D, Hinds G, Brickman A, Goldenberg D, Demitrack M, Blakely T, Wessely S, Sharpe M, Lloyd A (2001) What is chronic fatigue syndrome? Heterogeneity within an international multicentre study. Aust NZ J Psychiatry 35:520–527
17. Johnson SK, DeLuca J, Natelson BH (1996) Personality dimensions in chronic fatigue syndrome: a comparison with multiple sclerosis and depression. J Psychiat Res 30:9–20
18. Wearden AJ, Morriss RK, Mullis R, Strickland PL, Pearson DJ, Appleby L, Campbell IT, Morris JA (1998) Randomised, double-blind, placebo-controlled treatment trial of fluoxetine and graded exercise in chronic fatigue syndrome. Br J Psychiatry 172:485–490; correction 173:89
19. Levine P, Schwartz S, Furst G (2003) Medical intervention and management. In: Jason LA, Fennell PA, Taylor RR (eds) Handbook of chronic fatigue syndrome. Wiley, Hoboken, Chap 21, pp 441–454
20. Whiting P, Bagnall AM, Sowden AJ, Cornell JE, Mulrow CD, Ramirez G (2001) Interventions for the treatment and management of chronic fatigue syndrome: a systematic review. JAMA 286:1360–1368
21. Fulcher KY, White PD (1997) Randomised controlled trial of graded exercise in patients with chronic fatigue syndrome. BMJ 314:1647–1652
22. Powell P, Bentall RP, Nye FJ, Edwards RH (2001) Randomised controlled trial of patient education to encourage graded exercise in chronic fatigue syndrome. BMJ 322:1–5
23. Deale A, Chalder T, Marks I, Wessely S (1997) Cognitive behavior therapy for chronic fatigue syndrome: a randomized controlled trial. Am J Psychiatry 154:408–414
24. Deale A, Husain K, Chalder T, Wessely S (2001) Long-term outcome of cognitive behavior therapy versus relaxation therapy for chronic fatigue syndrome: a 5-year follow-up study. Am J Psychiatry 158:2038–2042
25. Sharpe M, Hawton K, Simkin S, Surawy C, Hackmann A, Klimes I, Peto T, Warrell D, Seagroatt V (1996) Cognitive behaviour therapy for chronic fatigue syndrome: a randomized controlled trial. BMJ 312:22–26
26. Ridsdale L, Godfrey E, Chalder T, Seed P, King M, Wallace P, Wessely S, Fatigue Trialists' Group (2001) Chronic fatigue in general practice: is counselling as good as cognitive behaviour therapy? A UK randomised trial. Br J Gen Pract 462:19–24
27. Prins JB, Bleijenberg G, Bazelmans E, Elving LD, de Boo TM, Severens JL, van der Wilt GJ, Spinhoven P, van der Meer JW (2001) Cognitive behaviour therapy for chronic fatigue syndrome: a multicentre randomised controlled trial. Lancet 357:841–847
28. Bleijenberg G, Prins J, Bazelmans E (2003) Cognitive–behavioral therapies. In: Jason LA, Fennell PA, Taylor RR (eds) Handbook of chronic fatigue syndrome. Wiley, Hoboken, pp 493–526
29. van der Werf SP, de Vree B, Alberts M, van der Meer JW, Bleijenberg G, Netherlands Fatigue Research Group Nijmegen (2002) Natural course and predicting self-reported improvement

in patients with chronic fatigue syndrome with a relatively short illness duration. J Psychosom Res 53:749–753

30. Pheley AM, Melby D, Schenck C, Mandel J, Peterson PK (1999) Can we predict recovery in chronic fatigue syndrome? Minnesota Med 82:52–56
31. Bell DS, Jordan K, Robinson M (2001) Thirteen-year follow-up of children and adolescents with chronic fatigue syndrome. Pediatrics 107:994–998
32. Anderson MM, Permin H, Albrecht F (2004) Illness and disability in Danish chronic fatigue syndrome patients at diagnosis and at 5-year follow-up. J Psychosom Res 56:217–229
33. Shimizu A, Okajima S, Takahashi R, Takahashi K, Kajimoto O, Kuratsune H, Yamaguti K (2000) The follow-up report on the prognosis of chronic fatigue syndrome (in Japanese). In: Kitani T (ed) 1999 annual report of research on the field survey and recovery methods of fatigue, Osaka, pp 156–168
34. Joyce J, Hotopf M, Wessely S (1997) The prognosis of chronic fatigue and chronic fatigue syndrome: a systematic review. Q J Med 90:223–233
35. Tiersky LA, Matheis RJ, Deluca J, Lange G, Natelson BH (2003) Functional status, neuropsychological functioning, and mood in chronic fatigue syndrome (CFS). J Nerv Ment Dis 5:324–331
36. Ciccone DS, Busichio K, Vickroy M, Natelson BH (2003) Psychiatric morbidity in chronic fatigue syndrome: are patients with personality disorder more physically impaired? J Psychosom Res 54:445–452

Some Patients with Chronic Fatigue Syndrome Have Brain Dysfunction

Benjamin H. Natelson

Chronic fatigue syndrome (CFS) is medically unexplained fatigue lasting at least 6 months and accompanied by infectious, rheumatological, and neuropsychiatric symptoms. CFS is primarily a problem in women's health because approximately 75% of patients seeking care for chronic fatigue are women. Because of complaints of muscle weakness and achiness, early work focused on peripheral mechanisms of fatigue via muscle dysfunction. However, those studies were unable to confirm any consistent anatomical or physiological abnormality. The lack of an obvious peripheral mechanism for fatigue led to a change in focus to central mechanisms. This change was supported by a set of studies, including those from this laboratory, which showed objective evidence of neuropsychological dysfunction.

Early work showed a specific problem in complex attentional processing using a test called the PASAT (paced auditory serial addition test). In this test, an audiotape reads numbers to the subject. The subject is asked to add the last two numbers they hear, and to continue doing so as new numbers are read. As the time between numbers shortens, even healthy subjects show a decrease in performance. However, CFS patients performed significantly slower and with more mistakes than healthy controls [1]. Unfortunately, subsequent studies failed to support the use of the PASAT as a diagnostic tool for CFS. We reasoned that this failure to replicate had to do with the specifics of the test itself, and that CFS patients had a subtle problem in the neuropsychological processes subsumed by the PASAT. To test this hypothesis, we asked CFS patients and controls to do a thorough neuropsychological battery evaluating memory, attention (concentration), speed of information processing, motor speed, and executive functioning [2]. CFS patients failed at least one test in each of the following domains: attention, speed of information processing, and motor speed. Their performance was worst on motor speed; 61% of patients failed tests of motor speed compared with 22% of healthy controls. In contrast, patients performed at control levels on tests of memory and executive functioning. This set of problems probably explains the common complaint of CFS patients

Pain and Fatigue Study Center, Department of Neurosciences, University of Medicine and Dentistry – New Jersey Medical School, Newark, NJ, USA

that they are unable to process information quickly. We are currently testing the hypothesis that CFS patients will perform as well as healthy controls in untimed tests. Importantly, when we separated the patients into groups based on the presence (or absence) of fibromyalgia in addition to CFS, we found that it was the CFS-only group that had the documented cognitive problems; those with both CFS and FM tested within the normal range [3]. Importantly, however, these results point to the brain as the site of the pathology in CFS.

As our subject pool of CFS patients increased, we were able to apply other stratification strategies to try to reduce the heterogeneity inherent in the use of a clinical case definition for diagnosis. We found that stratifying based on the presence or absence of current depression and/or anxiety was a successful strategy. Patients who had no prior history of any psychiatric diagnosis were the ones with the subtle problems on neuropsychological testing, while patients with co-morbid depression and/or anxiety had similar test results to healthy controls [4]. In addition, we found a step-wise decrement in functional status with progressive failures of individual neuropsychological tests [5]. This finding supported our interpretation that cognitive problems impact significantly on a patient's ability to live a normal life. Other work coming from the CDC (Centers for Disease Control) reports significant correlations between the existence of mental fatigue and impairment on cognitive testing [6].

Our finding of neuropsychological problems in CFS patients devoid of psychiatric illness led us to hypothesize that we would find that the same group had the most abnormalities on anatomical magnetic resonance imaging (MRI). We found this result in a study where MRIs were read separately by two neuroradiologists. Specifically, similar rates of abnormalities were found in healthy controls and CFS patients with co-morbid psychiatric diagnoses (32% and 22%). In contrast, the group with no psychiatric co-morbidity had a significantly higher rate of abnormalities (67%). The largest difference between groups was in subcortical white matter hyperintensities, as distinct from the ventricles. These were more frequent and more often smaller than 5 mm in diameter for the CFS group who were devoid of psychiatric diagnoses than in the other group. Subjects with these lesions tended to show them in frontal lobes. Importantly, we found that patients with MRI abnormalities reported poorer functional status than those with normal MRI studies [7]. As was the case for neuropsychological dysfunction, this study suggested that these lesions, although small in number and size, were impacting on functional status.

The finding of an increased rate of MRI abnormalities in the brains of CFS patients led us to hypothesize that these lesions were the tip of an encephalitic process. To test this hypothesis, we performed cerebral morphometrics to determine ventricular size in subjects participating in the MRI study described above. We found a trend toward bigger ventricles in the CFS group relative to healthy controls [8]. Unfortunately, we were unable to replicate this finding in a new data set of CFS patients without psychiatric co-morbidity (unpublished data). Nonetheless, two other groups mapped structural cerebral morphology and volume in CFS patients compared with controls. The first group looked at women only with no psychiatric co-morbidity. A global reduction in gray matter volume was found in two cohorts of CFS patients relative to controls [9]. A second group found focal reductions in gray matter volume in the bilateral frontal cortex [10]. Considering these results, we are not clear why we did not find significant ventricular enlargement in CFS patients in our follow-up study.

One possible mechanism for the development of lesions is cerebral hypoperfusion. Several methodologies have been used to evaluate brain blood flow (BBF), but the results have not been consistent. The majority of studies have employed single photon emission computed tomography (SPECT) to count the distribution of a radioactive marker throughout the brain. Early studies done in nonstratified patient samples revealed global decreases in cerebral flow [11,12], but later studies of twins [13] and of selected CFS patients without co-morbid psychiatric diagnoses did not confirm these generalized reductions in blood flow [14–16]. However, two of these studies did find changes in more basal brain structures, namely a reduction of flow in the brain stem [15] and actual increases in the thalamus [16]. These increases could reflect increased metabolism. Of interest were the results of another study that reported increased metabolism in basal ganglia of CFS patients without depression; the basal ganglia connect directly to the thalamus [17].

Two groups used positron emission tomography (PET) to study cerebral cellular metabolism in CFS patients without co-morbid psychiatric disorders. The first found normal metabolism in half their subjects, but hypometabolism in cingulate and adjacent mesial cortical areas [18]. The second study found reduced metabolism in the brain stem, thus supporting the earlier SPECT study [19]. A third PET study, in which the psychiatric status of the patients was not provided, used a novel radioactive marker and could not confirm brain stem hypometabolism, although global decreases in brain blood flow were noted [20].

One issue about using SPECT or PET to reflect BBF is that the values obtained are relative—either to the whole brain or to the cerebellum. Therefore, any regional abnormality found could reflect a more general underlying problem which would not be appreciated. To bypass this issue, we studied absolute brain blood flow using xenon–CT, a commercially available technique used in assessing stroke [21]. Although our results were somewhat limited by the small size of our healthy control group, we did find consistent and rather large decreases in BBF over broad regions of the brain. Furthermore, the decreases were most marked in patients with no psychiatric co-morbidity—again supporting our idea that this group may have an underlying encephalopathy.

There are data from other dimensions that also point to the brain as the organ involved in some cases of CFS. A number of groups have studied the brain correlates of the delayed reaction time seen in CFS. While early work suggested that the P300 cortical response to a cognitive task was abnormal in latency or amplitude in some CFS patients [22], later work found that variable to be normal, and instead found that the premovement readiness potential was reduced in CFS [23]. In contrast, potentials occurring before self-paced movements were normal. In addition, brain activity during the performance of a motor task was significantly greater than that for controls, and brain activity was even higher when the CFS patients performed fatiguing tasks [24]. The authors concluded that the patients had to work harder than the controls to perform the motor tasks. This result was very similar to one we found using functional neuroimaging [25]. Although one group of patients we studied had no measurable cognitive deficit, their brain acted as if the task was extremely hard. In other words, the same brain areas were activated as was the case in normal people doing a very difficult task. In another study, after a fatiguing task, areas of the brain outside of those activated by the task showed reduced responsiveness for patients compared with controls [26]. This suggests that blood might be being diverted to areas of higher need, and more so in patients than in controls.

In addition to "brain fog," CFS patients sometimes complain of altered balance. In fact, in my experience, the only abnormality I see (and permit without making a diagnostic exclusion) on neurological examination is some difficulty in balance. I test this by getting patients to try a military Romberg (i.e., with one foot in front of the other) as well as a classical Romberg. Approximately 15% of patients have problems with the more demanding military Romberg. This patient complaint led us to an early study in which we found that patients were found to have subtle differences in the dynamics of their gait [27]. Because of data suggesting vestibular function abnormalities in CFS [28], we did dynamic postural testing comparing CFS patients with age- and sex-matched healthy controls and found substantial group differences (unpublished data).

To further test the hypothesis that some CFS patients had an underlying encephalopathy, we did lumbar punctures on 44 patients who fulfilled the 1994 case definition for CFS and 13 healthy controls. None of the controls had elevations in cell counts or spinal fluid protein levels, but 30% of the patients did. Four patients had normal protein levels with elevated numbers of WBCs (6, 7, 9, and 20), one patient had an elevated protein level of 67 and 5 WBCs, and 8 patients had elevated proteins alone (range 46–93 mg/dl; median of all 8 with elevations, 51 mg/dl). The patient group with abnormal spinal fluid had increased levels of IL-10, an anti-inflammatory cytokine. We do not know if this finding relates to the symptoms of CFS or simply reflects the presence of immunologically active cells in the spinal fluid. Of interest was the fact that six subjects—all in the CFS group—developed post-spinal-tap headaches; only one of these had an abnormal spinal fluid result. The rates of current major depression were lower in those patients with abnormal spinal fluid than in those with normal spinal fluid (0% vs. 27%; one-tailed $P < 0.04$), but rates of lifetime depression or overall Axis I diagnoses did not differ between the groups (46.2% vs. 48.4% and 69.2% vs. 51.6%, respectively).

These accumulated data strongly support our major working hypothesis that some patients with CFS have their problem because of an underlying brain dysfunction. Continued work to support and extend this hypothesis should continue to use stratification stratagems to reduce the heterogeneity inherent in using a clinical case definition to diagnose CFS.

Acknowledgments. The preparation of this chapter was supported in part by NIH AI-54478.

References

1. DeLuca J, Johnson SK, Natelson BH (1993) Information processing efficiency in chronic fatigue syndrome and multiple sclerosis. Arch Neurol 50:301–304

2. Busichio K, Tiersky LA, DeLuca J, Natelson BH (2004) Neuropsychological deficits in patients with chronic fatigue syndrome. J Int Neuropsychol Soc 10:1–8
3. Cook DB, Nagelkirk PR, Peckerman A, Poluri A, Mores J, Natelson BH (2005) Exercise and cognitive performance in Chronic Fatigue Syndrome. Med Sci Sports Exerc 37:1460–1467
4. DeLuca J, Johnson SK, Ellis SP, Natelson BH (1997) Cognitive functioning is impaired in chronic fatigue syndrome patients devoid of psychiatric disease. J Neurol Neurosurg Psychiatr 62:151–155
5. Christodoulou C, DeLuca J, Lange G, Sisto S, Natelson BH (1998) Relation between neuropsychological impairment and functional disability in patients with chronic fatigue syndrome. J Neurol Neurosurg Psychiatr 64:431–434
6. Capuron L, Welberg L, Heim C, Wagner D, Solomon L, Papanicolaou DA, Craddock RC, Miller AH, Reeves WC (2006) Cognitive dysfuntion relates to subjective report of mental fatigue in patients with chronic fatigue syndrome. Neuropsychopharmacology 1–8
7. Cook DB, Lange G, DeLuca J, Natelson BH (2001) Relationship of brain MRI abnormalities and physical functional status in CFS. Int J Neurosci 107:1–6
8. Lange G, Holodny A, DeLuca J, et al. (2001) Quantitative assessment of cerebral ventricular volumes in CFS. Appl Neuropsychol 8:23–30
9. De Lange FP, Kalkman JS, Bleijenberg G, Hagoort P, van der Meer JW, Toni I (2005) Gray matter volume reduction in the chronic fatigue syndrome. Neuroimage 26:777–781
10. Okada T, Tanaka M, Kuratsune H, Watanabe Y, Sadato N (2004) Mechanisms underlying fatigue: a voxel-based morphometric study of chronic fatigue syndrome. BMC Neurol 4(10.1186/1471–2377/4/14)
11. Ichise M, Salit IE, Abbey SE, et al. (1992) Assessment of regional cerebral perfusion by $^{99}Tc^{m}$-HMPAO SPECT in chronic fatigue syndrome. Nucl Med Commun 13:767–772
12. Schwartz RB, Komaroff AL, Garada BM, et al. (1994) SPECT imaging of the brain: comparison of findings in patients with chronic fatigue syndrome, AIDS dementia complex, and major unipolar depression. Am J Roentgenol 162:943–951
13. Lewis DH, Mayberg HS, Fischer ME, et al. (2001) Monozygotic twins discordant for chronic fatigue syndrome: regional cerebral blood flow SPECT. Radiology 219:766–773
14. Fischler B, D'Haenen H, Cluydts R, et al. (1996) Comparison of ^{99m}Tc HMPAO SPECT scan between chronic fatigue syndrome, major depression and healthy controls: an exploratory study of clinical correlates of regional cerebral blood flow. Neuropsychobiology 34:175–183
15. Costa DC, Tannock C, Brostoff J (1995) Brainstem perfusion is impaired in chronic fatigue syndrome. Q J Med 88:767–773
16. MacHale SM, Lawrie SM, Cavanagh JTO, et al. (2000) Cerebral perfusion in chronic fatigue syndrome and depression. Br J Psychiatr 176:550–556
17. Chaudhuri A, Condon BR, Gow JW, Brennan D, Hadley DM (2003) Proton magnetic resonance spectroscopy of basal ganglia in chronic fatigue syndrome. Neuroreport 14:225–228
18. Siessmeier T, Nix WA, Hardt J, Schreckenberger M, Egle UT, Bartenstein P (2003) Observer independent analysis of cerebral glucose metabolism in patients with chronic fatigue syndrome. J Neurol Neurosurg Psychiatr 74:922–928
19. Tirelli U, Chierichetti F, Tavio M, Simonelli C, Bianchin G, Zanco P, Ferlin G (1998) Brain positron emission tomography (PET) in chronic fatigue syndrome: preliminary data. Am J Med 105(3A):54S–58S
20. Kuratsune H, Yamaguti K, Lindh G, et al. (2002) Brain regions involved in fatigue sensation: reduced acetylcarnitine uptake into the brain. Neuroimage 17:1256–1265
21. Yoshiuchi K, Farkas J, Natelson BH (2006) Patients with chronic fatigue syndrome have reduced absolute cortical blood flow. Clin Physiol Funct Imaging 26:83–86
22. Prasher D, Smith A, Findley L (1990) Sensory and cognitive event-related potentials in myalgic encephalomyelitis. J Neurol Neurosurg Psychiatr 53:247–253

23. Gordon R, Michalewski HJ, Nguyen T, Gupta S, Starr A (1999) Cortical motor potential alterations in chronic fatigue syndrome. Int J Molec Med 4:493–499
24. Siemionow V, Fang Y, Calabrese L, Sahgal V, Yue GH (2004) Altered central nervous system signal during motor performance in chronic fatigue syndrome. Clin Neurophysiol 115:2372–2381
25. Lange G, Steffener J, Bly BM, et al. (2005) Chronic fatigue syndrome affects verbal working memory: a BOLD fMRI study. Neuroimage 26:513–524
26. Tanaka M, Sadato N, Okada T, et al. (2006) Reduced responsiveness is an essential feature of chronic fatigue syndrome: a fMRI study. BMC Neurol 6(9):doi:10.1186/1471-2377-6-9
27. Boda WL, Natelson BH, Sisto SA, Tapp WN (1995) Gait abnormalities in chronic fatigue syndrome. J Neurol Sci 131:156–161
28. Ash-Bernal R, Wall C, Komaroff AL, et al. (1995) Vestibular test anomalies in patients with chronic fatigue syndrome. Acta Otolaryngol (Stockholm) 115:9–17

Neurobiology of Chronic Fatigue Syndrome

Abhijit Chaudhuri[1], John W. Gow[2], and Peter O. Behan[3]

Summary

Severe persistent or relapsing fatigue is the most disabling symptom in patients with chronic fatigue syndrome (CFS). Clinical and brain imaging studies with proton magnetic resonance spectroscopy support the view that fatigue in CFS is central, i.e., brain-derived. It seems likely that an interruption of the basal ganglia pathways integrating voluntary motor output to the afferent sensory input and cognitive processing is the neural basis of fatigue in CFS. A genome-wide microarray study in patients with CFS suggests significant changes in gene expression of pathways responsible for immune modulation, oxidative stress, and apoptosis. Altered neural cell membrane signalling in regional brain areas induced by downstream effects of these changes may explain the paroxysmal and fluctuating nature of symptom severity in many CFS patients. It is possible, but not yet proven, that CFS is due to a neurological channelopathy.

"When a man begins with certainty, he ends in doubt. When someone starts from doubt, he ends in certainty" (Francis Bacon, 1606)

Introduction

Chronic fatigue syndrome (CFS) is characterized by otherwise unexplained, overwhelming persistent or relapsing fatigue of new onset in variable combinations with postexertional malaise, unrefreshing sleep, self-reported impairment in short-term

Declaration of Conflict of Interest

The Court of the University of Glasgow has filed a patent entitled "Materials and Methods for Diagnosis and Treatment of Chronic Fatigue Syndrome" based on microarray work of John W. Gow and Abhijit Chaudhuri (Patent File Number GB0502042.5).

[1]Essex Centre for Neurological Sciences, Romford, Essex, UK

[2]Caledonian University, Glasgow, UK

[3]University of Glasgow, Glasgow, UK

memory, headache, and muscle and joint pain. For research purposes, the case definition of CFS is based on the modified international criteria proposed by the Center of Disease Control (CDC), Atlanta, in 1994 [1]. CFS is recognized worldwide and in all age groups, and usually affects more women than men. Because of its chronicity, lack of effective therapy, and consequent disability in adults, a diagnosis of CFS has a significant socioeconomic impact.

The precise aetiology of CFS and the mechanism(s) of its symptoms are unknown. New-onset fatigue and a limitation in physical endurance are two important defining characteristics. In the absence of a disease marker, the present case definition of CFS (modified CDC criteria) selects a heterogeneous population. This heterogeneity may explain the variability in research findings in CFS. The limitations and the pitfalls of many of the CFS studies are reminiscent of the well-known Indian tale of the six blind men and the elephant, where each observer's description of the elephant was as incomplete as any other.

Approach to Fatigue

A possible approach to conceptualizing the neurobiology of CFS is to apply existing knowledge of the mechanisms of fatigue in known neurological diseases. Fatigue may be peripheral, central, or both. In disorders of *peripheral fatigue,* as in myasthenia gravis, the inability to sustain a specified force or work rate is related to exercise or physical activity. However, patients with central fatigue experience difficulty in sustaining normal physical as well as mental activities. The failure to endure sustained mental tasks (e.g., a sequential digit span or mental arithmetic) is an important symptom in central fatigue. Many patients also experience difficulty in exerting or sustaining mental effort in tasks that require directed attention. Most CFS patients experience impairment in short-term memory or concentration, which has been verified in objective psychological assessments. As with multiple sclerosis, patients with CFS experience not only physical but also mental fatigue, and show impaired function in tests of verbal memory, attention, verbal fluency, and spatial reasoning [2].

Central fatigue represents a failure of physical and mental tasks that require self-motivation and internal cues in the absence of demonstrable cognitive failure or motor weakness. Patients with central fatigue have less difficulty in performing when stimulated externally or cued in advance, although they need a much higher perceived effort for the tasks executed. These patients may also fail to complete the execution of incremental or serial tasks that require sustained motivation and attention. This failure of focused attention, that normally provides the unconscious ("automatic") link between the self-guided voluntary effort, the performance of sequential motor or cognitive tasks, and sensory input, is a characteristic feature of central fatigue. It has been proposed that central fatigue, as defined above, is due to a failure of the nonmotor function of the basal ganglia [3].

Proton Magnetic Resonance Spectroscopy of Basal Ganglia in CFS

Proton magnetic resonance spectroscopy (^{1}H MRS) is a relatively new tool for imaging metabolic brain functions. Typically, ^{1}H MRS measures regional brain metabolite levels of N-acetyl aspartate (NAA), choline-containing compounds (Cho), and creatine-containing compounds (Cr). While NAA levels broadly correlate with the functional neuronal mass, Cr is generally considered to be an unvarying metabolic marker of brain function in ^{1}H MRS. In contrast, the Cho peak is considered to be largely derived from the cell membrane lipids. ^{1}H MRS of brain tumors shows high peaks of Cho, reflecting mobile brain lipids due to tissue degradation and necrosis. Cho is acutely elevated in relapsing multiple sclerosis, where lipid breakdown follows myelin injury. However, elevated [Cho] is also observed in the areas of reactive or reparative gliosis, probably as a result of increased membrane turnover [4].

In our study of regional ^{1}H MRS of basal ganglia [5], cases ($n = 8$) were selected carefully in order to identify neurologically defined CFS patients. While there was no evidence of significant loss of functional neuronal mass (reflected by reduced levels of NAA and low NAA/Cr ratio) in the basal ganglia of our CFS patients, the Cho peaks were uniformly increased in all CFS patients, irrespective of their age or the duration of illness, when compared with matched healthy controls (Fig. 1). The statistical strength of this association was extremely high ($P < 0.001$). In the only other ^{1}H MRS study of the basal ganglia in three children with CFS (ages 11, 12, and 13 years), a remarkable elevation of the Cho/Cr ratio was also observed [6]. None of these patients (ours and the three paediatric cases) had focal structural abnormalities of the basal ganglia on MRI.

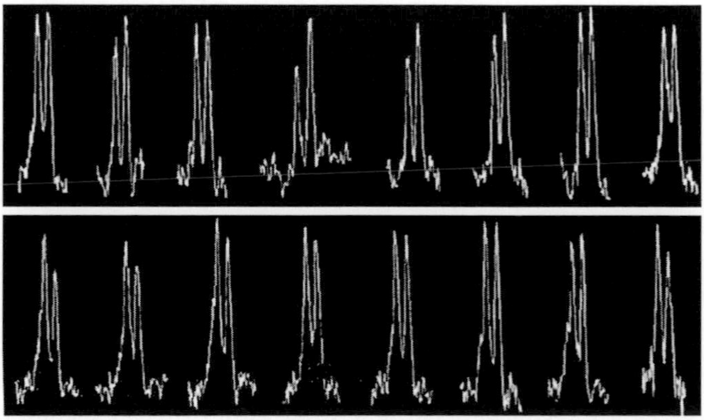

Fig. 1. Regional ^{1}H-MRS of basal ganglia in healthy subjects (*top panel*) compared with those in CFS patients (*bottom panel*). The first peak comes from choline (Cho) and the second from creatine (Cr)-containing compounds of largely glial cell membranes

In general, Cho peaks in ^{1}H MRS are influenced by specific structural changes (tumor or demyelination), certain viral infections (e.g., hepatitis C or HIV), and higher rates of cell turnover (as in reparative gliosis). From the results of this study [5], it appears that choline-containing compounds are elevated in the basal ganglia of CFS patients irrespective of the age of the patient or the duration of the symptoms. Glial cell membrane turnover due to reparative gliosis appears to be the most likely explanation for this observation, although the precise stimulus for this process could not be identified in the ^{1}H MRS study.

Neural Substrate of Central Fatigue: Role of Basal Ganglia

The proton magnetic spectroscopic signature of altered glial cell membrane metabolism in the basal ganglia suggested that fatigue is a centrally derived in CFS. In addition, this research supported a possible role of basal ganglia pathways in CFS in a way that is comparable to other disorders of central fatigue [3]. Under normal circumstances, the initiation and sequential performance of a task requires an internally driven mechanism integrated at the level of basal ganglia to prepare the emotive, motor, and sensory apparatus ("cues") responsible for next and the subsequent set of responses. Disruption of the normal basal-ganglia-derived algorithm of the sequential task-processing mechanism would not only delay the initiation, but also prevent the smooth execution of the intended task, a feature that is typical of patients with central fatigue. Observations have repeatedly confirmed that parts of the basal ganglia circuitry functionally involved in the nonmotor and emotional processes are linked to the frontal lobes. The caudate–dorsolateral prefrontal circuit and the ventral striatopallidal system, especially nucleus accumbens, are implicated in the cognitive and behavioral syndromes associated with basal ganglia diseases. The ventral striopallidal system has a more complex relationship involving the shell of nucleus accumbens (the ventral striatum) and the extended amygdala, incorporating connections with the olfactory tubercles, hypothalamus, and brain stem. Loss of the motivational influence of the striato-thalamic input to the frontal lobe (prefrontal, orbitofrontal, and cingulate region) is integral to the genesis of central fatigue.

Cell Membrane Changes After Infection

Changes in the property and function of host cell membranes are well known in the course of viral infections. What is not known is whether membrane changes may be sustained as a consequence of viral infection, but without ongoing, persistent infection or viral reactivation in the central nervous system. There is some evidence from in vivo studies that this may, indeed, be a possibility. The influenza virus is one of the well-studied models of membrane fusion. The protein responsible for influenza virus fusion is its well-characterized membrane hemagglutinin. Transmembrane domains of hemagglutinin are responsible for the merger of the lipid bilayers of the viral and host cells. Like the hemagglutinin of the influenza virus, a number of other viral fusion proteins promote mixing of the lipid components from two apposed bilayers. This fusion event is highly localized to the cell membrane, and fusion "pores" develop during viral and intracellular membrane fusion events. It appears from the experimental data that during membrane fusion, there is a "free mingling" of the lipids from the two bilayers (virus and host cells).

Since Cho resonance peaks in ^{1}H MRS primarily arise from phosphocholine and glycerophosphocholine, both of which are metabolites of membrane lipid (phosphatidylcholine), changes in neuronal membrane signalling in CFS is possibly related to localized cell membrane lipid breakdown. One could assume that changes in the surviving host cell membranes as a result of persistent membrane fusion proteins may persist long after symptomatic recovery in some cases. Indeed, if cell membrane lipid constituents are unstable, membrane-associated cell signalling functions will change. Glial cells inwardly rectifying potassium (Kir) channels are susceptible to changes, which may affect the excitability of the nervous system, depending on regional metabolic demands and functions.

Paroxysmal Symptoms in Neurological Channelopathies

Idiopathic epilepsy and common migraine are common, multifactorial episodic disorders of the central nervous system that are currently considered to be channelopathies. In epilepsy and migraine, paroxysmal neurological dysfunctions occur due the neuronal dysfunction affecting cortical and brain stem electrochemical activities. Complex changes in neurotransmitter release, cerebral blood flow, and the autonomic nervous system characterize the paroxysms of epilepsy and migraine, and cortical electrical activity may be suppressed for a considerable time after a typical attack. This neuronal depression is believed to be due to a shift in the electrochemical gradient of extracellular potassium ions. A rising level of extracellular potassium accompanied by increased intracellular calcium accounts for spreading depression [7].

Migraine-like symptoms are common in CFS, and conversely, fatigue similar to CFS can antedate, accompany, or follow an attack of migraine. CFS shares many features of migraine, such as headache, sensitization to foods and chemicals, photophobia, transient confusion, and serotonin sensitivity. Both recurrent and relapsing fatigue are common in migraineurs, who frequently report mood swings (irritability, tenseness, depression) during the attacks. Typically, migraine attacks in women are worst during a menstrual period, which is the same as fatigue symptoms in women with CFS. Stress, alcohol, and caffeine worsen fatigue in CFS and precipitate headache in migraineurs. Prodromes of muscle pain, tingling, numbness, dysequilibrium, sweating, flushes, and headache are common in both [8].

A genetic mutation affecting the voltage-gated calcium channel in the cell membranes has recently been identified in familial hemiplegic migraine (FHM), where attacks of headache and focal neurological abnormality can be triggered by stress or exercise, or following viral infections, and these are the same precipitants as for CFS. The same, or a closely related, genetic locus is postulated to have a role in nonhemiplegic migraine without aura. About 50% of patients with type 2 episodic ataxia, a calcium channelopathy, also suffer from migraine [9]. Indeed, ^{31}P NMR spectroscopy in the skeletal muscle of FHM has shown a reduced rate of phosphocreatinine recovery after exercise, and a similar abnormality is characteristic of CFS [8].

Neurotransmitters and neurohormones activate *second messengers* and *ion channels* (ionophores) located on cell membranes. In all cases, once neurotransmitters are released into the synapse, they bind to specific receptors on the postsynaptic target cell. There they exert a brief and decisive action, communicating as either an inhibitory or an excitatory message. This signal is usually transmitted across the membrane as an "electrical message" in the form of a membrane potential change, occurring as a result of the activation of selective ion gates or channels which exist in close physical association with these specific receptors. Clearly, cell membrane integrity is critical for neuronal excitation, which in turn can be influenced by modifications of receptors, ion channels, or membrane protein genes.

Gene Signature for Chronic Fatigue Syndrome

DNA chip microarray technology provides a method for examining the differential expression of mRNA from a large number of genes. We used whole-genome microarray technology to obtain a complete gene expression signature from patients with CFS, with the dual aims of identifying biochemical changes in patients with CFS compared with healthy controls, and also identifying potential biomarkers for the condition. Whole human genome-wide Affymetrix GeneChip arrays (39 000 transcripts derived from 33 000 gene sequences) were used to compare the levels of gene expression in the peripheral blood mononuclear cells of patients with postviral chronic fatigue (n = 8) and healthy control subjects (n = 7). Potential biomarkers identified by microarray data were subsequently verified by reverse transcriptase–polymerase chain reaction (RT–PCR)/Western blot/enzyme-linked immunosorbent assay (ELISA) assays in 20 consecutive adult, nonpsychiatric patients with chronic fatigue syndrome.

In this study, we aimed to obtain a complete "gene signature" for nonpsychiatric patients with persistent symptoms due to CFS. By using an Affymetrix GeneChip Human Genome U133 double-chip set that contains nearly 45 000 probe sets representing 39 000 transcripts derived from 33 000 human gene sequences, the entire human genome was encompassed in this work. Patients and healthy subjects differed significantly in the level of expression of 770 genes which showed a greater than two-fold change, and of 39 genes which showed a greater than three-fold change. Analysis of the differentially expressed genes indicated functional implications in immune modulation, oxidative stress, and apoptosis. Prototype markers were identified on the basis of the differential level of gene expression and possible biological significance. Defensin α-1 mRNA expression, β-tubulin, thrombospondin 1, and arginase protein levels were selectively increased in patients, and reliably distinguished patients from healthy control subjects by RT–PCR, Western blot, and ELISA assays. A number of the top-ranked up-regulated genes are listed in Table 1. In Table 2, up- or down-regulated genes are collated from the microarray data

Table 1. Up-regulated gene expression in CFS

NCBI accession number		Gene symbol
NM_002343	Defensin α-1	DEFA 1
AI 133353	Hemoglobin β	HBG2
L 01639	Chemokine (c-x-c) receptor 4	CXCR4
NM_002343	Lactotransferrin	LTF
NM_004226	Serine/threonine kinase 17B	STK17B
BC005312	Major histocompatibility complex Class II DR B4	HLA-DRB4
NM_030773	Tubulin β-1	TUBB1
NM_000558	Hemoglobin α-1	HBA1
NM_001925	Defensin α-4	DEFA 4
U13699	Caspase 1	CASP 1
NM_000419	Integrin α-2B, CD41B	ITGA2B
NM35999	Integrin β-3 CD61	ITGB3
NM_005764	Membrane-associated protein 17	MAP 17
NM_001828	Charcot Leyden crystal protein	CLC
S36219	Prostaglandin–endoperoxide Synthase 1	PTGS1
NM_000963	Prostaglandin–endoperoxide Synthase 2	PTGS2
M16276	Major histocompatibility complex Class II DQβ-1	HLA-DQB1
NM 87789	Immunoglobulin heavy constant γ-3	IGG3
NM_012062	Dynamin 1-like	DNM1L
NM_004657	Phosphatidyl serine-binding protein Serum deprivation response	SDPR
NM_000045	Arginase 1	ARG1
U75667	Arginase 2	ARG2
AI812030	Thrombospondin 1	THBS1
D32039	Chondroitin sulphate Proteoglycan 2 (versican)	CSPG2
NM_001693	ATPase H+ transporting Protein (vATPase)	ATP6V1B2
AI 133353	Hemoglobin γ	HBG1
M63310	Annexin	A3ANXA3
NM_00422	Serine/threonine kinase 17b	STK17B
AI 679555	Decay-accelerating factor CD55	DAF
U19970	Cathelicidin antimicrobial peptide	CAMP

Table 2. Three altered biosystems in CFS identified in a genome-wide microarray search

(a) Immune dysfunction genes (including markers of viral immunomodulation/evasion)	
Up-regulated:	DAF (CD55) & CD46
	Antigen processing via MHC class II (MHC II DP α1 and DR α)
	IL-12, IL-13, and IL-6 biosynthesis
Down-regulated:	The MHC-1 system, including:
	Natural killer cell receptors (Kir)
	TCR complex (T-cell receptors $\alpha,\beta,\delta,\gamma$)
	NO production (up-regulation of arginase I and II)
	Flavohemoprotein B5
	Leukocyte-derived arginine aminopeptidase (L-rap)
(b) Oxidative stress genes	
Up-regulated:	Prostaglandin synthase: Cox 1 and 2
	Hemoglobin $\alpha,\beta,\delta,\gamma$
Down-regulated:	Glutathion-s-transferase
(c) Apoptosis genes	
Up-regulated:	Annexin -A3, -A5
	Serine/threonine kinase 17b
	Histones 1 and 2
	Protein S-α
	Serum deprivation response (phosphatidylserine-binding protein)
	Caspase 1
	TGF β
	Death effector filament-forming CED-4-like apoptosis protein
	Complement 3a receptor 1
	Early growth response 1
	TNF-A1P3, -RSF17, -SF4

Table 3. Functional summary of the differentially expressed gene iterative group analyses

A shift of immune response with preferential antigen presentation to MHC class II receptors
Down-regulation of the MHC class I system
Suppression of natural killer inhibitory cell receptors
Suppression of the TCR (T-cell receptors)
Increased cell membrane prostaglandin–endoperoxide synthase activity with downstream changes in oxygen transport
Superoxide production
Macrophage activation
Suppression of nitric oxide synthesis
Evidence of apoptosis
Up-regulation of cytoskeletal proteins
Viral assembly and maturation genes up-regulated
Defensin and related genes up-regulated

to demonstrate that three main biological systems appear to be dysregulated in patients with CFS. In Table 3, a functional summary of the microarray data is presented.

The microarray data generated a genome-wide gene expression signature for CFS for the first time. Iterative group analyses of the genes suggest that the three pathways that are altered in fatigue patients relate to immune modulation after viral infection and viral immunosurveillance, oxidative stress, and apoptosis. Many of the higher expressed genes belong to the macrophage, monocyte, eosinophil, or basophil groups within the innate immune system. Within the top 100 up-regulated genes, there is a majority of innate immune proteins; one of the highest is α-defensin, an antiviral/bacterial protein, as well as the charcot leyden protein (expressed in eosinophils and basophils). Other up-regulated genes are involved in oxygen transport, apoptosis, platelet activation, prostaglandin–endoperoxide synthase activity, macrophage activation, viral assembly maturation, and release.

Altered Immune Surveillance

Highly up-regulated immune-related genes in patients were lactotransferrin, defensin-α-1, and integrin. Lactotransferrin is an iron-binding protein responsible for immunological reactions, while defensins are a family of microbicidal and cytotoxic peptides made by neutrophilic granules and released in response to viral and bacterial infections. The protein encoded by this gene is found in the microbicidal granules of neutrophils, and probably plays a role in phagocyte-mediated host defence. Defensins are also involved in the antimicrobial defence of the epithelial surfaces (respiratory tract, urinary tract, and vagina). Patients with CFS are known to have increased proneness to infections, and women with CFS frequently report vaginal candidiasis.

Integrins are extracellular matrix proteins involved in cell adhesion, and they also activate cytosolic signal cascades for cell growth and regulation. Arginase is a key enzyme considered to be active in immune modulation; arginase is also involved in NK cell function. Other notable up-regulated genes involved hemoglobin, and especially fetal hemoglobin, and this may suggest response to increased oxidative stress. Another family of up-regulated genes relate to cellular apopotosis, and serine–theronine kinase is a member of the brain kinase family of proteins implicated in neural apoptosis and the formation of corpora amylacea. Of the down-regulated genes, ribosomal protein genes and zinc finger protein genes are involved in cell cycle and cellular growth. The overall picture emerging from these results points to a significant perturbation of function in relation to microbial defence, viral immunosurveillance, and cell growth among patients with postviral chronic fatigue.

Oxidative Stress

Cell membrane oxidative stress may be important, and may contribute to the free Cho peaks observed in the ^{1}H MRS study of CFS patients [5]. The gene array confirms evidence of oxidative stress, with the highest changes (100%) in the genes for prostaglandin–endoperoxide synthase 1 and 2 (Table 2, b). These enzymes are responsible for the regulation of prostaglandin synthesis. The inducible form COX 2 leads to the release of prostanoids, which sensitize peripheral nociceptor terminals and produce localized pain hypersensitivity. More indirect evidence of oxidative stress comes from the up-regulation of fetal hemoglobin (Hb F), which is normally expressed in the fetus. Other up-regulated genes involved in oxidative stress on the array are leukotriene B4, cytochrome P 450, and superoxide dysmutase.

Apoptosis

Within the top up-regulated genes there was a large number of apoptosis-associated genes (Table 2, c). Many factors trigger apoptosis: cellular damage, infection with a virus, and homeostasis. The signal for apoptosis can be from within the cell, from surrounding tissue, or from a cell belonging to the immune system. Apoptotic cells and their nuclei shrink and often fragment, and are then efficiently phagocytosed by macrophages or neighboring cells. Tubulin β-1 is the major constituent of microtubules. Up-regulation of this gene supports the theory of increased cell breakdown and replacement in patients with CFS.

In summary, the microarray data illustrated important differences in gene expression between CFS patients and healthy subjects. While these differences in gene signatures may offer a rational explanation for the symptoms at the cellular level, the data do not imply that CFS is a genetic disorder, or that the differentially expressed genes are predisposing for the illness. We believe the data presented here is a first step forward toward the goal of identifying putative biomarkers to support a clinical diagnosis of CFS. However, a larger patient cohort, together with a wide range of control disease populations, including patients with clinical depression, is necessary to confirm the utility of the markers identified in this study.

Conclusions

> *"Life is the art of drawing sufficient conclusions from insufficient premises"* (Samuel Butler, 1912)

It is only in the past few years that neurological diseases caused by acquired modifications of ion channel functions have become recognized. Ciguatera fish poisoning and anti-VGKC antibody-associated disorders are some of the best examples. Despite the increasing numbers of "new" ion channel genes being discovered, more still remain to be uncovered. For many more, their precise physiological roles in health and disease remain unexplored and unanswered. We are only beginning to understand the rich variety of isoforms that are expressed with individual ion channels, but we still do not fully understand how tissue-specific expressions will act if these isoforms are controlled. We know very little about how ion channel numbers are up-regulated or down-regulated in response to stimuli. Yet we are aware that a large variety of physiological functions in the cells and cellular trafficking are regulated by ion channels, and any dysfunction of these channels produces significant disturbances in neurological function without demonstrable loss of structure. The list of ion channelopathies in neurological diseases is still growing, and at present we are only able to identify a minority of cases with known gene mutations with confidence.

Data from regional brain ^{1}H MRS clearly point to a role of central fatigue due to basal ganglia cell membrane changes in CFS. These changes could be secondary to altered gene signatures affecting immune surveillance, oxidative stress, and apoptosis. The differential expression of key genes identified in the genome-wide microarray study offers an insight into the possible cellular mechanism of chronic fatigue affecting the neural network, which in turn affects basal ganglia and the transbasal ganglionic connections of the limbic system and frontal cortex.

Based on our current understanding, we propose the following steps as possible pathogenic mechanisms of CFS.

Step 1. Selection of susceptible individuals. Genetically predisposed individuals are exposed to an initial, single precipitant and become "primed" or "conditioned."

Step 2. Changes in cell membrane function follow, due to a combination of increased oxidative stress and altered immune surveillance.

Step 3. "Primed" or susceptible persons are now hit by a second trigger: stress or a second infection. The second trigger operates by increasing metabolic demands. Cell membrane potassium channels (Kir) de-compensate in response to the humoral factors released. Neural excitability in the basal ganglia circuitry is altered as a consequence, leading to persistent fatigue symptoms.

As with idiopathic epilepsy and common migraine, CFS may be a channelopathy affecting a specific neural network in the brain. The growing number of transgenic studies, the rapid identification of missense mutations of ion channel genes, and in vivo experiments of ion channel disturbance in response to viral infections are expected to create a whole new world of knowledge about ion channels and their functions. Until then, the story of ion channelopathy in CFS will remain far from complete.

Dedication. This manuscript is dedicated to the memory of Prof. W.M.H. Behan (1939–2005).

Acknowledgments. We are also grateful to Pawel Herzyk, Stuart Keir, and Celia Cannon (University of Glasgow) for their expert assistance with the microarray work and its statistical analysis. We acknowledge the financial support of the Cunningham Trust, the Barclay Foundation, Scottish Enterprise, and the ME Association during the course of this work.

References

1. Fukuda K, Strauss SE, Hickie I, Sharpe MC, Dobbins JG, Komaroff A (1994) The chronic fatigue syndrome: a comprehensive approach to case definition and study. Ann Intern Med 121:953–959
2. Krupp LB, Elkins LE (2000) Fatigue and decline in cognitive functioning in multiple sclerosis. Neurology 55:934–939
3. Chaudhuri A, Behan WH, Behan PO (2000) Fatigue and basal ganglia. J Neurol Sci 179:34–42
4. Brand A, Reichter-Landsberg C, Leibfritz D (1993) Multinuclear NMR studies on the energy metabolism of glial and neuronal cells. Dev Neurosci 15:289–298
5. Chaudhuri A, Condon BR, Gow JW, Brennan D, Hadley DM (2003) Proton magnetic resonance spectroscopy of basal ganglia in chronic fatigue syndrome. NeuroReport 14:225–228
6. Tomoda A, Miike T, Yamada E, Honda H, Moroi T, Ogawa M, Ohtami Y, Morishita S (2000) Chronic fatigue syndrome in childhood. Brain Dev 22:60–64
7. Ptacek LJ (1998) The place of migraine as a channelopathy. Curr Opin Neurol 11:217–226
8. Chaudhuri A, Behan PO (1999) Chronic fatigue syndrome is an acquired neurological channelopathy. Hum Psychopharmacol Clin Exp 14:7–17
9. Greenberg DA (1997) Calcium channels in neurological disease. Ann Neurol 42:275–282

Chronic Fatigue Syndrome and Herpesvirus Infection

Kazuhiro Kondo

Summary

Chronic fatigue syndrome (CFS) is a disease of unknown etiology which is accompanied by severe fatigue as a main complaint. The prominence of the acute onset of illness, the persistent symptoms consistent with a viral infection, and the increased titers of viral antibodies and enhanced activity of the interferon-induced enzyme suggest the role of viruses in CFS. In other words, in CFS patients, it is suggested that there may be some kind of "postinfectious fatigue syndrome" following any infection by a virus. Among the variety of viruses evaluated to date are enteroviruses, retroviruses, and human herpesviruses.

CFS is a disease which lasts far longer than postinfectious fatigue. It is considered, accordingly, that the infection causing CFS is a latent infection with some herpesvirus. Human herpesvirus 6 (HHV-6) has exhibited the most promise as a candidate for a CFS-associated virus. As there may be an unusual latent infection with HHV-6, which may be an etiology of CFS in CFS patients, a study of latent infection is considered to be important in understanding CFS.

Introduction

Fatigue is caused by many different factors, of which infection is one of the most important. Fatigue, which not only lessens work efficiency but also constitutes the cause of various diseases as well as death from overwork, poses a serious health problem for sufferers. In spite of this importance, however, the mechanisms of fatigue, by which fatigue is caused and felt, are barely known.

In the spectrum of fatigue, chronic fatigue syndrome (CFS) is the most complicated disorder, characterized by extreme fatigue that does not improve with bed rest, and may worsen with physical or mental activity. Of all chronic illnesses,

---

Department of Virology, The Jikei University School of Medicine, 3-25-8 Nishi-Shimbashi, Minato-ku, Tokyo 105-8461, Japan

chronic fatigue syndrome is one of the most mysterious because, unlike infections, it has no clear cause.

It is easy to identify the presence of fatigue which is caused by bacterial or viral infection, because the time and cause of fatigue are known. Therefore, postinfectious fatigue attracts attention as an important subject in studies of the mechanism of fatigue. Also, in view of the fact that many cases of CFS, in which severe fatigue of unknown etiology continues for long time, occur following an infectious disease, the relationship between infection and CFS is considered to be very important.

Mechanism of Fatigue

In general, "fatigue" is defined as decreased physical functions attributable to prolonged physical and/or mental stresses, while "tiredness" indicates the condition in which the brain recognizes decreased physical functions. Tiredness is an important biological signal, as are pain and drowsiness, in the need to maintain biofunctions.

Becoming fatigued or feeling tired might indicate the presence of substances which increase or accumulate through fatigue, and/or a fatigue-transmitting substance which transmits fatigue to the brain. Lactic acid has long been considered as a major fatigue-causing substance. However, it was reported recently that lactic acid is not a fatigue-causing but a fatigue-preventing substance [1]. At present, therefore, there is no proven fatigue-causing substance or fatigue-transmitting substance.

However, the most probable candidates for such fatigue-inducing or fatigue-transmitting substances are cytokines, including interferon. This is shown by the fact that patients undergoing treatment for hepatitis virus using interferon or other cytokines feel severe tiredness [2–4]. It has also been reported that TGF-β is associated with the occurrence of fatigue [5, 6]. However, because the mutual interaction and association of multiple cytokines are involved in the production and activation of cytokines, it is not yet known which cytokine plays a central role in causing or transmitting fatigue.

On the other hand, it is well known that a viral infection such as flu often leads to the intense expression of cytokines and then to severe fatigue. These facts suggest that infection and immunity are closely related to fatigue, and are important for the investigation into CFS.

Chronic Fatigue

Fatigue is usually cured with rest, although sometimes fatigue without recovery may accumulate. The latter is defined as chronic fatigue, and is divided roughly into two categories. One is the accumulation of physiological fatigue because of continuous labor without rest, and the other is the continuation of morbid fatigue accompanying disease. At worst, accumulated physical fatigue may result in the tragic outcome known as "death from overwork" so it should not be neglected, although it is only the extension of the physical phenomena.

Major morbid fatigue includes postinfectious fatigue and CFS. Although the etiology of CFS is unknown, the involvement of infection with some pathogenic organism is suspected. Therefore, postinfectious fatigue and CFS are not unconnected.

Diagnostic criteria to define CFS can be simplified as follows.

1. A condition with serious tiredness which forces absence from school or work for several days per month, and continues for over 6 months or recurs many times.
2. No other disease is identified.

Patients with eight or more of the following symptoms, which are often observed in CFS, are definitively diagnosed as having CFS: (1) slight fever or chill, (2) throat pain, (3) swollen lymph nodes, (4) feeling of exhaustion of unknown etiology, (5) muscle pain, (6) general weariness, (7) headache, (8) joint pain, (9) psychoneurotic symptoms (memory impairment, confusion, impaired concentration, depression), (10) sleep disorders (insomnia, hypersomnia), and (11) sudden onset of symptoms (within several hours to a few days).

Of these symptoms, 1, 2, 3, 5, 8, and 11 are often observed in virus infections. The clinical features of some cases of CFS, such as abrupt onset with fever, adenopathy, and influenza-like symptoms, in combination with epidemiologic studies consistent with outbreaks [7,8], have suggested that CFS may be the result of a virus infection or immune dysfunction and/or activation.

The reasons why such symptoms are included in the diagnostic criteria are that patients suspected of having CFS very frequently display symptoms which are similar to those of infectious diseases, and that CFS is considered to be caused by continuous fatigue following infection with some infecting factor. As a result, the study of postinfectious fatigue is also important for identifying the unestablished etiology of CFS.

Examples of Postinfectious Fatigue

There have been many reports of cases of postinfectious fatigue and, as shown in Table 1, the pathogenic organisms or infecting factors associated with the fatigue are wide-ranging. This chapter identifies some cases which have an important meaning for subsequent studies and the understanding of postinfectious fatigue.

Acquired Immunodeficiency Syndrome (AIDS)

Postinfectious fatigue is caused by various pathogenic organisms, and a mass outbreak of postinfectious fatigue suggests an epidemic of some pathogenic infection.

Table 1. Pathogens reported to be causing postinfectious fatigue. Organisms which have been reported to be the causes of postinfectious fatigue are listed

Organisms causing persistent or latent infection	Virus	Epstein–Barr virus, human herpesvirus 6, human herpesvirus 7, herpes simplex virus, human immunodeficiency virus, hepatitis C virus, parvovirus B19, influenza virus
	Bacteria, etc.	*Coxiella burnetii*, *Helicobacter pylori*
Organisms causing no persistent or latent infection	Virus	Polio virus, Coxsackie B virus, West Nile virus, smallpox vaccine, hemorrhagic fever with renal syndrome viruses
	Bacteria, etc.	*Borrelia burgdorferi*, *Streptococcus pneumoniae*, *Trichinella spiralis*, *Trichinella pseudospiralis*, *Staphylococcus*, Legionnaires

This is often an epidemic of a known pathogenic organism, such as influenza, but an unknown or unreported pathogen in the area can sometimes be discovered and identified as a cause of postinfectious fatigue. For example, until human immunodeficiency virus (HIV) was established as a cause, acquired immunodeficiency syndrome (AIDS) had attracted attention as a disease accompanied by fatigue of unknown etiology [9].

Post-Rickettsia Infectious Fatigue

Coxiella burnetii is an organism which causes Q-fever, belongs to the family Rickettsiaceae, and infects humans via cattle and pet animals. Many patients with Q-fever complain of symptoms such as fever, headache, muscle pain, respiratory symptoms, and strong systemic weariness. Infection with *Coxiella burnetti* often ends as an acute infectious disease, whilst in about 5% of the patients *Coxiella burnetti* remains in the body long after the acute infection, and progresses to chronic Q fever.

Chronic Q fever accompanied by *Coxiella burnetii* infection for over 6 months is often more severe than acute Q fever. Chronic Q fever occurs in acute Q-fever patients from 1 year to 20 years after the first infection, and is often accompanied by infectious endocarditis [10,11]. Chronic Q-fever patients complain of symptoms such as weariness, insomnia, and joint pain. As these symptoms can continue for a few years to over 10 years, they may be diagnosed as CFS.

Chronic Active Epstein–Barr Virus (EBV) Infection

It has been reported that some patients suffering from infectious mononucleosis remained ill for up to 28 months, and persistently manifested the presence of antibodies to EA-R and elevated levels of IgG anti-VCA antibody titres, suggesting continued Epstein–Barr virus (EBV) activity [12]. Since some patients with severe persistent fatigue have high antibody titers to EBV, EBV has been considered to be one of the causes of CFS-like disease. However, most patients suffering from EBV infection and showing CFS-like symptoms are now recognized as having chronic active EBV infection (CAEBV) [13,14], and EBV infectious diseases other than CAEBV are considered to be unrelated to CFS [15,16]. CAEBV is a disease in which the symptoms of infectious mononucleosis (IM), such as fever, pharyngitis, swollen lymph nodes, and hepatosplenomegaly, appear with the first EBV infection and continue for over 3 months, and CAEBV patients complain of severe fatigue. IM is a disease which is often observed in acute EBV infection, and which subsides with the disappearance of symptoms in 1–3 months. One of the reasons why IM-like symptoms continue for a long time in CAEBV is the different pattern of EBV latent infection. EBV latently infects B cells in general, and this latent infection progresses asymptomatically in many cases, but it may cause various diseases depending on the pattern of latent infection (Table 2). In the case of CAEBV, EBV latently infects NK cells and T cells, and induces active virus gene expression [17]. It is believed that this produces abnormal immunoreactions and causes fever and intense weariness.

Of the three cases mentioned above, chronic Q fever and CAEBV in particular show CFS-like symptoms, and can be said to be the cause of CFS. However, according to the present diagnostic criteria, diseases of known etiology are not CFS

Table 2. Various latent infection forms of Epstein–Barr virus (EBV)

Type of latent infected cell	Form of latent infection	Manifested latent infected gene	Associated morbidity
B cell	Latency 0	EBER1, EBER 2, BARTs	Latent infection in healthy people
	Latency I	EBER1, EBER2, BARTs, EBNA 1	Burkitt's lymphoma, etc.
	Latency II	EBER1, EBER2, BARTs, EBNA 1, LMP-1, LMP-2A, LMP-2B	Nasopharyngeal carcinoma, etc.
	Latency III	EBER1, EBER2, BARTs, EBNA 1, EBNA2, EBNA 3A, EBNA 3B, EBNA 3C, EBNA-LP, LMP-1, LMP-2A, LMP-2B	In vitro immortalization or reactivation (?)
NK cell/T cell	Latency II	EBER1, LMP-1, LMP-2A	CAEBV

and so they are not categorized as such. This means that the identification of a pathogenic organism such as chronic Q fever or chronic active EBV infection is most important for identifying the etiology of the CFS that occurs following infection. Also, the example of CAEBV suggests that infection with the same EBV may present completely different symptoms depending on the pattern of the EBV presence, particularly the pattern of latent EBV infection, and lead to persistent fatigue.

Causes of Chronic Fatigue Syndrome

As previously mentioned, the fact that infection with various organisms causes postinfectious fatigue has been known for decades. However, it appears that morbidities such as "postinfectious fatigue" and "postviral infectious fatigue" came to the attention of the public following an outbreak known as the "Lake Tahoe mystery," in which CFS-like symptoms affected a large number of people in the geographical area around Lake Tahoe in Nevada, USA. At this time, the concept of a "fatigue epidemic" was proposed [18]. This condition posed a serious social problem, and many infection specialists launched investigations into its etiology. The concept of CFS was also proposed for this Lake Tahoe incident.

The morbidity named "Gulf War syndrome" made the public aware of the importance of postinfectious fatigue. Gulf War syndrome is a disorder which has been observed in many veterans who have been discharged from military service in the Gulf War, which started in 1991. Their main symptoms are muscle pain, night sweats, skin rashes, headache, and diarrhea, and central nervous symptoms such as impairment in memory or concentration [19,20]. Many researchers consider that Gulf War syndrome is caused by infection from some factors which are included in biological weaponry [21]. Gulf War syndrome is considered to be a type of CFS, which supports the argument that an identification of the infectious factor is most important in examining the etiology of CFS.

In fact, the observation of an abnormal production of 2-5A synthetase and RNase L, indicators of interferon production in CFS patients, suggests that tiredness, a symptom seen in CFS, is associated with the abnormal production of interferon [22]. This is one of the reasons why CFS is considered to be a type of postinfectious fatigue.

The diagnostic criteria for defining CFS include those which are known as the symptoms of infectious disease, such as slight fever or chill, sore throat, swollen lymph nodes, and the sudden onset of disease. In other words, it cannot be denied that these criteria were established on the assumption that the most probable cause of CFS was postinfectious fatigue.

Herpesvirus and Chronic Fatigue Syndrome

The prominence of the acute onset of illness, the persistent symptoms consistent with a viral infection, and early reports of increased titers of viral antibodies and enhanced activity of the interferon-induced enzyme 2′5′-oligoadenylate synthetase [23,24] has led to an examination of the role of viruses in CFS.

Moreover, CFS is a disease which lasts far longer than postinfectious fatigue. Accordingly, it is considered that the infection causing CFS is a persistent or latent infection with some virus. It is known that once infecting herpesvirus establishes latent infection, it then produces some symptoms by frequent reactivation. Since these properties of herpesvirus can explain why the symptoms of CFS patients show cycles of remission and exacerbation, the theory that herpesvirus is a cause of CFS is supported by many people. The viruses which have been the object of the most intensive scientific inquiry are the herpes viruses, including EBV [24–26] and HHV-6 [7,27], the entero-viruses [28–33] particularly Coxsackie B, and a putative novel retrovirus [34].

HHV-6 was isolated in 1986 from patients with AIDS and malignant lymphoma. This was at the time when many patients who were presenting with CFS-like symptoms were found in the area near Lake Tahoe (USA), leading to the recognition of CFS as a disease. Since this newly discovered virus was detected in patients with the "fatigue epidemic," HHV-6 was considered to be the most probable candidate for the causative virus of CFS [18]. As EBV was frequently detected in patients presenting with CFS symptoms, an association of EBV with CFS was also strongly suspected. However, in many cases, CFS-like diseases associated with EBV were categorized as "chronic active EBV infection," and this was defined as a different disease from CFS of unknown etiology.

An initial infection with HHV-6 in early childhood, causing exanthem subitum, is followed a by life-long latent infection in peripheral blood. As the rate of infection of this virus is almost 100% in almost all countries, the antibody-positive rate in adults is also almost 100%. Whether or not a virus is associated with a particular disease is generally examined by checking whether a patient has been infected with the virus, based on the presence of serum antibody, and whether the patient's past history is correlated with the occurrence of the disease. However, this examination cannot be applied to HHV-6, since the HHV-6 incidence rate is 100% (Fig. 1B).

However, if HHV-6 infection follows a special pattern which is similar to that of CAEBV infection, it may possibly present CFS-like symptoms. To examine such a special-pattern latent infection, it is important to identify an HHV-6 gene specific to the latent EBV infection and its encoded protein, which appears specifically in the latent EBV infection and plays an important role in the diagnosis and research of latent infection, such as a gene corresponding to Epstein–Barr nuclear antigen (EBNA).

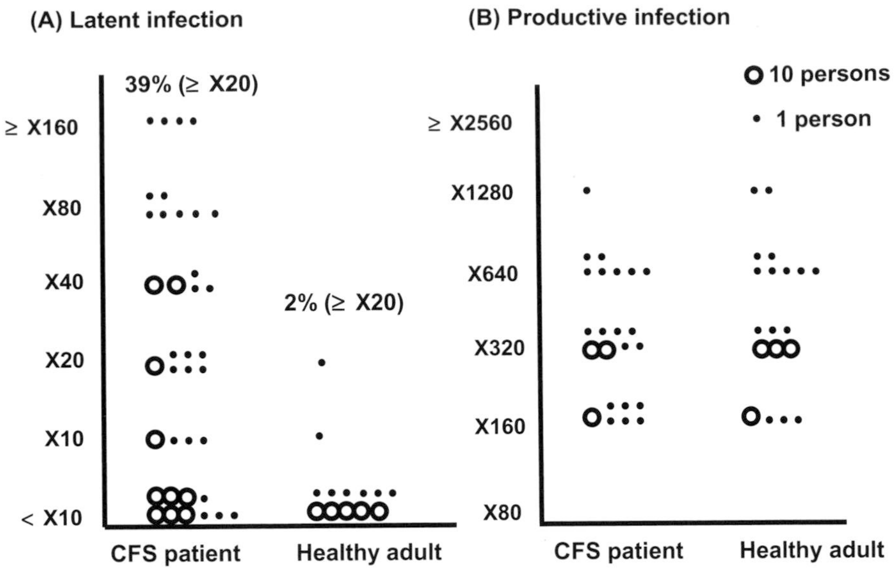

Fig. 1. Antibody titers to HHV-6 latent infection protein and structural protein. **A** Antibody against latent infection. **B** Antibody against productive infection. Antibody (**A**) to latency-associated proteins, which specifically appears in the latent HHV-6 infection, and the antibody titers (**B**) to virus structural protein, which mainly appear in the productive infection, were examined in CFS patients and healthy adults. The antibody to structural protein often used in regular examinations shows no significant difference between CFS patients and healthy adults, but that to latency-associated protein shows substantial differences

Latent Infection of HHV-6

HHV-6 belongs to the Roseolovirus genus of the β-herpesviruses subfamily that consists of human cytomegalovirus (HCMV), HHV-6, and HHV-7. HHV-6 species are divided into two variants: HHV-6A and HHV-6B. In almost all studies, HHV-6B has emerged as the predominant strain, and is found in both normal and immunocompromised hosts. In this section, HHV-6B is called HHV-6. HHV-6 is capable of establishing a life-long latent infection in its host, is reactivated frequently, and the reactivated virus is shed into the saliva [35,36].

As for the sites of latency, viral DNA is detected predominantly in the peripheral blood monocytes/macrophages of seropositive healthy adults [37]. Furthermore, primary cultured macrophages support HHV-6 latent infection, and viral reactivation is induced in them by treatment with 12-0-tetradecanoylphorbol-13-acetate (TPA) [37]. It has also been reported that HHV-6 establishes latency in myeloid cell lines [38], and that HHV-6 is detectable in CD34 (+) peripheral blood progenitor cells [39]. Therefore, HHV-6 might establish latency in hematopoietic progenitor cells.

Several lines of evidence suggest that latent HHV-6 infection in the brain may be involved in the pathology of some neurological diseases, such as recurrent febrile convulsion [40–42], multiple sclerosis (MS) [43,44], and encephalitis [45]. The site of HHV-6 latency in the brain is assumed to be glia cells.

Latency-Associated Transcripts of HHV-6

The investigation of latency-associated transcripts is important for understanding the molecular basis of herpesvirus persistence. Two types of HHV-6 latency-associated transcripts (H6LTs) have been identified in the gene locus of the immediate early (IE) 1/2 genes [46]. They are detected only in latently infected cells in vitro and in vivo. Although they are encoded in the same direction as the immediate early (IE) 1/2 genes and share their protein-coding region with IE1/2, their transcription start sites and exon(s) are different from those of the productive-phase transcripts [47,48] (Fig. 2). Type I H6LTs originate at the latent start site (LSS) 1, which is located 9.7 kilobases upstream of the IE1/2 start site, and Type II H6LTs originate at LSS2, which is located between exons 2 and 3 of IE1/2 (Fig. 2). In

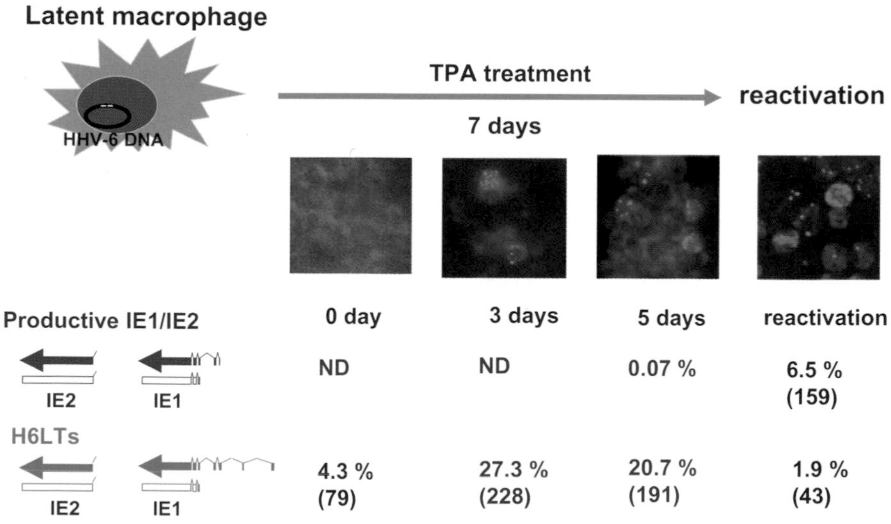

Fig. 2. mRNA and protein expression in latently infected macrophages. Latently infected macrophages were treated with 12-0-tetradecanoylphorbol-13-acetate (*TPA*) for 3, 5, and 7 days (reactivation). Cells were then stained with a monospecific antibody against IE1. Percentage of H6LT-expressing cells during viral latency and reactivation: the percentages of H6LT-positive cells during viral reactivation were estimated. The copy number of each type of transcript in one H6LT-positive cell is shown in parentheses. The percentage of cells that showed the productive IE1/IE2 is also shown

addition, novel short ORFs with latency-associated exons are encoded at the 5′ proximal region of the H6LTs (Fig. 2) [46].

The structures of the H6LTs are similar to those of HCMV latency-specific transcripts [49,50]; the latter encode IE1/IE2 ORFs, and short ORFs appear in the latency-specific exon. Furthermore, in the case of the HCMV latent transcripts, the translation of the IE1/IE2 protein is probably prevented by the existence of latency-specific ORFs upstream of the IE1/IE2 ORFs. Similarly, the HHV-6 IE1/IE2 protein is not detectable in latently infected macrophages. These findings suggest that viral replication of HCMV and HHV-6 may be suppressed at the point of the translation of major immediate early proteins during latency. The function of these upstream ORFs is discussed below.

Consistent with these findings, HHV-6 and HCMV exhibit similarities in their latent infections: (i) both viruses can establish latency in cells of the monocyte/macrophage lineage [37,51–53]; (ii) both viruses tend to persist in the latent state but are reactivated frequently, and the reactivated viruses are shed into the saliva [35,36]; (iii) HCMV as well as HHV-6 is a possible candidate for the causative agent of CFS [54].

Intermediate Phase of HHV-6 Latency

In order to identify the first molecular event of HHV-6 reactivation, the latent infection system of HHV-6 was used. In this system, macrophages are infected with HHV-6 and cultured for 4 weeks. At 4 weeks postinfection, no macrophage shows any signs of viral replication, such as viral protein expression or infectious virus production. Viral reactivation is induced by treatment with TPA (20 ng/ml) for 7 days [37].

At the early stage of the induction (3 and 5 days after the treatment with TPA), the proportion of cells that express the type I H6LTs significantly increases; however, transcription of productive-phase IE1/IE2 is not detected at days 0, 3, and 5 (Fig. 2). In this phase, IE1 protein is detectable in the cells without the production of infectious virus. Because productive-phase IE1 mRNAs are not detectable, the H6LTs, which contain the IE1 ORF (Fig. 3) are thought to be translated into IE1 protein at the first stage of viral reactivation. A similar molecular event has been observed in transplant patients: approximately two-thirds of reactivation-positive patients express the type I H6LTs 1–3 weeks before the onset of HHV-6 reactivation [55]. This intermediate phase of viral reactivation is different from the complete reactivation phase that is characterized by the expression of productive-phase IE1/IE2 transcripts [56,57], and this intermediate phase seems to be relatively stable [55].

Transfection of an IE1-expression vector into latent macrophages stimulates the viral reactivation. As described above, H6LTs have latency-associated small ORFs upstream of the IE1/IE2 ORFs (Fig. 3). For certain other mRNAs that have small upstream ORFs (uORFs) that restrict the translation of the downstream ORFs,

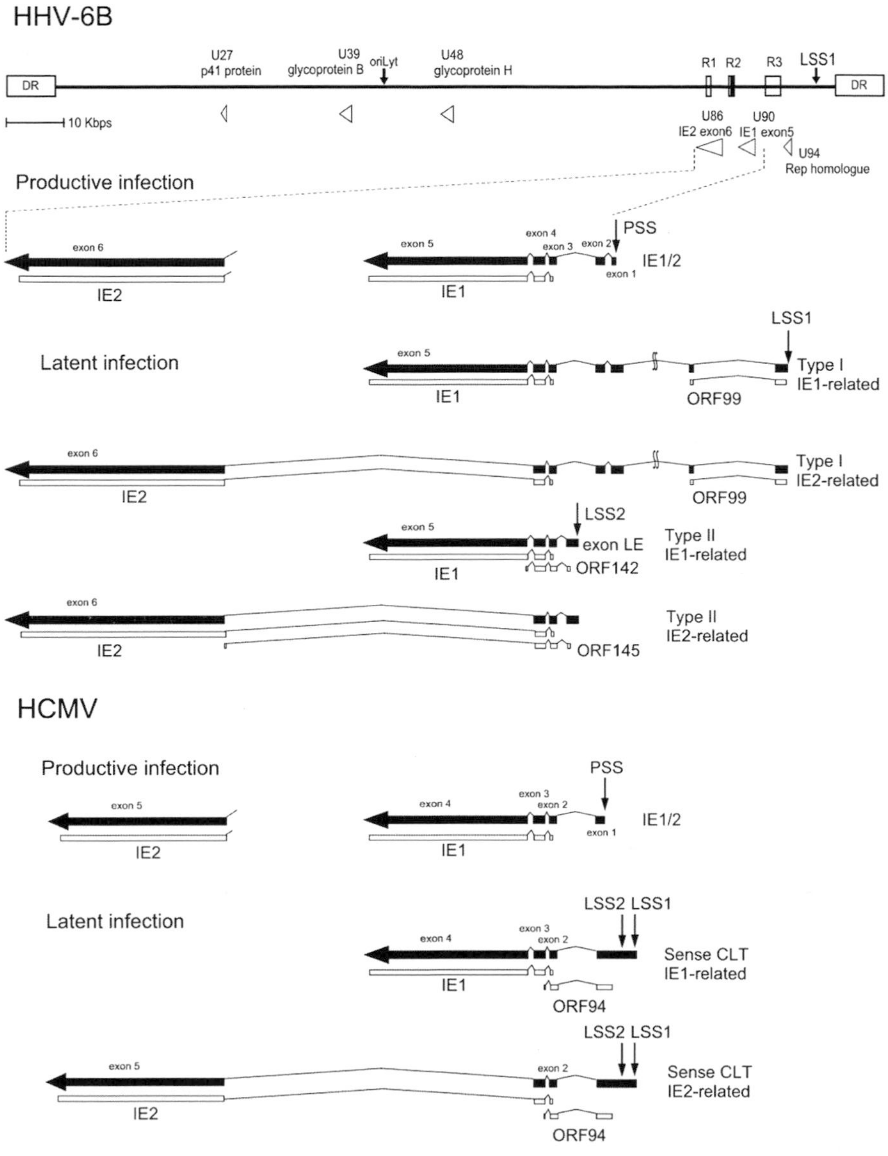

Fig. 3. Structures of the HHV-6 and human cytomegalovirus (*HCMV*) latency-associated transcripts. Schematic drawings of the H6LT structures are shown. Productive-phase transcripts are also shown. The drawings of the mRNAs are in the same orientation relative to the viral genome. *Thin lines* represent introns; *thick arrows* represent exons. All exons and introns are drawn to scale. Latency-associated exons starting from latent start site 1 (*LSS1*) and *LSS2* are depicted. The position of the productive start site (*PSS*) is also shown. In HHV-6, exon 1 of the type I latent transcript is 138-bp longer than that of IE1/2. Two additional exons of the type I latent transcripts are located approximately 7.8 kb and 9.7 kb upstream from the PSS. ORFs of IE1, IE2, and putative latency-associated proteins ORF99, ORF142, and ORF145 are depicted. In HCMV, exon 1 of the cytomegalovirus latency-associated transcript (*CLT*) is longer than that of IE1/2. Latency-associated exons starting from LSS1 and LSS2 are depicted. ORFs of IE1, IE2, and putative latency-associated proteins ORF94 are depicted

regulation at the translational and mRNA levels is important for release from the uORF control [58,59]. An alteration in the regulation of translation as well as the increase in H6LTs might contribute to the increased IE1 protein expression and viral reactivation [55].

Latent HHV-6 Infection and Chronic Fatigue Syndrome

HHV-6 establishes latent infection in macrophages and in the brain, and manifests latency-associated gene mRNA specific to latent infection. In order to understand the mechanism by which CFS is contracted, we attempted to identify a special latent HHV-6 infection state named "intermediate phase," as described above. In this phase, a few types of HHV-6 latency-associated protein corresponding to EBNAs might be expressed. This intermediate phase is observed in the first phase where HHV-6 commences reactivation, but is completely different from the reactivation because no virus is produced (Fig. 4).

In order to examine the relationship between latent infection protein, whose manifestation is promoted in the intermediate phase, and disease, CFS patients' serum antibody titers to the cells in which latent infection protein is well manifested were examined. This examination revealed that about 40% of the CFS patients showed antibody reaction to intermediate phase HHV-6 latent infection, as shown

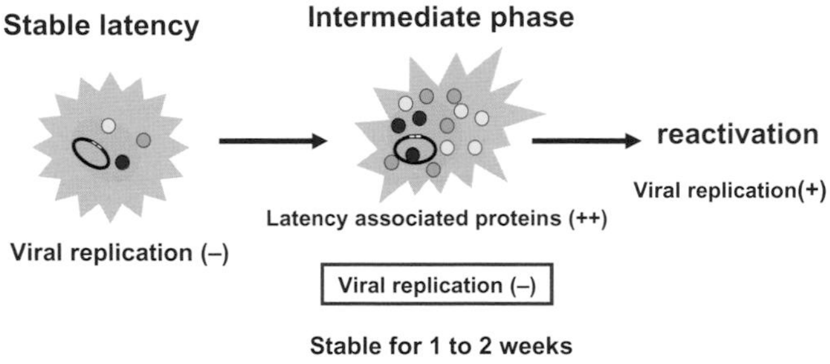

Fig. 4. Intermediate phase of HHV-6. HHV-6 shows the expression of mRNA from the gene s(latency-associated genes) which appear specifically in a stable latent infection phase. However, the mRNA does not produce protein, because its translation to protein is inhibited. However, the enhancement of transcription of latency-associated genes and the removal of the inhibition of the translation in the intermediate phase leads to an active manifestation of the latency-associated virus protein, but no virus production (reactivation). It is thought that this phase lasts from a few days to a few weeks, followed by virus production in those progressing to reactivation. It is estimated that the intermediate phase is important for the virus to prepare efficient reactivation, and to the reproduction and maintenance of virus genes. In view of the fact that CFS patients show abnormal immunoreaction to the latency-associated proteins, which appear in this phase, it is considered that the presence of a large number of cells in this intermediate phase for a long period of time is associated with the onset of CFS

in Fig. 4, whereas healthy subjects showed virtually no reaction (Fig. 1). It is possible that what is reacting with the infection is a virus protein which appears specifically in the latent HHV-6 infection, and has EBNA-like functions and diagnostic significance that is important in the diagnosis of latent infection and reactivation of EBV. We considered that such immunoreaction, which is clearly different between CFS patients and healthy subjects, is undoubtedly associated with CFS morbidities. On the other hand, what is examined usually by using serum antibody titers against HHV-6 is the antibody that appears when HHV-6 proliferates, particularly the antibody to structural protein required in virus formation. As shown in Fig. 1B, the antibody titers to the protein involved in the HHV-6 productive infection show no significant difference between CFS patients and healthy subjects. This explains why no difference in HHV-6 infection between CFS patients and healthy subjects is observed in a regular examination.

It is considered that the higher antibody titers to the protein that appears and increases in the intermediary phase in latent HHV-6 infection in CFS patients suggest the presence of cells in this intermediate phase in the body of CFS patients. The cells constituting latent HHV-6 infection and the intermediate phase are macrophage and glia cells. This is consistent with the fact that CFS presents immunological and psychiatric symptoms.

Conclusions

Since the demonstration that elevated antibody titers and other evidence of viral infection has been inconsistent, the abnormalities observed have typically been modest, and results have not been stratified by patient subgroups most likely to have viral involvement, the usefulness of viral serologies in CFS has yet to be fully resolved. It is considered that the issue of persistent and latent virus infection is critical for investigating the etiology of CFS. However, knowledge about persistent and latent infection with a pathogenic organism is indispensable for the investigation, and further progress in the investigation is required.

References

1. Pedersen TH, Nielsen OB, Lamb GD, Stephenson DG (2004) Intracellular acidosis enhances the excitability of working muscle. Science 305:1144–1147
2. Katafuchi T, Kondo T, Yasaka T, Kubo K, Take S, Yoshimura M (2003) Prolonged effects of polyriboinosinic:polyribocytidylic acid on spontaneous running wheel activity and brain interferon-alpha mRNA in rats: a model for immunologically induced fatigue. Neuroscience 120:837–845
3. Neri S, Pistone G, Saraceno B, Pennisi G, Luca S, Malaguarnera M (2003) L-carnitine decreases severity and type of fatigue induced by interferon-alpha in the treatment of patients with hepatitis C. Neuropsychobiology 35:94–97

4. Schwartz AL, Thompson JA, Masood N (2002) Interferon-induced fatigue in patients with melanoma: a pilot study of exercise and methylphenidate. Oncol Nurs Forum 26 Spec No. 2: E85–E90
5. Arai M, Yamazaki H, Inoue K, Fushiki T (2001) Effects of intracranial injection of transforming growth factor-beta relevant to central fatigue on the waking electroencephalogram of rats: comparison with effects of exercise. Prog Neuropsychopharmacol Biol Psychiatr 8:307–312
6. Tomoda A, Joudoi T, Rabab e-M, Matsumoto T, Park TH, Miike T (2005) Cytokine production and modulation: comparison of patients with chronic fatigue syndrome and normal controls. Psychiatr Res 288:101–104
7. Buchwald D, Cheney PR, Peterson DL, Henry B, Wormsley SB, Geiger A, Ablashi DV, Salahuddin SZ, Saxinger C, Biddle R, Kiknus, R, Jolesz FA, Folks T, Balachandran N, Peter JB, Gallo RC, Komaroff AL (1992) A chronic illness characterized by fatigue, neurologic and immunologic disorders, and active human herpesvirus type 6 infection. Ann Intern Med 116:103–113
8. Levine PH, Jacobson S, Pocinki AG, Cheney P, Peterson D, Connelly RR, Weil R, Robinson SM, Ablashi DV, Salahuddin SZ, Pearson GR, Hoover R (1992) Clinical, epidemiologic, and virologic studies in four clusters of the chronic fatigue syndrome. Arch Intern Med 152:1611–1616
9. Morin SF, Charles KA, Malyon AK (1984) The psychological impact of AIDS on gay men. Am Psychol 39:1288–1293
10. Ayres JG, Flint N, Smith EG, Tunnicliffe WS, Fletcher TJ, Hammond K, Ward D, Marmion BP (1998) Post-infection fatigue syndrome following Q fever. QJM 91:105–123
11. Hatchette TF, Hayes M, Merry H, Schlech WF, Marrie TJ (2003) The effect of *C. burnetii* infection on the quality of life of patients following an outbreak of Q fever. Epidemiol Infect 4:491–495
12. Horwitz CA, Henle W, Henle G, Schmitz H (1975) Clinical evaluation of patients with infectious mononucleosis and development of antibodies to the R component of the Epstein–Barr virus-induced early antigen complex. Am J Med 58:330–338
13. Buchwald D, Goldenberg DL, Sullivan JL, Komaroff AL (1987) The "chronic, active Epstein–Barr virus infection" syndrome and primary fibromyalgia. Arthritis Rheum 30:1132–1136
14. Hotchin NA, Read R, Smith DG, Crawford DH (1989) Active Epstein–Barr virus infection in post-viral fatigue syndrome. J Infect 18:143–150
15. Soto NE, Straus SE (2000) Chronic fatigue syndrome and herpesviruses: the fading evidence. Herpes 7:46–50
16. Swanink CM, van der Meer JW, Vercoulen JH, Bleijenberg G, Fennis JF, Galama JM (1994) Epstein–Barr virus (EBV) and the chronic fatigue syndrome: normal virus load in blood and normal immunologic reactivity in the EBV regression assay. Clin Infect Dis 19:1390–1392
17. Kimura H, Hoshino Y, Hara S, Sugaya N, Kawada J, Shibata Y, Kojima S, Nagasaka T, Kuzushima K, Morishima T (2005) Differences between T cell-type and natural killer cell-type chronic active Epstein–Barr virus infection. J Infect Dis 191:531–539
18. Barnes DM (1986) Mystery disease at Lake Tahoe challenges virologists and clinicians. Science 234:541–542
19. Eisen SA, Kang HK, Murphy FM, Blanchard MS, Reda DJ, Henderson WG, Toomey R, Jackson LW, Alpern R, Parks BJ, Klimas N, Hall C, Pak HS, Hunter J, Karlinsky J, Battistone MJ, Lyons MJ (2005) Gulf War veterans' health: medical evaluation of a US cohort. Ann Intern Med 142:881–890
20. Hotopf M, David AS, Hull L, Nikalaou V, Unwin C, Wessely S 2003.Gulf war illness: better, worse, or just the same? A cohort study. BMJ 183:1370
21. Roffey R, Lantorp K, Tegnell A, Elgh F (2002) Biological weapons and bioterrorism preparedness: importance of public-health awareness and international cooperation. Clin Microbiol Infect 8:522–528

22. Snell CR, Vanness JM, Strayer DR, Stevens SR (2002) Physical performance and prediction of 2-5A synthetase/RNase L antiviral pathway activity in patients with chronic fatigue syndrome. In Vivo 16:107–109
23. Morag A, Tobi M, Ravid Z, Revel M, Schattner A (1982) Increased (2′-5′)-oligo-A synthetase activity in patients with prolonged illness associated with serological evidence of persistent Epstein–Barr virus infection. Lancet 1:744
24. Straus SE, Tosato G, Armstrong G, Lawley T, Preble OT, Henle W, Davey R, Pearson G, Epstein J, Brus I, Blaese RM (1985) Persisting illness and fatigue in adults with evidence of Epstein–Barr virus infection. Ann Intern Med 102:7–16
25. Holmes GP, Kaplan JE, Gantz NM, Komaroff AL, Schonberger LB, Straus SE, Jones JF, Dubois RE, Cunningham-Rundles C, Pahwa S, Tosato G, Zegans LS, Purtilo DT, Browh N, Schooles RT, Brus I (1988) Chronic fatigue syndrome: a working case definition. Ann Intern Med 108:387–389
26. Jones JF, Ray CG, Minnich LL, Hicks MJ, Kibler R, Lucas DO (1985) Evidence for active Epstein–Barr virus infection in patients with persistent, unexplained illnesses: elevated anti-early antigen antibodies. Ann Intern Med 102:1–7
27. Josephs SF, Henry B, Balachandran N, Strayer D, Peterson D, Komaroff AL, Ablashi DV (1991) HHV-6 reactivation in chronic fatigue syndrome. Lancet 337:1346–1347
28. Archard LC, Bowles NE, Behan PO, Bell EJ, Doyle D (1988) Postviral fatigue syndrome: persistence of enterovirus RNA in muscle and elevated creatine kinase. J R Soc Med 81:326–329
29. Bell EJ, McCartney RA, Riding MH (1988) Coxsackie B viruses and myalgic encephalomyelitis. J R Soc Med 81:329–331
30. Calder BD, Warnock PJ, McCartney RA, Bell EJ (1987) Coxsackie B viruses and the post-viral syndrome: a prospective study in general practice. J R Coll Gen Pract 37:11–14
31. Cunningham L, Bowles NE, Lane RJ, Dubowitz V, Archard LC (1990) Persistence of enteroviral RNA in chronic fatigue syndrome is associated with the abnormal production of equal amounts of positive and negative strands of enteroviral RNA. J Gen Virol 71:1399–1402
32. Halpin D, Wessely S (1989) VP-1 antigen in chronic postviral fatigue syndrome. Lancet 1:1028–1029
33. Yousef GE, Bell EJ, Mann GF, Murugesan V, Smith DG, McCartney RA, Mowbray JF (1988) Chronic enterovirus infection in patients with postviral fatigue syndrome. Lancet 1:146–150
34. Khan AS, Heneine WM, Chapman LE, Gary Jr HE, Woods TC, Folks TM, Schonberger LB (1993) Assessment of a retrovirus sequence and other possible risk factors for the chronic fatigue syndrome in adults. Ann Intern Med 118:241–245
35. Jordan MC (1983) Latent infection and the elusive cytomegalovirus. Rev Infect Dis 5:205–215
36. Krueger GR, Wassermann K, De Clerck LS, Stevens WJ, Bourgeois N, Ablashi DV, Josephs SF, Balachandran N (1990) Latent herpesvirus-6 in salivary and bronchial glands [letter; comment]. Lancet 336:1255–1256
37. Kondo K, Kondo T, Okuno T, Takahashi M, Yamanishi K (1991) Latent human herpesvirus 6 infection of human monocytes/macrophages. J Gen Virol 72:1401–1408
38. Yasukawa M, Ohminami H, Sada E, Yakushijin Y, Kaneko M, Yanagisawa K, Kohno H, Bando S, Fujita S (1999) Latent infection and reactivation of human herpesvirus 6 in two novel myeloid cell lines. Blood 93:991–999
39. Luppi M, Barozzi P, Morris C, Maiorana A, Garber R, Bonacorsi G, Donelli A, Marasca R, Tabilio A, Torelli G (1999) Human herpesvirus 6 latently infects early bone marrow progenitors in vivo. J Virol 73:754–759
40. Hall CB, Long CE, Schnabel KC, Caserta MT, McIntyre KM, Costanzo MA, Knott A, Dewhurst S, Insel RA, Epstein LG (1994) Human herpesvirus-6 infection in children. A prospective study of complications and reactivation. N Engl J Med 331:432–438
41. Kimberlin DW, Whitley RJ (1998) Human herpesvirus-6: neurologic implications of a newly described viral pathogen. J Neurovirol 4:474–485

42. Kondo K, Nagafuji H, Hata A, Tomomori C, Yamanishi K (1993) Association of human herpesvirus 6 infection of the central nervous system with recurrence of febrile convulsions. J Infect Dis 167:1197–1200
43. Challoner PB, Smith KT, Parker JD, MacLeod DL, Coulter SN, Rose TM, Schultz ER, Bennett JL, Garber RL, Chang M, Schad PA, Stewart PM, Nowinski RC, Brown JP, Burmer GC (1995) Plaque-associated expression of human herpesvirus 6 in multiple sclerosis. Proc Natl Acad Sci USA 92:7440–7444
44. Sola P, Merelli E, Marasca R, Poggi M, Luppi M, Montorsi M, Torelli G (1993) Human herpesvirus 6 and multiple sclerosis: survey of anti-HHV-6 antibodies by immunofluorescence analysis and of viral sequences by polymerase chain reaction. J Neurol Neurosurg Psychiatry 56:917–919
45. Caserta MT, Hall CB, Schnabel K, McIntyre K, Long C, Costanzo M, Dewhurst S, Insel R, Epstein LG (1994) Neuroinvasion and persistence of human herpesvirus 6 in children. J Infect Dis 170:1586–1589
46. Kondo K, Shimada K, Sashihara J, Tanaka-Taya K, Yamanishi K (2002) Identification of human herpesvirus 6 latency-associated transcripts. J Virol 76:4145–4151
47. Mirandola P, Menegazzi P, Merighi S, Ravaioli T, Cassai E, Di Luca D (1998) Temporal mapping of transcripts in herpesvirus 6 variants. J Virol 72:3837–3844
48. Schiewe U, Neipel F, Schreiner D, Fleckenstein B (1994) Structure and transcription of an immediate-early region in the human herpesvirus 6 genome. J Virol 68:2978–2985
49. Kondo K, Mocarski ES (1995) Cytomegalovirus latency and latency-specific transcription in hematopoietic progenitors. Scand J Infect Dis Suppl 99:63–67
50. Kondo K, Xu J, Mocarski ES (1996) Human cytomegalovirus latent gene expression in granulocyte–macrophage progenitors in culture and in seropositive individuals. Proc Natl Acad Sci USA 93:11137–11142
51. Kempf W, Adams V, Wey N, Moos R, Schmid M, Avitabile E, Campadelli-Fiume G (1997) CD68+ cells of monocyte/macrophage lineage in the environment of AIDS-associated and classic-sporadic Kaposi sarcoma are singly or doubly infected with human herpesviruses 7 and 6B. Proc Natl Acad Sci USA 94:7600–7605
52. Kondo K, Kaneshima H, Mocarski ES (1994) Human cytomegalovirus latent infection of granulocyte-macrophage progenitors. Proc Natl Acad Sci USA 91:11879–11883
53. Taylor-Wiedeman J, Sissons JG, Borysiewicz LK, Sinclair JH (1991) Monocytes are a major site of persistence of human cytomegalovirus in peripheral blood mononuclear cells. J Gen Virol 72:2059–2064
54. Lerner AM, Dworkin HJ, Sayyed T, Chang CH, Fitzgerald JT, Beqaj S, Deeter RG, Goldstein J, Gottipolu P, O'Neill W (2004) Prevalence of abnormal cardiac wall motion in the cardiomyopathy associated with incomplete multiplication of Epstein–Barr virus and/or cytomegalovirus in patients with chronic fatigue syndrome. In Vivo 18:417–424
55. Kondo K, Sashihara J, Shimada K, Takemoto M, Amo K, Miyagawa H, Yamanishi K (2003) Recognition of a novel stage of beta-herpesvirus latency in human herpesvirus 6. J Virol 77:2258–2264
56. Hummel M, Zhang Z, Yan S, DePlaen I, Golia P, Varghese T, Thomas G, Abecassis MI (2001) Allogeneic transplantation induces expression of cytomegalovirus immediate-early genes in vivo: a model for reactivation from latency. J Virol 75:4814–4822
57. Soderberg-Naucler C, Streblow DN, Fish KN, Allan-Yorke J, Smith PP, Nelson JA (2001) Reactivation of latent human cytomegalovirus in CD14(+) monocytes is differentiation-dependent. J Virol 75:7543–7554
58. Hoffmann B, Valerius O, Andermann M, Braus GH (2001) Transcriptional autoregulation and inhibition of mRNA translation of amino acid regulator gene cpcA of filamentous fungus *Aspergillus nidulans*. Mol Biol Cell 12:2846–2857
59. Nomura A, Iwasaki Y, Saito M, Aoki Y, Yamamori E, Ozaki N, Tachikawa K, Mutsuga N, Morishita M, Yoshida M, Asai M, Oiso Y, Saito H (2001) Involvement of upstream open reading frames in regulation of rat V(1b) vasopressin receptor expression. Am J Physiol Endocrinol Metab 280:E780–E787

Chronic Fatigue Syndrome in Childhood and Adolescence

Teruhisa Miike[1] **and David S. Bell**[2]

Summary

Chronic fatigue syndrome (CFS) in children and adolescents is a complex clinical condition with severe morbidity. It is common, with up to 8% of children and adolescents experiencing fatigue for more than 1 month, and nearly 2% having a CFS-like illness. The hallmark of the condition is activity limitation due to fatigue/exhaustion, and a pattern of somatic symptoms, including headache, sore throat, lymph node tenderness, cognitive difficulties, abdominal pain, and muscle and joint pain. While this pattern may be similar to adult CFS, the expression of these symptoms may differ because of developmental factors and identity formation. A physical examination typically demonstrates minor abnormalities only despite the sometimes marked activity limitation. Routine laboratory studies are similar to those carried out for adult CFS. New research demonstrating abnormalities with cerebral blood flow and tilt-table testing link pediatric CFS with pediatric orthostatic intolerance.

Treatment begins with extensive support in nutrition, education, and social and psychosocial domains, along with symptom reduction, particularly in the areas of pain and sleep. Overall the prognosis is favorable for the majority of children and adolescents with CFS, but complete recovery is rare. It is probable that 20% of pediatric CFS cases evolve into a chronic, lifelong disability.

Research areas include the relation of infection to the development of the syndrome, the differences in symptom patterns in younger children, immunological abnormalities, and blood flow abnormalities, particularly cerebral blood flow. Increased medical-provider education is essential for early recognition and treatment of the condition.

[1]Faculty of Medical and Pharmaceutical Sciences, Kumamoto University Graduate School, 1-1-1 Honjyo, Kumamoto 860-8556, Japan

[2]State University of New York at Buffalo, 77 South Main Street, Lyndonville, New York 14098, USA

Introduction

Chronic fatigue syndrome (CFS) in children and adolescents is a complex illness characterized by fatigue and/or exhaustion that significantly limit daily activities, along with numerous somatic symptoms. It has been described in clusters or "outbreaks" as well as in isolated cases. Recent research has made considerable progress in understanding the pathophysiology, and this progress is described throughout this text. While the majority of studies on CFS have been in adults, pediatric reviews have also been published [1–8].

As with chronic fatigue syndrome in adults, CFS in children has been embroiled in controversy. Arguments have ranged over the possibilities that CFS is an organic illness, a psychiatric illness, an "illness behavior," or even a factitious illness. The simple paradox which generates this controversy is that the child or adolescent with CFS looks well, and a physical examination and routine laboratory findings are relatively normal. Medical providers, who are used to severe fatigue in patients with a terminal illness, may not believe that a patient who looks well could have such a severe debility. This difficulty is particularly pronounced in pediatrics, as children and adolescents may not be able to express the complex pattern of symptoms, and lack an activity reference point to describe changes.

The symptom pattern of pediatric CFS is broad and overlaps with other conditions. The reduction in levels of activity, such as the inability to go to school, is attributed primarily to severe fatigue. The accompanying somatic symptoms may also limit activity, and fatigue is not always the most severe symptom. While it is invariably present, it was the most severe symptom in only 49 of 100 adolescents with chronic fatigue for which alternative explanations could not be found (D.S.B., unpublished observation).

CFS is also closely related to conditions such as fibromyalgia, chemical sensitivities, and orthostatic intolerance. It is possible that these conditions represent the same underlying pathophysiology, but they are described differently because of reporter bias or interest. Conversely, it is also possible that they may represent separate illnesses. However, it is unlikely that this debate will be decided until appropriate markers and/or diagnostic criteria for children are established.

An example of this is primary juvenile fibromyalgia syndrome (PJFS). In practice, an adolescent evaluated because of activity-limiting fatigue and widespread musculoskeletal symptoms would receive a diagnosis of CFS if the activity-limiting fatigue was the most severe symptom. On the other hand, if the musculoskeletal pain was the most severe symptom, a diagnosis of PJFS would probably be made. PJFS is a common illness, with up to 6% of school children having tender points on examination [9], but both CFS and PVFS show a common pattern of presenting symptoms [10]. In one study of adolescents with CFS, 75% met criteria for PJFS [11].

Of critical concern for future studies of CFS and related illnesses is the development of specific pediatric diagnostic criteria. Adult criteria are most commonly used in pediatric settings [12–15], but these criteria may not be appropriate for children and adolescents. A case definition was proposed in the Netherlands, which was designed to help define CFS in the pediatric population [16]. In all CFS case definitions, no alternative condition can explain the activity limitation and/or symptom pattern. However, variations exist in the different adult criteria as to the length and severity of the activity limitation, the severity of the symptoms, the relative importance of different aspects of the symptom pattern, and whether the symptoms began suddenly or insidiously.

A case definition which is specifically for children and adolescents is essential in order to further research into these conditions. A lack of ability to diagnose young people with CFS or other forms of unexplained fatigue has caused medical practitioners to doubt the presence or importance of the symptoms. An inability to make a diagnosis may suggest to the pediatric patient and their family that the symptoms are trivial, unimportant, or even imaginary. This social attitude, which is prevalent at the current time, erodes the self-confidence and health identity of the pediatric patient at a critical time of identity formation.

In clinical pediatric practice, we have evaluated adolescents with the referral diagnosis of chronic fatigue syndrome, primary juvenile fibromyalgia syndrome, chronic Lyme disease, postural tachycardia syndrome, delayed orthostatic hypotension, somatization disorder, and Munchausen's syndrome by proxy, all of whom appear to have the same illness. A laboratory evaluation was not helpful in establishing diagnostic lines, and in these adolescents, the referral diagnosis seemed almost arbitrary. No diagnostic opinion expressed by even an experienced clinician will be acceptable as long as there are no agreed pediatric diagnostic criteria.

Historical Review

Modern descriptions of chronic fatigue syndrome-like illnesses have extended back over the past century. Because of the complexity of the symptom pattern, widespread recognition did not occur until somewhat later, when similarities with poliomyelitis led to the term "atypical poliomyelitis" [17]. Among the symptoms which accompanied fatigue were headache, cognitive difficulties, muscle weakness, autonomic symptoms, and paresthesiae. However, the muscle weakness did not evolve into paralysis, and with the more widespread use of virological testing, poliovirus types one through three were not found in those affected.

From the 1950s until the mid-1980s, medical providers commonly called the illness "chronic mononucleosis" because of the clinical similarities with Epstein–Barr virus infection. This term was clinically appropriate, as CFS often followed mononucleosis or appeared to be a "glandular fever" which did not resolve appropriately. As mononucleosis was, and still is, a common occurrence in the pediatric population, extension into a chronic phase was a reasonable explanation. In addition, it served the practical purpose of explaining an apparent viral illness which could persist for years.

In the 1950s, however, the concept of mass hysteria was proposed, and with the inability to isolate Epstein–Barr virus in the form of chronic-active infection, the concepts of somatization, variant depression, hysteria, and malingering became the prominent view. Even in the 21st century there are medical providers and educators who doubt the validity of CFS as a specific illness. The difficulty has been more acute for adolescents than for adults because of developmental issues and the often-smoldering clinical course. The history of CFS has been reviewed [18].

Nearly fifty outbreaks or epidemics of CFS-like illnesses have been described over the past fifty years [19]. Because of symptom complexity and reporter bias, it has not been clear whether these illnesses were the same as that which is currently defined as CFS. However, these outbreaks have prominently involved children and adolescents, and have had similar symptom patterns and prevalence rates as the descriptions of current isolated cases of CFS. In community-wide epidemics, it was rare to note the illness in children under the age of five [20], but the attack rates for adolescents were often the highest of any 10-year age group.

A CFS-like outbreak of illness on the north coast of Iceland in 1950 involved more than 1200 people, 194 of whom were children. These patients developed severe fatigue, widespread musculoskeletal pain, and other symptoms which were similar to CFS [17]. Because of the concern about poliomyelitis that was prevalent at that time, an emphasis was placed on the evaluation of neurological symptoms, and autonomic symptoms were noted to be prominent.

In 1985, a community-wide outbreak occurred in Lyndonville, New York, affecting 137 adults (67%) and 65 children (33%) under the age of 18 [21]. The illness was assumed to have an infectious onset, although the specific organism was never ascertained. Studies done at the time implied that Epstein–Barr virus was not responsible [22]. As this study was done prior to the publication of the current diagnostic criteria, specific criteria were employed [23]. In following these children clinically for the past 20 years, it is possible to say that the illness they experienced was clinically indistinguishable from what would be considered sporadic CFS (D.S.B., personal observation).

There have been many lessons to be learned from the historical view of CFS. Because it may occur in clusters or outbreaks, either an infectious agent or a shared environmental factor is likely to be involved. Because of our inability to discover a simple infectious agent causing CFS, the role of an infectious agent has been questioned. However, with the emergence of the concept of CFS being a post-infectious phenomenon [24], it would be appropriate to re-examine previous clusters.

Incidence/Prevalence

The epidemiology of CFS in childhood and adolescence has been hampered by the lack of diagnostic criteria which are specific for children. Which symptoms to assess, how to measure fatigue severity, and the length of time the fatigue persists are all critical factors for epidemiological study. Prevalence estimates of simple chronic fatigue in the pediatric population range from 0.2% to 8% [25,26].

In a 1990 Australian study, an overall prevalence of 37 cases of CFS per 100 000 children was estimated, with the highest incidence being in the fourth decade. The prevalence in children under the age of 10 was 5.5 per 100 000, and the incidence in years 10–19 was 47.9 per 100 000 [27]. A surveillance study from the Centers for Disease Control found a chronic fatigue prevalence of 8.7 per 100 000 for children between the ages of 12 and 17, and a prevalence of CFS-like illness of 2.7 per 100 000. However, this study required physician participation, and thus may have been seriously flawed [28]. A UK study estimated the prevalence of adolescent CFS-like illness at 70 per 100 000 [29], and a rural New York state study estimated 23 per 100 000 [21]. A more recent CDC telephone survey in San Francisco suggested that for children aged 2 through 11, 71.9 per 100 000 experienced chronic fatigue and none had CFS-like illnesses. However, for older adolescents, 465.7 per 10 000 had chronic fatigue and 116.4 per 100 000 had a CFS-like illness [30]. In a recent UK study, the prevalence of fatigue lasting more than 3 months was 2.34% and the presence of a CFS-like illness was 1.29% [31].

Perhaps the most comprehensive fatigue prevalence study was a telephone survey of 28 673 American households. Adult household members were asked about fatigue and other symptoms present in the children of the households. In children aged from 5 to 17, 4.4% were reported to experience persistent fatigue, and 2.05% experienced a CFS-like illness, i.e., fatigue and somatic symptoms suggestive of CFS. Further analysis showed that 2.91% (2910 per 100 000) of adolescents had a CFS-like illness, and 1.96% (1960 per 100 000) of children under the age of 13. These figures are considerably higher than others which have been reported, particularly in regards to younger children with chronic fatigue. The sex distribution for the entire pediatric group was 47.5% male and 52.5% female [25].

There are numerous possible explanations for the wide variation in prevalence figures for CFS in the pediatric population. Most pediatricians who are familiar with CFS would agree that the illness is less common in children under the age of ten. However, chronic fatigue, as defined by parental reports of decreased activity, is much more frequent, and it is in these children that the entire symptom complex of CFS may not become manifest until adolescence, frequently following a flu-like or mononucleosis-like infection (T.M., D.S.B., personal observations). These children would be assumed to have had an adolescent onset, when in fact they would have had a gradual onset beginning in childhood. While this hypothesis has never been studied, if it is correct it would help explain the wide disparity in prevalence figures.

Moreover, there are many children seen in clinical practice who have what appears to be lifelong fatigue, because caregivers report excessive sleepiness and rest requirements extending back to young childhood. These children do not complain of fatigue, perhaps because they are so used to experiencing the symptom. Currently, children who cannot date the onset of their chronic fatigue are specifically excluded from a diagnosis of CFS.

In summary, both chronic fatigue and chronic fatigue-like illnesses are common in pediatric practice. Children and adolescents meeting the adult CFS criteria appear to be about half as common as those with unexplained chronic fatigue, and the incidence and prevalence of both increases at puberty. This observation suggests that pubertal hormones may play a role in the genesis of symptoms.

Clinical Presentation

The clinical presentation of CFS has been extensively described [12,13,32,33; and other chapters in this volume], but clinical reviews are rare in the pediatric literature [1,2,4,6,8,34]. Because of the lack of pediatric criteria, even two experienced pediatricians may disagree over the diagnosis in a child or adolescent with chronic fatigue.

Onset

The onset of CFS is usually acute, such as an abrupt onset following an upper respiratory or gastrointestinal infection. Clinicians who evaluate children and adolescents at the time of this acute onset are not usually overly concerned about this initiating infection, suggesting that it does not differ markedly from "normal" day-to-day illnesses in pediatric practice. In our experience, children with CFS began their illness with an upper respiratory infection that was experienced by other family members, an infection that resolved normally in the family members but not in the CFS patient. The initiating infection could be marked by an unusual severity of exhaustion (D.S.B., T.M., personal observations). The role of pre-illness stresses such as chronic sleep deprivation may increase the child's vulnerability (T.M., personal observation).

Acute onset is estimated to occur in three-quarters of pediatric CFS cases, but ranges from 58% to 100% [2,4,35–37]. However, the assessment of acute or gradual onset is subject to many potential errors. Many young persons will have a gradual onset of symptoms, including fatigue noted by parents, but "remember" the onset as following a flu-like illness. Secondly, children, unlike adults, are not aware of baseline activity levels and may not articulate perceived changes in energy status. Furthermore, children may be more adaptable to these changes in functional status. Lastly, the reporting of an acute onset may be biased by the social stigma associated with tiredness and fatigue. There is a wide range of estimates of sex distribution, but it appears to be nearly equal in children before puberty, and is more common in adolescents [1,2,6,7,33,38].

Symptoms

The symptoms of pediatric CFS in children fall into two broad categories: activity limitation (fatigue and post-exertional malaise) and somatic symptoms (headache, sore throat, lymph node pain, muscle pain, joint pain, sleep disturbance, cognitive difficulties, and abdominal pain).

The first category, activity limitation, is the more difficult to describe, but is responsible for most of the morbidity of the illness [2,33]. It is nearly impossible for the younger child to describe or articulate the symptom of fatigue. Instead they say that they feel "sick" and are noticed to reduce their activity. Adolescents are more likely to describe the activity limitation in the same manner as adults. They use the words "fatigue," "exhaustion," and "weakness," not referring to specific muscle weakness but to an overwhelming sensation. Observations from family members indicate reduced activities, including enjoyable activities, social events, and school. Frequent yawning and a nearly constant desire to rest or lie down are noted by family members.

However, closer questioning of the adolescent about the nature of their tiredness may point out differences between the fatigue of CFS and "normal" fatigue. This is particularly true of articulate adolescents who have been athletes. The fatigue or activity limitation of CFS is often combined with a flu-like malaise or dysphoria, in contrast to the more positive sensation experienced with fatigue following strenuous exercise. In addition, a post-exertional malaise is described, where the young person feels particularly sick for days following a previously tolerated exertion. This post-exertional malaise may be the most important marker of the illness, but unfortunately, the language is not sufficiently subtle to express this symptom correctly.

Direct inquiry involves asking an adolescent about their favorite activities, such as walking in an amusement park or being with friends in the mall. If they say it would make them "sick," we would inquire how long they would feel ill following an 8-hour day of activity. Mild CFS would cause a single day of feeling ill, while more severe CFS would cause the adolescent to be in bed for a week or more. The longer the post-exertional malaise persists following a previously tolerated activity, the more severe the illness and the worse the prognosis (T.M., D.S.B., personal observations).

The somatic symptoms of CFS in children are, in general, similar to the pattern in adults. Headache, recurrent sore throat, lymph node tenderness, and muscle and joint pain are very similar to the symptoms described in adults. In one report [2], the three most common complaints, besides fatigue, were headache, sleep disturbance, and cognitive difficulties. However, there may be differences in the symptom pattern, with more prominent abdominal pain, pallor, and flushing [21,39]. Pediatric patients with fatigue may display more irritability, and in younger patients may cause confusion with behavior disorders [40].

Disturbed learning, memorizing, and maintenance of attention may be primary manifestations of CFS in children [41], and is more difficult to elucidate in their history because of confusion with attention deficit disorder. In one recent study of event-related potentials, children and adolescents with CFS could be separated into three distinct patterns suggesting abnormal cognitive function (T.M., submitted for publication). Single photon emission computed tomography (SPECT) and magnetic resonance studies (MRS) have shown lower cerebral blood flow and elevated choline concentrations, again implying abnormal cognitive functions [42,43].

In adults with an established fund of knowledge and learning style, the symptoms of cognitive difficulty can be elicited because of the abrupt changes experienced. Adults complain of difficulties with short-term memory, maintaining attention, double-tasking, and word-finding (see review in this volume). There are now several adult studies showing abnormal verbal memory processing in fMRI studies [44,45]. In children, however, clinical symptoms are more difficult to elicit due to changing learning patterns and a changing fund of knowledge.

A proportion of children with an acute onset of chronic fatigue in adolescence have a history suggestive of attention deficit disorder in early childhood. Because many of the same problems exist in defining attention deficit as in defining chronic fatigue, this subject has not been definitively studied.

Another striking feature of chronic fatigue syndrome in children and adolescents is the individuality of symptom patterns and the fluctuations in symptom severity. These variations in severity are difficult for the young person because they may consider themselves to be improving and make plans for activities only to find themselves unsuccessful in accomplishing them. The pattern of feeling well enough to go to school one day followed by feeling very ill (post-exertional malaise) is stressful for both patient and family. Friends, family, and classmates may see them on "good days," and thus become confused or skeptical about the seriousness and debilitating effects of the illness.

The skepticism of medical and educational providers may lead to social service referrals because of excessive school absence without a medical diagnosis. Munchausen's-by-proxy syndrome has been inappropriately diagnosed with an assumption that the child's symptoms reflect the parents' unconscious desire that the child should stay at home (T.M., D.S.B., personal observations). It should be noted, however, that the diagnosis of Munchausen's-by-proxy cannot be made without proof of the proxy's intent to harm the child. The diagnosis should not be made if the parent is "over-protective." However, all too often the parent appears to be excessively over-protective because they see an illness in their child when the medical providers do not. It is an irony that they are accused of child neglect by not sending their child to school when they may, in fact, be being excessively harsh if they do.

Physical Examination

Children and adolescents experiencing activity-limiting fatigue should be given a thorough physical examination with attention to small details. Any abnormality that could imply an alternative diagnosis should be followed with appropriate laboratory evaluations. In pediatric CFS, with its significant morbidity, cursory physical examinations are not only medically inappropriate, but they undermine the pediatric patient's confidence that their symptoms will be taken seriously.

Because of the lack of pediatric diagnostic criteria, formal studies on physical examination findings are rare. The most important finding on examination is the appearance of good health. Children and adolescents with debilitating CFS look well, and can even look "robust" if they have facial flushing causing "rosy cheeks." This healthy appearance is important, as it represents the principal paradox of the illness; it should not generate the assumption that the symptoms are fabricated. In a pediatric patient who appears to be chronically ill, the examination should be directed at finding signs of organ failure that would suggest an alternative diagnosis.

Minor abnormalities that may be found on examination include red throat, photophobia on fundoscopic examination, lymph node tenderness (but not enlargement), muscle tenderness in the fibromyalgia distribution, flushing and/or pallor, tachycardia at rest, dermatographism, and occasional hyper-reflexia. In more severe cases, calf muscle atrophy and a change in muscle contour verify the marked activity limitation and correspond to the length of time the activity limitation has been present. Joint laxity may be present, and this has suggested abnormal connective tissue as a predisposing condition [46–48].

Careful attention should be paid to an assessment of the patient's psychosocial state as well as to the assessment of family dynamics [4]. In the older patient a full expression of emotions is usual, but this may not occur until a bond of trust has been established with the medical provider. Adolescent autonomy should be explored, with attention to the relationship between autonomy and activity limitation. In families struggling with CFS for a prolonged period of time, and particularly with skeptical physicians, parents may get into the habit of relating the history in order to include details and to emphasize severity. This should not automatically be interpreted as enmeshment causing symptom magnification. A separate session so that the pediatric patient can relate their symptoms and how they are coping with these symptoms is helpful. Pediatricians are, in general, well suited to family assessment and can usually distinguish between appropriate, normal parental concern and the artificial concern that could encourage activity limitation. This family assessment is no different from that which is done on each visit for a pediatric patient with any chronic condition.

Another area of the physical examination that should be assessed is the response to simple standing, or orthostatic stress. While research studies use the tilt-table to conduct formal tests, the following simple test may have value. The subject lies recumbent for 15 min while their blood pressure is measured and their pulse recorded, along with a symptom assessment. Then the subject stands at the bedside without moving and continuous or frequent pulse and blood pressure readings are taken. During this "simple standing," symptom progression can be noted, along with observations of pallor or dependent cyanosis [49]. Of particular value has been the observation of how the patient copes with increasing orthostatic stress. Many pediatric CFS patients will be remarkably stoic as the symptoms progress to pre-syncope and even syncope, presumably because they are quite accustomed to these symptoms. This information can be correlated to the activity limitation, and is useful in activity planning and educational management.

Roughly one-third of normal adolescents have light-headedness or dizziness on simple standing [50]. Children with CFS may have measurable neurally mediated hypotension (NMH) [51], postural orthostatic tachycardia (POTS) [52], delayed hypotension [52], or immediate hypotension [53]. The combination of increasing pulse and narrowing of the pulse pressure as the symptoms progress has been frequent (D.S.B., personal observation).

Laboratory Evaluation

Routine laboratory evaluations are generally normal, and are of value to exclude alternative causes of fatigue. Glucose pathways may be abnormal [54], antinuclear antibodies may be elevated [55] and serum pyruvate levels may also be elevated (T.M., unpublished observations).

Research evaluations, described in other chapters in this volume, have not been systematically applied in pediatric CFS, except in the area of orthostatic intolerance, which will be described in the next section.

Orthostatic Intolerance

One of the many advances in understanding CFS in recent years has been the increasing awareness of the relationship between CFS and orthostatic intolerance. The term "orthostatic intolerance" refers to the inability to tolerate orthostasis, the upright position. The term may signify a general symptom, or a specific type of intolerance such as NMH. Much of the new literature on this subject relates to the pediatric population, and it may be that orthostatic intolerance plays a greater role in pediatric CFS than in the adult condition. On careful questioning of a patient with pediatric CFS, a discrepancy between the term fatigue and orthostatic intolerance becomes apparent. Some young persons will define the disabling symptom of CFS as "having to lie down."

Orthostatic intolerance is assumed to be related to reduced blood flow to the brain, and a recent adult study has addressed this directly [56]. In milder forms of pediatric CFS, participation in sports will actually make the subject feel better, possibly because of improved circulation secondary to muscle contraction. Other details characteristic of the concept of orthostatic intolerance are the drug sensitivities to vasodilating medications, sensitivity to heat, and increased exhaustion following a hot shower. Patients with CFS read lying down, while healthy persons usually read sitting up, so the cognitive dysfunction of the illness may have an orthostatic component (D.S.B., personal observation).

Knowledge of the relationship between CFS and orthostatic intolerance dates to 1994, when investigators studying NMH noted an association with CFS. They also noted that treatment with plasma expanders improved the symptoms [51,57]. More recent studies have looked at the role of the autonomic nervous system in general, as well as specific studies on heart rate variability [52,58]. An overlap exists between pediatric CFS and POTS [59], as well as immediate orthostatic hypotension [53] and delayed orthostatic hypotension. In reviews of adolescent POTS, the pattern of disabling fatigue is described in terms similar to descriptions of CFS [60].

The common end factor in these studies is hypoperfusion of the brain in the upright position. Pediatric syncope and presyncope is associated with reduced cerebral blood flow velocity, presumably due to increases in cerebral vascular resistance. The sustained reduction in cerebral blood flow velocity can occur in the absence of hypotension [61]. The increased cerebral resistance combined with reduced circulating blood volume [62] may account for the increase in orthostatic symptoms. Regional cerebral blood flow has been evaluated in children with CFS by SPECT [42] combined with magnetic resonance spectroscopy, and has demonstrated reduced cerebral blood flow [1,43]. One intriguing developmental detail is that adolescents have orthostatic symptoms far more frequently than younger children [50], which correlates to data on the age of onset of CFS.

Differential Diagnosis

Many fatigue-causing illnesses are readily apparent on physical examination combined with basic laboratory screening. Examples of this would include anemia, hypothyroidism, and subclinical hepatitis. Disease entities that should be considered in the differential diagnosis of a child or adolescent with debilitating fatigue would include malignancies, HIV infection, lupus erythematosis, rheumatoid arthritis, inflammatory bowel disease, drug abuse, and pregnancy, and appropriate laboratory testing can confirm these diagnoses. Other illnesses that are more difficult to exclude by simple history and laboratory testing would include those described below.

Depressive Illness

Some symptoms seen in both CFS and adolescent depression include sleepiness, mood changes, and sleep disturbance. However CFS patients were more likely to report somatic complaints such as headache, arthralgia, sore throat, myalgia, dizziness, concentration difficulties, and autonomic symptoms. As expected, affective symptoms were more severe in adolescents with primary depression than in those with CFS [63]. The presence of post-exertional malaise also distinguishes the two illnesses [6].

School Phobia

School avoidance because of psychosocial stressors at school or separation anxiety is characterized by symptoms that culminate with the avoidance of school in the morning, and are usually resolved in the evenings or at weekends. Observation of the overall activity levels of children with true school phobia do not usually show reduced activity, although they may express somatic complaints. Inquiring about leisure and social activities is important in distinguishing school (social) phobia and CFS. The former will maintain their hobbies and social activities, while the latter will have a marked reduction in social activities [4,35]. Moreover, there is usually a history of a precipitating event at school [64]. Evaluation during the history for "secondary gain" is an essential part of the evaluation of fatigue in children. Children and adolescents with CFS are eager to return to school, and may eagerly accept partial days when offered and when this is within their capabilities [6].

Anorexia Nervosa

In some pediatric patients, continuous nausea and abdominal symptoms may be so prominent as to cause weight loss and suggest anorexia. The decreased appetite persists for years in some of the more severely affected patients with CFS [36]. However, a careful diet history and observations during discussions of eating and body image readily distinguish the two conditions.

Somatoform Disorders

The criteria for somatization disorder do not include the symptom of fatigue [65]. Also, the colorful and sensational description of symptoms is different from that in CFS. The difficulty with the diagnosis of somatization disorder is that judgments as to symptom validity are subjective and arbitrary. In one adult review, the rate of somatization disorder in adult patients with CFS without a history of psychiatric disease ranged from 0% to 98% [66].

Sleep Phase Disorders

Virtually all patients with CFS have abnormal sleep patterns, and sleep phase abnormalities are common. Adolescents frequently say that they feel better in the late evening and may be unable to sleep until daybreak. There has been some concern that this may represent an alternative diagnosis. However, with medication and appropriate sleep hygiene this may be reversed while not significantly improving the activity limitation. Increased melatonin has been noted in the first part of the night in adolescents with CFS [67]. In general, it is our view that the sleep abnormalities of CFS are secondary to the underlying pathophysiology, and are not the cause of the illness.

Treatment, Education, and Socialization

Treatment for the child or adolescent with CFS should be aggressive, and include both symptom alleviation and extensive support. Appropriate treatment is rarely possible without a correct diagnosis. In adults, it has been estimated that 80% of persons with CFS have never received a diagnosis, and this is likely to be higher for children. Early recognition and diagnosis should be a priority for those involved in pediatric medical education [1,2,68].

Treatment in pediatric CFS also requires a strong bond between provider and patient regardless of whether the provider views CFS as an organic or psychiatric illness. As with any chronic illness, components of both may exist. It is not appropriate to assume a benign course or to suggest hypochondriasis, with the implication of the symptoms being unimportant. A long-term approach to the pediatric CFS patient can be a rewarding experience for the pediatrician and other providers, but requires a sustained effort. Cognitive behavioral therapy, which may be of value [69], and specific symptomatic treatments follow the pattern for adults, and will not be discussed in this chapter.

Widespread agreement exists for the need for aggressive educational support [1,2,6]. Arguments that home tutoring will reinforce the sick role or illness behavior [70] must be weighed against the loss of educational opportunities and the critical need for education should the illness persist and prevent future full-time activity. In one study, CFS was the leading cause of long-term school sickness absence [29]. Education plans should be individualized to the specific limiting symptoms, and should encourage independent study with flexible time available for rest. Special services or accommodation from the school are important to maximize the amount of time the pediatric patient will be able to stay in the classroom setting.

One of the important considerations in educational planning is preparing for the possibility of poor functional return. Should the symptoms, particularly activity limitation, resolve, future occupational considerations would not be affected. However, should activity limitation persist, a future occupation with flexibility, limited continuous orthostatic stresses, and a minimum of sustained physical labor will be necessary for self-sufficiency.

The role of exercise and rest has been debated extensively, yet simple prescribed regimens are impossible because of the wide range of illness severity. In general, a gradual increase of activity is appropriate, but the medical provider must watch for signs of post-exertional malaise. If this increased activity is tolerated, it may be combined with increased attendance at school and social functions. However, it is important to remember that CFS is a relapsing/remitting illness, and common sense and flexibility are essential in assessing activity goals. If exercise, or the increase in simple activity, directly limits education, then the amount of physical upright activity should be reduced.

Coping skills are also of importance in the long-term management of children and adolescents with CFS. The most important coping skill learned by the pediatric patient is not to exceed the level of activity which precipitates post-exertional malaise. Most adolescents begin to employ this skill within the first 2 years of illness. Because of the success of management through coping, it is often difficult to distinguish improvement due to a reduced degree of illness from improvement due to coping.

In terms of emotional adjustment, depression is a constant threat and should be treated aggressively whenever noted. Anxiety may also be frequent, due to both emotional and physiological factors. Blood testing for elevated catecholamines during orthostatic stress may show elevation in a pattern suggestive of hyperadrenergic orthostatic intolerance (D.S.B., unpublished observations). This mechanism is presumably an attempt at improving cerebral circulation during the dependent pooling which occurs during orthostasis.

Frequent diagnostic re-evaluation is important, as in any chronic illness, but the appearance of other illnesses is rare. Symptomatic management of pain and sleep disorder happens to be my preference in symptomatic treatment, but no data are available. Restructuring the sleep/wake cycle is a priority [6,68].

Prognosis

As in adults, an understanding of the prognosis of childhood and adolescent CFS has suffered because of the lack of pediatric criteria. However, some of the more recent studies have made progress in defining both recovery and stages of recovery, which is a critical issue in understanding prognosis. Complete recovery would be defined as the absence of both daily activity limitations and post-exertional malaise, so that the young adult could participate in vigorous activities and sports without the re-appearance of the symptom pattern of CFS. Fatigue which follows stress and exercise should not be associated with malaise or flu-like symptoms. Partial recovery is defined by the degree of improvement in activity limitation (fatigue) and the severity of post-exertional malaise, as well as the somatic symptoms.

It has become clear that complete recovery from childhood or adolescent CFS is rare, despite early assumptions to the contrary [71]. The majority of young people with CFS do improve after several years, often to the degree that they can return to normal or near normal activity [6,72]. In a telephone survey 1–3 years after the initial evaluation, 4 of 15 subjects were well, 4 had improved, and 7 were unimproved or worse [4]. In another study, improvement or resolution occurred in over 90% of pediatric subjects [73]. In a study that underlines the difficulty in defining recovery, Marshall reported that 76% of subjects reported improvement or recovery, although 38% of these had periods of fatigue that interfered with daily activities [74]. In a 1998 pediatric CFS prognosis study, 58 patients were evaluated several years after onset. Forty-three percent were considered to be cured, 52% had improved, and 5% were worse [75]. In another study, 31 pediatric patients with "persistent unexplained fatigue" were followed for 17 months. Seventy-seven percent had either "returned to normal or improved with occasional relapses" [36]. In a more recent study, 44% were unimproved or worse, and only 25% were completely or nearly completely recovered [72].

In a recent article, twenty-eight pediatric patients who were between the ages of 7 and 17 at illness onset were diagnosed by the Oxford Criteria and followed for a mean of 3 years. All symptoms had a trend toward improvement, but recovery was variable. Seventy-nine percent returned to full-time education or employment, but the majority required 3 months or more out of school. Sixty-eight percent stated that their illness significantly affected their education and/or future plans [68].

In an unpublished study of one hundred pediatric CFS patients followed for 5–10 years, 70% were functioning well, although half of these continued to have symptoms, and 30% were withdrawn from society and had more severe symptoms (T.M., unpublished observations). In the longest published pediatric follow-up study, 35 children and adolescents were followed for an average of 13 years from illness onset. Twenty-two percent missed at least 2 years of school. At follow-up, 80% were functioning well. Of this 80%, half appeared to have complete illness resolution, and the other half had persistence of both mild symptoms and mild activity limitation which could be managed by coping skills [76].

This same group of children was restudied in 2005, representing a follow-up of nearly twenty years. While the overall positive response remained high, severe disability persisted in the 20% identified earlier. There was also a suggestion that some of those previously doing well experienced increased activity limitation. If true, this would imply a slowly progressive illness for some. This topic has been only incompletely studied, and much more research is needed (study presented at the International Conference on Fatigue Science, Karuizawa, Japan, 2005). Furthermore, until adequate markers for the illness are identified, this subject will remain difficult to explore.

It is clear from the literature that pediatric and adolescent CFS is an illness that may be benign with a short course (2 years or less), but in the majority of cases it is a long-term illness with severe morbidity. Even when it resolves either completely or partially, it occurs at a vulnerable time of identity formation and educational accomplishment, thus disrupting both. It should be noted that children with lifelong fatigue or an inability to date the onset of their fatigue clearly are usually not included in the prognosis studies, thus underestimating the morbidity experienced from chronic fatigue.

Conclusions

CFS in children and adolescents is an illness that causes great morbidity that can be life-long. While the focus in evaluating the illness has often been the question of whether it is organic or psychosomatic, the harm done in underestimating the difficulties posed can be enormous. Regardless of whether the etiology turns out to be infectious, immunological, autoimmune, psychosomatic, or some combination of all these, it is an illness that requires all the skill and training of the pediatrician. It is not an illness that can be dismissed. Oversimplification is perceived by the pediatric patient as rejection, and is poor pediatric practice.

References

1. Tomoda A, Miike T, Yamada E, Honda H, Moroi T, Ogawa M, Ohtani Y, Morishita S (2000) Chronic fatigue syndrome in childhood. Brain Dev 22:60–64
2. Bell DS (1995) Chronic fatigue syndrome in children and adolescents: a review. Focus Opinion: Pediatrics 1:412–420
3. Rowe KS, Rowe KJ (2002) Symptom patterns of children and adolescents with chronic fatigue syndrome. In: Singh NN, Ollendick TH, Singh AN (eds) International perspectives on child and adolescent mental health, vol 2. Elsevier Science, Oxford, pp 395–421
4. Oleske JM, Palumbo D, Sterling J, Evans TL (2002) CFS in children and adolescents. In: John JF, Oleske JM (eds) A consensus manual for the primary care and management of chronic fatigue syndrome. Academy of Medicine of New Jersey, Lawrenceville, pp 51–56
5. Smith MS, Carter BD (2003) Chronic fatigue syndrome in adolescence. In: Jason LA, Fennell PA, Taylor RR (eds) Handbook of chronic fatigue syndrome. Wiley, New York, pp 693–712
6. Jordan KM, Landis DA, Downey MC, Osterman SL, Thurm AE, Jason LA (1998) Chronic fatigue syndrome in children and adolescents: a review. J Adolescent Health 22:4–18
7. Arav-Boger R, Spirer Z (1995) Chronic fatigue syndrome: pediatric aspects. Isr J Med Sci 31:330–334
8. Tomoda A, Jhodoi T, Miike T (2001) Chronic fatigue syndrome and abnormal biological rhythms in school children. J Chronic Fatigue Syndrome 8:29–37
9. Buskila D, Press J, Gedalia A, Klein M, Neuman L, Boehm R, Sukenik S (1993) Assessment of nonarticular tenderness and prevalence of fibromyalgia in children. J Rheumatol 20:368–370
10. Kulig JW (1991) Chronic fatigue syndrome and fibromyalgia in adolescence. Adolescence Med: State Art Rev 2:473–484
11. Bell D, Bell K, Cheney P (1994) Primary juvenile fibromyalgia syndrome and chronic fatigue syndrome in adolescents. Clin Inf Dis 18(Suppl 1):S21–S23
12. Fukuda K, Straus SE, Hickie I, Sharpe MC, Dobbins JG, Komaroff A, and the International Chronic Fatigue Syndrome Study Group (1994) The chronic fatigue syndrome: A comprehensive approach to its definition and study. Ann Intern Med 121:953–959
13. Carruthers B, Jain AK, De Meirlier KL, Peterson DL, Klimas NG, Lerner AM, Bested AC, Flor-Henry P, Joshi P, Powles ACP, van de Sande M (2003) Myalgic encephalomyelitis/chronic fatigue syndrome: clinical working case definition, diagnostic and treatment protocols. J Chronic Fatigue Syndrome 11:1–12
14. Sharpe MC, Archard LC, Banatuala JE, Borysecwicz LK, Clare AW, David A, Edwards RH, Hawton KE, Lambert HP, Lane R (1991) A report. Chronic fatigue syndrome: guidelines for research. J R Soc Med 84:118–121

15. Reeves WC, Lloyd A, Vernon SD, Klimas NG, Jason LA, Bleijenberg G, Evengard B, White PD, Nisenmbaum R, Unger ER (2003) Identification of ambiguities in the 1994 chronic fatigue syndrome research case definition and recommendations for resolution. BMC Health Services Research 3:25. http://www.biomedcentral.com/a472-6963/3/25
16. De Jong IWAM, Prins JB, Fiselier THJW, Weemaes CMR, Meijer-Van Den Bergh EMM, Bleijenberg G (1997) Chronic fatigue syndrome in youngsters. (Het chronisch vermoeidheidssyndroom bij jongeren.) Ned Tijdschr Geneeskd [Dutch J Med] 141:1513–1516
17. Sigurdsson B, Sigurjonsson J, Sigurdsson J, Thorkelsson J, Gudmundsson KA (1950) Disease epidemic in Iceland simulating poliomyelitis. Am J Hyg 52:222–238
18. Bell DS (1992) Children with ME/CFIDS: overview and review of the literature. In: Hyde B, Goldstein J, Levine P (eds) Myalgic encephalomyelitis. Nightingale Research Foundation, Ottawa, pp 209–218
19. Parish J (1974) Epidemic neuromyasthenia: a reappraisal. J Int Res Commun Med Sci 2:22–26
20. Acheson ED (1959) The clinical syndrome variously called benign myalgic encephalomyelitis, Iceland disease, and epidemic neuromyasthenia. Am J Med 26:569–595
21. Bell K, Cookfair D, Bell D, Reese P, Cooper L (1991) Risk factors associated with chronic fatigue syndrome in a cluster of pediatric cases. Rev Inf Dis 13(Suppl 1):S32–38
22. Bell D, Bell K (1989) Chronic fatigue syndrome in childhood: relation to Epstein–Barr virus. In: Ablashi D (ed) Epstein–Barr virus and human disease. Humana Press, Rome, pp 412–417
23. Bell D, Bell K (1988) The post-infectious chronic fatigue syndrome: diagnosis in childhood (Letter). Ann Intern Med 109:167
24. Vernon SD, Whistler T, Cameron B, Hickie I, Reeves W, Lloyd A (2006) Preliminary evidence of mitochondrial dysfunction associated with post-infectious fatigue after acute infection with Epstein–Barr virus. BMC Infect Dis 6 http://www.biomedcentral.com/1471-2334/1476/1416
25. Jordan KM, Ayers PM, Jahn SC, Taylor KK, Huang CF, Richman J, Jason LA (2000) Prevalence of fatigue and chronic fatigue syndrome-like illness in children and adolescents. J Chronic Fatigue Syndrome 6:3–21
26. Mears CJ, Taylor RR, Jordan KM, Binns HJ, Pediatric Research Group (2004) Sociodemographic and symptom correlates of fatigue in an adolescent primary care sample. J Adolescent Health 35:528–533
27. Lloyd AR, Hickie I, Boughton CR, Spencer O, Wakefield D (1990) Prevalence of chronic fatigue syndrome in an Australian population. Med J Austr 153:522–528
28. Dobbins JG, Randall B, Reyes M, Steele L, Livens EA, Reeves WC (1997) The prevalence of chronic fatiguing illnesses among adolescents in the United States. J Chronic Fatigue Syndrome 3:15–27
29. Dowsett EG, Colby J (1997) Long-term sickness absence due to ME/CFS in UK schools: an epidemiological study with medical and educational implications. J Chronic Fatigue Syndrome 3:29–42
30. Jones JF, Nisenbaum R, Solomon L, Reyes M, Reeves WC (2004) Chronic fatigue syndrome and other fatiguing illnesses in adolescents: A population-based study. J Adolescent Health 35:34–40
31. Farmer A, Fowler T, Scourfield J, Thapar A (2004) Prevalence of chronic fatigue in children and adolescents. Br J Psychiatr 184:477–481
32. Komaroff AL, Buchwald D (1991) Symptoms and signs of chronic fatigue syndrome. J Rev Infect Dis 13(Suppl 1):S8–S11
33. Jason L, King CP, Frankenberry EL, Jordan KM, Tyron WW, Rademaker F, Huang CF (1999) Chronic fatigue syndrome: assessing symptoms and activity level. J Clin Psychol 55: 411–424
34. Smith MS, Mitchell J, Corey L, Gold D, McCauley EA, Glover D, Tenover F (1991) Chronic fatigue in adolescents. Pediatrics 88:195–202

35. Walford GA, Nelson WM, McCluskey DR (1993) Fatigue, depression, and social adjustment in chronic fatigue syndrome. Arch Dis Child 68:384–388
36. Carter BD, Edwards JF, Kronenberger WG, Michalczyk L, Marshall GS (1995) Case control study of chronic fatigue in pediatric patients. Pediatrics 95:179–186
37. Saidi G, Haines L (2006) The management of children with chronic fatigue syndrome-like illness in primary care: a cross-sectional study. Br J Gen Pract 56:43–47
38. Gunn WJ, Connell DB, Randall B (1993) Epidemiology of chronic fatigue syndrome: the centers for disease control study. In: Bock G, Whelan J (eds) Chronic fatigue syndrome. Wiley, New York, pp 83–101
39. Jordan KM, Kolak AM, Jason LA (1997) Research with children and adolescents with chronic fatigue syndrome: methodologies, designs, and special considerations. J Chronic Fatigue Syndrome 3:3–13
40. Van Hoof E, Maertens M (2002) No, I am not lazy! A guide for adolescents with CFS/ME and their primary caregivers. (Neen, ik ben niet lui! Een gids voor jongeren met CVS/ME en hun opvoeders.) VUB Press, Brussels
41. Miike T, Tomoda A, Jhodoi T, Iwatani N, Mabe H (2004). Learning and memorization impairment in childhood chronic fatigue syndrome manifesting as school phobia in Japan. Brain Dev 26:442–447
42. Tomoda A, Miike T, Honda T, Fukuda K, Kai Y, Nabeshima M, Takahashi M (1995) Single-photon emission computed tomography for cerebral blood flow in school phobias. Curr Ther Res 56:1088–1093
43. Furusawa M, Morishita S, Kira M, Takahashi M, Tomoda A, Miike T, Arai N (1998) Evaluation of school refusal with localized proton MR spectroscopy. Asia Ocean J Radiol 3:170–174
44. de Lange F, Kalkman JS, Bleijenberg G, Hagoort P, Werf SP, van der Meer JW, Toni I (2004) Neural correlates of the chronic fatigue syndrome: an fMRI study. Brain 127:1948–1957
45. Lange G, Streffner J, Cook D, Bly B, Christodoulou C, Liu W, De Luca J, Natelson BH (2005) Objective evidence of cognitive complaints in chronic fatigue syndrome: a BOLD fMRI study of verbal working memory. NeuroImage 26:513–524
46. Barron DF, Cohen BA, Geraghty MT, Violand R, Rowe PC (2002) Joint hypermobility is more common in children with chronic fatigue syndrome than in healthy controls. J Pediatr 141:421–425
47. Rowe PC, Barron DF, Calkins H, Maumenee IH, Tong PY, Geraghty MT (1999) Orthostatic intolerance and chronic fatigue syndrome associated with Ehlers–Danlos syndrome. J Pediatr 135:494–499
48. van de Putte EM, Uiterwaal CSPM, Bots ML, Kuis W, Kimpen JLL, Engelbert RHH (2005) Is chronic fatigue syndrome a connective tissue disorder? A cross-sectional study in adolescents. Pediatrics 115:e415–e422
49. Spence V, Stewart J (2004) Standing up for ME. Biologist 51:65–70
50. Yamaguchi H, Tanaka H, Adachi K, Mino M (1996) Beat-to-beat blood pressure and heart rate responses to active standing in Japanese children. ACTA Paediatr 85:577–583
51. Rowe P, Bou-Holaigh I, Kan J, Calkins H (1995) Is neurally mediated hypotension an unrecognized cause of chronic fatigue? Lancet 345:623–625
52. Stewart JM, Gewitz MH, Weldon A, Munoz J (1999) Patterns of orthostatic intolerance: the orthostatic tachycardia syndrome and adolescent chronic fatigue. J Pediatr 135:218–225
53. Tanaka H, Yamaguchi H, Matushima R, Tamai H (1999) Instantaneous orthostatic hypotension in children and adolescents: A new entity of orthostatic intolerance. Pediatr Res 46:691–696
54. Iwatani N, Miike T, Kai Y, Kodama M, Mabe H, Tomoda A, Fukuda K, Jhodoi T (1997) Gluco-regulatory disorders in school refusal students. Clin Endocrinol 47:273–278
55. Itoh Y, Fukunaga Y, Igarashi T, Imai T, Yoshida J, Tsuchiya M, Fujino O, Murakami M, Yamamoto M (1998) Autoimmunity in chronic fatigue syndrome in children. Jpn J Rheumatol 8:429–437

56. Yoshiuchi K, Farkas J, Natelson BH (2006) Patients with chronic fatigue syndrome have reduced absolute cortical blood flow. Clin Physiol Funct Imaging 26:83–86
57. Bou-Holaigh I, Rowe P, Kan J, Calkins H (1995) The relationship between neurally mediated hypotension and the chronic fatigue syndrome. JAMA 274:961–967
58. Stewart J, Weldon A, Arlievsky N, Li K, Munoz J (1998) Neurally mediated hypotension and autonomic dysfunction measured by heart rate variability during head-up tilt testing in children with chronic fatigue syndrome. Clin Autonom Res 8:221–230
59. Stewart J (2001) Orthostatic intolerance: a review with application to the chronic fatigue syndrome. J Chronic Fatigue Syndrome 8:45–64
60. Grubb B, Karas B (1999) Clinical disorders of the autonomic nervous system associated with orthostatic intolerance: an overview of classification, clinical evaluation and management. Pacing Clin Electrophysiol 22:798–810
61. Rodriguez R, Snider K, Cornel G, Teixeira OHP (1999) Cerebral blood flow velocity during tilt-table test for pediatric syncope. Pediatrics 104:237–242
62. Streeten D, Thomas D, Bell D (2000) The roles of orthostatic hypotension, orthostatic tachycardia, and subnormal erythrocyte volume in the pathogenesis of the chronic fatigue syndrome. Am J Med Sci 320:1–8
63. Carter BD, Kronenberger WG, Edwards JF, Michalczyk L, Marshall GS (1996) Differential diagnosis of chronic fatigue in children: behavioral and emotional dimensions. J Dev Behav Pediatr 17:16–21
64. Solnit AJ, Provence S, Schowalter M (1987) Psychological development: from health to illness. In: Rudolphe AM, Hoffman JIE (eds) Pediatrics, 18th edn. Appleton & Lange, Norwalk, pp 53–54
65. American Psychiatric Association (1994) Diagnostic and statistical manual of mental disorders, 4th edn. American Psychiatric Association, Washington, DC
66. Johnson S, DeLuca J, Natelson B (1996) Assessing somatization disorder in the chronic fatigue syndrome. Psychosom Med 58:50–57
67. Knook L, Kavelaars A, Sinnema G, Kuis W, Heijnen C (2000) High nocturnal melatonin in adolescents with chronic fatigue syndrome. J Clin Endocrinol Metab 85:3690–3692
68. Sankey A, Hill C, Brown J, Quinn L, Fletcher A (2006) A follow-up study of chronic fatigue syndrome in children and adolescents: symptom persistence and school absenteeism. Clin Child Psychol Psychiatr 11:126–138
69. Stulemeijer M, de Jong L, Fiselier T, Hoogveld S, Bleijenberg G (2005) Cognitive behavior therapy for adolescents with chronic fatigue syndrome: randomized controlled trial. BMJ 330:14–25
70. Richards J (2000) Chronic fatigue syndrome in children and adolescents: a review article. Clin Child Psychol Psychiatr 5:31–51
71. Dale JK, Straus SE (1992) The chronic fatigue syndrome: considerations relevant to children and adolescents. Adv Pediatr Infect Dis 7:63–83
72. Gill AC, Dosen A, Ziegler JB (2004) Chronic fatigue syndrome in adolescents: a follow-up study. Arch Pediatr Adolescent Med 158:225–229
73. Feder HM, Dworkin PH, Orkin C (1994) Outcome of 48 pediatric patients with chronic fatigue: a clinical experience. Arch Fam Med 3:1049–1055
74. Marshall GS, Gesser RM, Yamanishi K, Starr SE (1991) Chronic fatigue in children: clinical features, Epstein–Barr virus, and human herpes virus 6 serology and long-term follow-up. Pediatr Inf Dis J 10:287–290
75. Krilov LR, Fisher M, Friedman SB, Reitman D, Mandel FS (1998) Course and outcome of chronic fatigue in children and adolescents. Pediatrics 102:360–366
76. Bell D, Jordan K, Robinson M (2001) Thirteen-year follow-up of children and adolescents with chronic fatigue syndrome. Pediatrics 107:994–998

Physical or Mental Fatigue and Immunodepression

Linda M. Castell

Summary

Fatigue is an integral component of illness and sickness behavior. This chapter reviews possible links between fatigue, mood states, immunodepression, and the incidence of illness, particularly upper respiratory tract infections. In terms of fatigue, our work has focused mainly on the biochemical markers (tryptophan, branched chain amino acids) involved in central fatigue in endurance athletes (with/without unexplained underperformance syndrome) in chronic fatigue syndrome, and in postoperative fatigue. We have also looked at tryptophan from a different perspective by undertaking a functional magnetic resonance imaging (fMRI) study on the brain in healthy humans, with/without tryptophan supplementation, undertaking a cognition function task. The availability of tryptophan has consequences for immune function. In prolonged exercise, mucosal protection may be impaired as a consequence of oronasal breathing. Individuals involved in our studies have often had a high incidence of minor illnesses, particularly upper respiratory tract infections (URTI), after prolonged, exhaustive exercise such as a marathon race, or intensive training. A concomitant decrease in plasma glutamine has been a frequent feature of these studies. Mood profiles and other parameters were assessed in military personnel undertaking intensive training in harsh environments: fatigue and other negative mood states were increased at the same time as the highest incidence of URTI. Sleep deprivation was a factor in this study, and a subsequent investigation of one night's sleep loss demonstrated changes in some parameters involved in immune function concomitant with decreased cognitive ability. As well as a variety of metabolites, the cytokines, both pro- and anti-inflammatory, clearly have an important role in all the circumstances mentioned above.

Nuffield Department of Anaesthetics, University of Oxford, Radcliffe Infirmary, Woodstock Road, Oxford OX2 6HE, UK

Introduction

Central Fatigue

The links between fatigue, immunodepression, and the incidence of illness, particularly upper respiratory tract infections, have long been of interest to our group. The biochemical markers involved in central fatigue have been investigated in endurance athletes (with/without unexplained underperformance syndrome) in chronic fatigue syndrome patients, and in patients after major surgery.

The central fatigue hypothesis was first proposed in the mid-1980s [1]. It centers around the competition between tryptophan and the branched chain amino acids (leucine, isoleucine, and valine) for entry across the blood–brain barrier [2]. A small amount of tryptophan is converted in the brain to the neurotransmitter 5-hydroxytryptamine (5-HT), which is involved in fatigue, sleep, and mood. Thus an increase in neuronal 5-HT may make it harder mentally to maintain, for example, endurance exercise [3].

An increased level of brain tryptophan can increase the rate of formation, and hence the level, of 5-HT in some areas of the brain, as observed by [4]. Tryptophan is unique among the amino acids in that it is bound to albumin in the blood. Stress, such as strenuous exercise, causes fatty acid mobilization via a surge in catecholamines. Fatty acids also bind to albumin, and an increase in free fatty acids decreases the affinity for tryptophan, which leads to an increase in plasma free tryptophan (p[FT]).

Despite increased rates of mobilization, the p[FA] may be only slightly increased in exercise: the rates of fatty acid uptake and oxidation by active muscle are well regulated [5]. However, E.A. Newsholme (personal communication) suggests that the p[FA], and thus p[FT], may increase markedly in exercise in unfit subjects, when control of fatty acid mobilization may not be precisely regulated in relation to the demand and control of oxidation within the muscle.

The branched-chain amino acids (leucine, isoleucine, and valine) are largely oxidized by muscle. The plasma concentration ratio of free tryptophan to BCAA (p[FT/BCAA]) governs the rate of entry of tryptophan into the brain, the level of tryptophan in the brain, and hence that of 5-HT [2]. The p[FT/BCAA] ratio is increased in humans after prolonged exhaustive exercise, and in the rat, the brain levels of tryptophan and 5-HT are increased [4,6]. Jakeman et al. [7] used prolactin release from the hypothalamus as an indirect marker of 5-HT activity. They observed that the increase in blood prolactin was much smaller in well-trained endurance athletes, compared with controls, in response to d-fenfluramine, the administration of which increased 5-HT levels in the hypothalamus. They suggested that this could be due to decreased numbers of 5-HT receptors as a result of chronic elevation of the 5-HT level in this part of the brain. Using a 5-HT$_{2C}$ agonist, m-chlorphenylpiperazine, Budgett et al. [8] observed a larger increase in the production of prolactin release (as a measure of 5-HT activity) in athletes with unexplained underperformance syndrome (UUPS) as opposed to well-trained, elite athletes who were not ill.

In chronic fatigue syndrome (CFS) patients, p[FT], and consequently the p[FT/BCAA] ratio, was 30% higher than in sedentary controls at rest [9]. However, unlike the controls, these parameters did not alter during subsequent exercise, despite the perception of the CFS patients that the exercise was extremely hard. This might denote an increased sensitivity of 5-HT receptors. An investigation into postoperative fatigue demonstrated a close correlation between p[FT/BCAA] and fatigue scores after major surgery [10].

In the past few years, supplementary feeding with BCAA has produced some results supporting the central fatigue hypothesis and some which showed no effect [11]. Many of the reported studies have not attempted to measure mental fatigue. In a laboratory-based, cross-over study, seven endurance cyclists were monitored for perceived effort and mental fatigue (using the Borg scale), with and without BCAA supplementation. In subjects receiving BCAA, compared with a placebo, a lower perception of effort was required to sustain the level of exercise required [12].

Calders et al. [13] observed an increase in the time to fatigue, as well as an increase in plasma ammonia, in fasting rats injected with 30 mg branched chain amino acids 5 min before exercise, compared with those injected with placebo. Injection of BCAA not only increased the time to fatigue of exercising rats, but also prevented the normal increase in brain tryptophan level caused by exhaustive exercise (T. Yamamoto, personal communication). Yamamoto and Azechi [14] observed a decreased performance in spatial learning in rats injected with L-tryptophan. Interestingly, rats injected with tryptophan but subjected to musical stimuli increased the time to exhaustion compared with a group subjected to white noise! Yamamoto and Azechi [14] extended their work to humans by giving BCAA and measuring both their profile of mood states (POMS) and the multiple mood scale after the Uchida–Kraepelin psychodiagnostic test: they observed a significant improvement in the group who received BCAA compared with those who received placebo. They consider that central fatigue can be diminished by inhibiting the L-system transporter for uptake of tryptophan. Therefore, they propose a tryptophan–serotonin hypothesis to explain the mechanisms of central fatigue, rather than just a serotonin hypothesis.

Tryptophan also has a role in immune function. Its degradation is linked with immune cell activity via the induction by IFN-γ of indolamine (2,3)–dioxygenase (IDO, tryptophan catabolism rate-limiting enzyme) [15,16].

In military personnel, plasma free tryptophan (p[FT]) was markedly decreased within 24 h of arriving at altitude: this decrease was maintained during 1 month's intensive mountain winter training, and reached above baseline levels upon their return to the desert. This decrease in p[FT] observed during winter field training may be associated with increased cellular immune activation, inducing the enzyme IDO to catabolize tryptophan. IDO also has antioxidant properties owing to its use of the superoxide anion (produced in greater quantity at altitude) as an oxygen source [17]. The ambient temperature may also have been a factor.

Tryptophan and Functional Magnetic Resonance Imaging in the Brain

More recently, we studied one of the markers of central fatigue from a different perspective by undertaking functional magnetic resonance imaging (MRI) of the brain (fMRIB) in healthy humans with/without tryptophan supplementation [18]. Participants were given a bolus dose of tryptophan (30 mg/kg body wt) or placebo, and subjected to fMRIB while undertaking a cognitive function task (modified Stroop counting test). Although reaction times were longer after tryptophan, the Stroop effect was not significantly different between placebo and tryptophan. Compared with placebo, L-tryptophan administration was associated with decreased activation in some regions of the brain, including the left postcentral, angular, inferior frontal, and the lateral orbital gyri, while increased activation occurred in the left precuneus and the posterior cingulate gyrus. These findings suggest that subcortical changes may have contributed to central fatigue, but that changes in neocortical activity were associated with the experience itself.

Prolonged, Exhaustive Exercise

Immunodepression in an endurance athlete appears to be firmly linked to intensity and duration of exercise [19]. Heath et al. [20] and Nieman et al. [21] observed a correlation between prolonged strenuous exercise and the frequency of URTI. The higher the mileage, the more frequent the incidence (and often severity) of URTI [20]. More than twice as many participating marathon runners suffered from a URTI in the weeks after a race compared with those who had trained and not participated. This bears out the perception of O'Connor et al. [22], who observed that the stress of competition more than doubled the risk of a URTI. The exhausted athlete is vulnerable to opportunistic infections for 3–4 h after an event such as a marathon. There is an increased incidence of illness in athletes undertaking prolonged, exhaustive exercise such as an endurance event or intensive training [23,24]. The individuals involved in our studies on endurance exercise had a notably high incidence of minor illnesses, in particular URTI [25]. Athletes undertaking repeated bouts of training without sufficient recovery time between sessions will show cumulative effects of fatigue and thus can become immunodepressed, which is likely to lead to an increased incidence of infection.

Lakier Smith [26] reviewed the changes which occur in immune cell function after intense, long-duration exercise. These changes include decreased circulating numbers of lymphocytes, decreased natural killer (NK) cell activity, and reduced secretory IgA levels in the mucosa. She also referred to the importance of the T-helper lymphocytes, Th_1 and Th_2, suggesting that tissue trauma leads to the suppression of cell-mediated immunity via the Th_2 response. NK cells are particularly responsive to prolonged stress such as hypoxia and hyperthermia [27], and to running a marathon. Markedly decreased circulating numbers of NK cells 1 h after a race were still 50% below normal the next morning (16 h later) [28]. The proportion of CD4 (helper cells) to CD8 (cytotoxic/suppressor cells) is also decreased after prolonged, exhaustive exercise. This ratio has been proposed both as a marker and a cause of immunodepression [29]. Decreased lymphocyte and neutrophil function also occur as a result of strenuous exercise [30]. A marked neutrophilia is responsible for the well-known leucocytosis which occurs in response to strenuous exercise. There is evidence that the provision of glutamine in both exercise and clinical situations effects a decrease in the cytokine IL-8, a major chemoattractant for neutrophil recruitment [30]. It has recently been established that human neutrophils use glutamine, via the presence of glutaminase on the secondary granules [31]. In view of this, the well-documented decrease in plasma glutamine which occurs after such stress as major surgery (ca. 35%) and prolonged, exhaustive exercise, (ca. 25%) may affect the ability of neutrophils to function fully in their role as first-line defenders against an immune challenge.

Intensive training in harsh environments over a prolonged period resulted in both immunodepression and fatigue in military personnel [32]. Glutamine, free tryptophan, and branched chain amino acids are possible markers of immunodepression and/or fatigue. The plasma concentration of these amino acids, linked with immune function, was found to be decreased after intensive training at altitude in winter. This coincided with increased URTI. In addition, the plasma concentrations of nonesterified fatty acids, leptin, and total antioxidant capacity were decreased at the end of the sojourn at altitude. Plasma antioxidant capacity was significantly increased 1 month after return to the desert [33]. It is thought this was due to residual infections following on from the high incidence observed at the end of mountain winter training.

The most striking finding was that plasma glutamine decreased by 14%–21% in these individuals after an overnight fast. This decrease is comparable to several studies which have shown a relatively transient decrease (20%–25%, maintained for 5–6 h) 1–2 h *after* a bout of prolonged exercise. However, the importance of this observation relates to the fact that these particular samples were taken at rest, early in the morning. This clearly suggests a cumulative effect of exhaustive exercise on plasma glutamine levels, which is potentially more serious in terms of providing fuel for the successful function of those immune cells that require circulating glutamine to be readily available in response to local demand at times of an immune challenge [34]. Interestingly, individuals with the highest illness scores also had the greatest decrease in plasma glutamine concentration. This finding was similar to that found in a study on elite athletes in an altitude training camp [35].

These military personnel also completed the profile of mood states (POMS) at multiple time points before and after the sojourn at high altitude. Significant increases in POMS scores were reported after the sojourn. Their anger and fatigue scores were comparable to adult male psychiatric outpatient norms, and lasted well beyond the completion of mountain winter training [36]. It was suggested that the negative moods observed in these circumstances and environments approached levels of clinical significance, and that they may affect the individual's ability to perform critical tasks. In a study on elite triathletes toward the end of a competitive season, our findings revealed a high incidence of both fatigue and URTI: there was a concomitant increase in anger and depression [37].

A study of army recruits looked at samples and questionnaires from the time the recruits arrived in camp, through mid-training, to the end of training 12 weeks later. By week 6 (mid-training), recruits had a high increase and duration of URTI [38]. They also had changes in mood states in an adverse direction, and in particular they had very high fatigue in week 6.

In another longitudinal study, elite female university rowers were studied over 8 weeks of winter training [39]. Changes were observed in the incidence of illness and mood state, as well as plasma glutamine and glutamate concentrations (p[Gln], p[Glu]), and rate of perceived exertion (RPE). There was a significant increase in the incidence and duration of gastrointestinal disturbances in open-weight rowers halfway through the training period. Although this was not assessed clinically, it is highly likely that this was some kind of communal infection of normal virulence (R. Baskerville, personal communication 2006).

The p[Glu] increased significantly over 8 weeks [39]. This finding is similar to those of Halson et al. [40] and Smith and Norris [41]. Parry-Billings et al. [42] observed that elevated [Glu] had no effect on the rate of T-lymphocyte proliferation in vitro. This suggests that p[Glu] neither plays a role in the mechanism nor is it a potential marker of the immunodepression seen in exercise, unlike p[Gln]. Smith and Norris [41] observed p[Gln/Glu] to be 25% lower in athletes classified as over-trained compared with those who were not. In rowers, the p[Gln/Glu] decreased significantly by 29% over 8 weeks (weeks 1–8 [39]). A negative correlation, which was close to significance, was observed between URTI and p[Gln/Glu], suggesting that p[Gln/Glu] ratio may be a possible marker of immune status.

RPE correlated significantly with the incidence/duration of URTI, fatigue, stress, motivation, and depression [39]. This suggests that RPE could be a potential marker of both immunodepression and mood state in athletes, and thus of over-reaching/over-training. This confirms the findings of Rietjens et al. [43], who postulated that RPE could be a sensitive parameter of over-reaching.

Mucosal Protection

Several observations in the 1970s and 1980s suggested that those who undertook a good deal of strenuous exercise appeared to be more vulnerable to opportunistic infections, such as polio, hepatitis B, and echoviral meningitis, than the general population [19]. In a comprehensive review, Maree Gleeson [54] examined more than 40 studies on a wide variety of sports. In the majority of these, salivary IgA was decreased as a result of intense exercise. Mackinnon and Hooper [55] observed a consistent decrease in salivary IgA in endurance athletes with UUPS. One of the symptoms of athletes with UUPS is a high incidence of URTI. With regard to moderate exercise, Klentrou et al. [56] showed an increase in resting salivary IgA in subjects exercising moderately for 12 weeks; this coincided with a decrease in URTI symptoms and days of sickness.

Salivary IgA in mucosal surfaces is the first line of defence against infections via bacterial and viral agents. The trapped organisms are cleared by mucociliary transport. As well as enabling cell mobility, cilia cover the cell surface with mucous [57]. In strenuous exercise, mucosal secretions dry up, particularly when mouth-breathing takes over from nasal breathing [58]. This is clearly more of a problem in endurance events, where a large majority of athletes (96%) were observed to breathe oronasally rather than nasally [59], and it may be that it is at this point that athletes become most vulnerable to opportunistic infections. Oronasal breathing may very well dry up mucosal secretions. This should result in an increased concentration of secretory IgA, provided that it does not result in a greater loss of measurable IgA due to binding to mucin (P. Brandtzaeg, personal communication). Muns et al. [60] observed a reduction in nasal mucociliary clearance in marathon runners for several days after a race, and suggested that ciliated cells with abnormal function were partly to blame.

Sleep Deprivation and Immunodepression

The role of sleep in immunocompetence is difficult to assess. However, both acute and chronic sleep loss have been found to be associated with decreased antibody response to vaccinations and increased levels of infections [44–46]. Other than the possible detrimental effects of sleep deprivation on performance, the risk of increased susceptibility to illness is also of importance to the athlete. Decreased IL-6 and IL-8 production by T lymphocytes in response to Con A [47] may represent an inability to respond to infectious stimuli, or in the case of IL-6, impaired humoral immunity. The observed decrease in IL-6 production the morning after sleep deprivation conflicts with the study by Robson [48], in which over-production of IL-6 is named as a causal factor in UUPS. However, the cell type responsible for over-production was not specified. Decreased IL-6 production by T lymphocytes may have implications of its own. It may represent the dominance of a Th1 response, meaning that although cellular immunity is not impaired, humoral immunity might be. Thus, in circumstances requiring antibody production, the infection may be prolonged and re-occurring if sleep deprivation occurs, as is typical in athletes suffering from UPS. Although IL-8 has not previously been implicated in UPS, a decrease in T lymphocyte production of IL-8 after sleep deprivation might increase the chance of contracting an opportunistic infection. Frequent minor infections are common in UPS and CFS.

Data from Brown and Castell [39] appears to support the suggestion that sleep plays a role in immune status. In particular, one individual reported regular sleep duration of at least 8 h per night during the 8-week study. Her incidence of illness appeared to be significantly less than the other subjects, and her mood states appeared much more stable. The restorative properties of sleep on the immune system remain elusive.

Leptin (the obesity hormone related to appetite control) has a role in UUPS [49] and in sleep. Gough et al. [47] observed that in some individuals, acute sleep deprivation can result in decreased p[Lep] the morning after. This agrees with observations made in a pilot study on sleep deprivation, where 8 out of 12 subjects had a mean decrease of 24% in plasma leptin the morning after the loss of one night's sleep (L.M. Castell, unpublished observations 2001). Mullington et al. [50] observed that the normal, nocturnal, appetite-suppressant rise in circulating leptin was reduced during one night of sleep deprivation. Given that sleep is perceived as a restorative process, then maybe there is more to the nocturnal enhancement of leptin than simply to suppress appetite during the night. Coupled with recent demonstrations of the effect of leptin on some immune parameters [51,52], the frequently reported sleep disturbances in UPS, and the consequences of a negative energy balance, it is possible that decreased concentrations of leptin during the night may contribute to the frequent infections reported by these athletes and their continuing fatigue [47].

Individual differences in the capacity to tolerate sleep loss in athletes, particularly endurance athletes, might compromise their immune function. The additive effect of sleep loss and already present immunodepression may be different from that observed in healthy individuals. It has long been considered that there is a high incidence of minor infections in obesity. This was investigated in a pilot study by Taylor and Castell [53] and looked at the incidence and duration of URTI in a different range of bodyweights over several weeks. There was an increased incidence of URTI, which appeared to be concomitant with increased body mass index (BMI). The incidence of URTI correlated with BMI; in turn, BMI correlated with p[Lep] (the obesity hormone related to appetite control, and which also has a role in immune function). It would be tempting to extrapolate, and speculate that an increased URTI incidence is thus related to increased plasma leptin concentration. However, this would be somewhat premature. It is interesting to note that obese individuals have a high incidence of sleep disturbance, which is to do with an enlargement of the soft palate; they tend to snore because they sleep with their mouths open. This has similarities with endurance athletes switching to oronasal breathing and the drying of the mucosa-producing cilia, as discussed above.

Role of Some Cytokines

Fatigue is an integral part of sickness behavior, which is mediated in the brain by pro- and anti-inflammatory cytokines [61] (see also Laye et al., this volume); they also enhance cortisol production. Uhlig and Kallus [62] state that in patients with inflammation, elevated cytokines, and fatigue, it is impossible to distinguish which is causing the other. In terms of exercise studies, IL-6 may well be an important player since, as proposed by Pedersen and Febbraio [63], it is primarily released by muscle. Nybo et al. [64] have proposed that IL-6 is also released from the brain during prolonged exercise, and that this is affected mainly by the duration of the exercise. However, they observed that IL-6 does not appear to have a role in central fatigue.

Cannon and Kluger [65] obtained plasma from humans immediately after prolonged exercise and injected it into rats: this produced symptoms compatible with pyrexia, i.e., substantially raised rectal temperature. Interestingly, injecting plasma obtained 3 h after the exercise produced even greater temperature elevations. This suggests that higher circulating levels of a cytokine or chemokine, such as one of the pro-inflammatory cytokines, may be stimulating the thermal increase. However, plasma IL-6 in humans is returning to normal by 1 h after an endurance event [28], its marked increase being more noticeable immediately after the cessation of exercise. Plasma IL-1β (pro-inflammatory) and IL-4 (anti-inflammatory) are elevated at 2 h after exercise [66]. A recent paper by Carmichael et al. [67] has emphasized the importance of brain IL-1β in fatigue after exercise-induced muscle damage. The injection of IL-1b significantly decreased the run-time to fatigue in male mice as opposed to IL-1ra, which increased the run-time. Plasma IL-8, the chemoattractant for neutrophils (also regarded as pro-inflammatory), is increased about 2-fold after 2 h in female rowers after an ergotest lasting about 12 min, and in marathon runners after a race (L. M. Castell, unpublished observations 1996).

Concluding Remarks

In contrast to the extremely positive effects that moderate exercise appears to have on psychological well being [68–70], intense training periods show a negative effect on mood states [40,36,71,72]. Stress is known to be a powerful modulator of immune function [73,74]. The relations between the immune, endocrine, and nervous systems, cytokines, and sleep are complex: they interact, affect, and are affected by one another. The high incidence of URTI and other illnesses resulting from stressful conditions is a clear indicator of immunodepression. Many factors are involved. A healthy lifestyle can best be promoted by good and varied nutrition, and by moderation in all things, including physical activity.

Acknowledgments. I am indebted to all my students, whose work has added fresh impetus to my thoughts. In particular, I thank Liz Gough who has discussed several aspects of this manuscript with me, and Professor Takanobu Yamamoto for his contribution to the section on central fatigue. There were no conflicts of interest in relation to this review.

References

1. Acworth I, Nicholass S, Morgan B, Newsholme EA (1986) Effect of sustained exercise on concentrations of plasma aromatic and branched-chain amino acids and brain amines. Biochem Biophys Res Commun 137:149–153

2. Fernstrom JD (1990) Aromatic amino acids and monoamine synthesis in the CNS: influence of the diet. J Nutr Biochem 1:508–517
3. Blomstrand E, Celsing F, Newsholme EA (1988) Changes in plasma concentrations of aromatic and branched-chain amino acids during sustained exercise in man and their possible role in fatigue. Acta Physiol Scand 133:115–121
4. Blomstrand E, Perrett D, Parry-Billings M, Newsholme EA (1989) Effect of sustained exercise on plasma amino acid concentrations and on 5-hydroxytryptamine metabolism in six different brain regions of the rat. Acta Physiol Scand 136:473–481
5. Winder WW (1996) Malonyl CoA as a metabolic regulator. In: Maughan RJ, Sherriffs SM (eds) Biochemistry of exercise, vol 9. Human Kinetics, Champaign, pp 173–184
6. Blomstrand E, Hassmen P, Ekblom B, Newsholme EA (1991) Administration of branched-chain amino acids during sustained exercise: effects on performance and on plasma concentration of some amino acids. Eur J Appl Physiol 63:83–88
7. Jakeman PM, Hawthorne JE, Maxwell SRJ, Kendall MJ, Holder G (1994) Evidence for down-regulation of hypothalamic 5-hydroxytryptamine function in endurance-trained athletes. Exp Physiol 79:461–464
8. Budgett RA, Castell LM, Hiscock N, Arida R (2003) The effects of 5-HT antagonist m-chlorophenylpiperazine on elite athletes with unexplained underperformance (overtraining). Med Sci Sport Exerc (Proceedings of the ACSM Congress) p S38
9. Castell LM, Phoenix J, Edwards RHT, Newsholme EA (1998) Plasma amino acid measurement in exercise-related chronic fatigue syndrome. J Physiol 509:206
10. McGuire J, Ross G, Price H, Mortensen N, Evans J, Castell LM (2003) Biochemical markers for post-operative fatigue after major surgery. Brain Res Bull 60:125–130
11. Newsholme EA, Castell LM (2000) Amino acids and nutrition in exercise. In: Maughan R (ed) Encyclopaedia of nutrition in sports medicine. Blackwell Scientific. Oxford, Chap 11, pp 153–170
12. Blomstrand E, Hassmen P, Ekblom B, Newsholme EA (1997) Influence of ingesting a solution of branched-chain amino acids on perceived exertion during exercise. Acta Physiol Scand 159:41–49
13. Calders P, Pannier JL, Matthys D, Lacroix EM (1997) Pre-exercise branched-chain amino acid administration increases endurance performance in rats. Med Sci Sports Exerc 29: 1182–1186
14. Yamamoto T, Azechi H (2005) Tryptophan–serotonin hypothesis for psychological links with fatigue. International Conference on Fatigue Science, pp 61–62
15. Widner B, Laich A, Spenrer-Unterweger B, Ledowski M, Fuchs D (2002) Neopterin production, tryptophan degradation and mental depression: what is the link? Brain Behav Immun 16:590–595
16. Wirleitner B, Rudzite V, Neurauter G, Murr C, Kalnins U, Erglis A, Trusinskis K, Fuchs D (2003) Immune activation and degradation of tryptophan in coronary heart disease. Eur J Clin Invest 33:550–554
17. Sun Y (1989) Indoleamine 2,3-dioxygenase – a new antioxidant enzyme. Mater Med Pol 21:244–250
18. Morgan RM, Parry AM, Arida RM, Matthews PM, Davies B, Castell LM (2007) Effects of plasma tryptophan on brain activation associated with the Stroop task. Psychopharmacology 190:383–389
19. Sharp C, Parry-Billings M (1992) Can exercise damage your health? New Sci, August 15, 33–37
20. Heath GW, Ford ES, Craven TE, Macera CA, Jackson KL, Pate RR (1991) Exercise and the incidence of upper respiratory tract infections. Med Sci Sports Exerc 23:152–157
21. Nieman D, Johanssen LM, Lee JW, Arabtzis K (1990) Infectious episodes before and after the Los Angeles marathon. J Sports Med Phys Fitness 30:289–296
22. O'Connor SA, Jones DP, Collins JV, Heath RB, Campbell MJ, Leighton MH (1979) Am Rev Respir Dis 120:1087–1090

23. Nieman D (1994) Exercise, upper respiratory tract infection and the immune system. Med Sci Sports Exerc 26:128–139
24. Weidner T (1994) Literature review: upper respiratory tract illness and sport and exercise. Int J Sports Med 15:1–9
25. Castell LM, Poortmans JR, Newsholme EA (1996) Does glutamine feeding affect the incidence of infection in athletes? Eur J Appl Physiol 73:488–490
26. Lakier Smith L (2003) Overtraining, excessive exercise, and altered immunity: is this a T-helper-1 versus T-helper-2 lymphocyte response? Sports Med 33:347–364
27. Pedersen BK, Kappel M, Klokker M, Nielsen HB, Secher NH (1994) The immune system during exposure to extreme physiologic conditions. Int J Sports Med 15:S116–121
28. Castell LM, Poortmans JR, Leclercq R, Brasseur M, Duchateau J, Newsholme EA (1997) Some aspects of the acute phase response after a marathon race, and the effects of glutamine supplementation. Eur J Appl Physiol 75:47–53
29. Nash HL (1986) Can exercise make us immune to disease? Physician Sportsmed 14:251–253
30. Castell LM (2003) Glutamine supplementation in vitro and in vivo, in exercise and in immunodepression. Sports Med 33:323–345
31. Castell LM, Vance C, Abbott R, Marquez J, Eggleton P (2004) Granule localization of glutaminase in human neutrophils and the consequence of glutamine utilization for neutrophil activity. J Biol Chem 279:13305–13310
32. Ensign W, Castell LM (2004) Intensive training in harsh environments. Proc 75th Aerospace Medical Conference, May, Anchorage, AL
33. Castell LM, Ensign W, Hudig D, Knight J, Roberts D, Thake D (2003) The stress of intensive training at altitude in winter after training in the desert. Proc 6th International Conference Exercise Immunology, Copenhagen
34. Newsholme EA (1994) Biochemical mechanisms to explain immunosuppression in well-trained and overtrained athletes. Int J Sports Med 15:S141–147
35. Bailey DM, Castell LM, Newsholme EA, Davies B (2000) Continuous and intermittent exposure to the hypoxia of altitude: implications for glutamine metabolism and exercise performance. Br J Sports Med 34:210–212
36. Bardwell WA, Ensign WY, Mills PJ (2005) Negative mood endures after completion of high-altitude military training. Ann Behav Mood 29:64–69
37. Dimitriou L, Jaques R, Maw G, Whyte G, Castell LM (2003) A longitudinal study on some potential markers of incidence of illness and immunodepression in triathletes. Proceedings 6th International Conference, Exercise Immunology, Copenhagen
38. Dimitriou L, Castell LM (2004) Possible immunodepression in military personnel undertaking twelve weeks training. Proceedings 9th European College of Sports Science Congress, Clermont-Ferrand, July, 2004
39. Brown D, Castell LM (2006) Fatigue and illness in endurance athletes during prolonged training. Proceedings 13th Oxford Nutrition Group Meeting, October 2006
40. Halson SL, Lancaster GI, Jeukendrup AE, Gleeson M (2003) Immunological responses to overreaching in cyclists. Med Sci Sports Exerc 35:854–861
41. Smith DJ, Norris SR (2000) Changes in glutamine and glutamate concentrations for tracking training tolerance. Med Sci Sports Exerc 32:684–689
42. Parry-Billings M, Budgett R, Koutedakis Y, Blomstrand E, Brooks S, Williams C, Calder PC, Pilling S, Baigrie R, Newsholme EA (1992) Plasma amino acid concentrations in the overtraining syndrome: possible effects on the immune system. Med Sci Sports Ex 24:1353–1358
43. Rietjens GJ, Kuipers H, Adam JJ, Saris WHM, van Breda E, van Hamont D, Keizer HA (2005) Physiological, biochemical and psychological markers of strenuous training-induced fatigue. Int J Sports Med 26:16–26
44. Spiegel K, Leproult R, Van Cauter E (2003) Impact of sleep debt on physiological rhythms. Rev Neurol (Paris) 159:6S 11–20

45. Mohren DC, Jansen NW, Kant IJ, Galama J, van den Brandt PA, Swaen GM (2002) Prevalence of common infections among employees in different work schedules. J Occup Environ Med 44:1003–1011
46. Lange T, Perras B, Fehm HL, Born J (2003) Sleep enhances the human antibody response to hepatitis A vaccination. Psychosom Med 65: 831–835
47. Gough L, Castell L, Miller J (2005) Cytokines, acute sleep deprivation and glutamine intervention. Proceedings 10th International Congress of the European College of Sports Science, Belgrade
48. Robson P (2003) Elucidating the unexplained underperformance syndrome in endurance athletes: the interleukin-6 hypothesis. Sports Med 33:771–781
49. Petibois C, Cazorla G, Poortmans JR, Deleris G (2002) Biochemical aspects of overtraining in endurance sports: a review. Sports Med 32:867–878
50. Mullington JM, Chan JL, Van Dongen HP, Szuba MP, Samaras J, Price NJ, Meier-Ewert HK, Dinges DF, Mantzoros CS (2003) Sleep loss reduces diurnal rhythm amplitude of leptin in healthy men. J Neuroendcrinol 15:851–854
51. Lord GM, Matarese G, Howard JK, Baker RJ, Bloom SR, Lechler RI (1998) Leptin modulates the T-cell immune response and reverses starvation-induced immunosuppression. Nature 394:897–901
52. Najib S, Sanchez-Margalet V (2002) Human leptin promotes survival of human circulating blood monocytes prone to apoptosis by activation of p42/44 MAPK pathway. Cell Immunol 220:143–149
53. Taylor A, Castell LM (2006) Leptin and incidence of minor illness at different body mass indices. Oxford Nutrition Group Meeting, October 2006, Proceedings
54. Gleeson M (2000) Mucosal immune responses and risk of respiratory illness. Exerc Immunol Rev 6:5–42
55. Mackinnon LT, Hooper S (1994) Mucosal (secretory) immune system responses to exercise of varying intensity and during overtraining. Int J Sports Med 15:S179–183
56. Klentrou P, Cieslak T, MacNeil M, Vintinner A, Plyley M (2002) Effect of moderate exercise on salivary immunoglobulin A and infection risk in humans. Eur J Appl Physiol 87:153–158
57. Rylander R (1968) Pulmonary defence mechanisms to airborne bacteria. Acta Physiol Scand 72: Suppl. 306, 6–85
58. Niinimaa V, Cole P, Mintz S, Shephard RJ (1980) The switching point from nasal to oronasal breathing. Respir Physiol 42:61–71
59. Niinimaa V (1983) Oronasal airway choice during running. Respir Physiol 53:129–133
60. Muns G, Singer P, Wolf F, Rubinstein I (1995) Impaired nasal mucociliary clearance in long-distance runners. Int J Sports Med 16:209–213
61. Dantzer R (2004) Cytokine-induced sickness behaviour: a neuroimmune response to activation of innate immunity. Eur J Pharmacol 500:399–411
62. Uhlig T, Kallus KW (2005) The brain: a psychoneuroimmunological approach. Curr Opinion Anaesth 18:147–150
63. Pedersen BK, Febbraio M (2005) Muscle-derived interleukin-6. A possible link between skeletal muscle, adipose tissue, liver and brain. Brain Behav Immun 19:371–376
64. Nybo L, Nielsen B, Pedersen BK, Moller K, Secher NH (2002) Interleukin-6 release from the human brain during prolonged exercise. J Physiol 542:991–995
65. Cannon JG, Kluger MJ (1983) Endogenous pyrogen activity in human plasma after exercise. Science 220:617–619
66. Suzuki K, Nakaji S, Yamada M, Totsuka M, Sato K, Sugawara K (2002) Systemic inflammatory response to exhaustive exercise. Cytokine kinetics. Ex Immunol Rev 8:6–48
67. Carmichael MD, Davis JM, Murphy EA, Brown AS, Carson JA, Mayer EP, Ghaffar A. Role of brain IL-1β on fatigue after exercise-induced muscle damage. Am J Physiol Regul Integr Comp Physiol 291:R1344–R1348
68. Fox KR (1999) The influence of physical activity on mental well-being. Public Health Nutr 2:411–418

69. Dimeo F, Bauer M, Varahram I, Proest G, Halter U (2001) Benefits from aerobic exercise in patients with major depression: a pilot study. Br J Sports Med 35:114–117
70. Galper DI, Trivedi MH, Barlow CE, Dunn AL, Kampert JB (2006) Inverse association between physical inactivity and mental health in men and women. Med Sci Sports Exerc 38:173–178
71. Hooper SL, Mackinnon LT, Howard A, Gordon RD, Bachmann AW (1995) Markers for monitoring overtraining and recovery. Med Sci Sports Exerc 27:106–112
72. Dimitriou L, Castell LM (2004) Possible immunodepression in military personnel undertaking twelve weeks training. Proceedings, 9th European Coll Sports Sci Congress, Clermont-Ferrand, July, 2004
73. Kiecolt-Glaser JK, Glaser R, Strain EC, Stout JC, Tarr KL, Holliday JE, Speicher CE (1986) Modulation of cellular immunity in medical students. J Behav Med 9:5–21
74. Kiecolt-Glaser JK, Glaser R (2002) Depression and immune function: central pathways to morbidity and mortality. J Psychosom Res 53:873–876

Exercise Fatigue

Kazuo Inoue and Tohru Fushiki

Summary

The mechanisms of the manifestation of central fatigue were studied. In the cerebrospinal fluid (CSF) from exercise-fatigued rats there was a factor that depressed the spontaneous motor activity (SMA) of the animals and caused the kind of behavior that is observed in exhausted animals. A bioassay which utilized hydra, a freshwater coelenterate, strongly suggested the existence of transforming growth factor-β (TGF-β) in the CSF. Because the immunoneutralizing treatment of the CSF from fatigued rats with anti-TGF-β antibody eliminated the factor that depresses the SMA of animals, the identity of this factor was shown to be TGF-β. The findings that the intracisternal administration of purified TGF-β depressed the SMA in a dose-dependent manner, and that the concentration of TGF-β in the CSF increased with an increase in the intensity of the exercise which was being used to cause fatigue, supported the speculation that this factor was responsible for the manifestation of central fatigue. In addition, we also demonstrated that TGF-β acted on the brain and modulated the activities of neurons, and that this changed the whole body metabolism to utilize more fat and enhanced the oxidation of fatty acid.

Introduction

In the study of exercise fatigue, some mechanisms, such as the decrease in the contractile force of skeletal muscles and the decline in performance with the reduction of the energy substrate store, are relatively well understood. In comparison, the mechanisms of the manifestation of the central component of exercise fatigue, in other words, a feeling of fatigue during exercise, has not yet been elucidated. Because feelings of fatigue during exercise are usually manifest long before the

Laboratory of Nutrition Chemistry, Division of Food Science and Biotechnology, Graduate School of Agriculture, Kyoto University, Kitashirakawa Oiwake-cho, Sakyo-ku, Kyoto 606-8502, Japan

body's physical limit is reached, the central component of exercise fatigue is thought to be the type of signal that alerts the body to the possibility of physical impairment by continuing that exercise. It would be very interesting if this kind of feeling of fatigue is generated by the same mechanism which produces similar sensations after suffering from lack of exercise or strong psychological stress. This section describes the involvement of transforming growth factor-β (TGF-β) (one of the cytokines) in the brain, with the manifestation of a feeling of fatigue.

Hypotheses of the Generation Mechanisms of Central Fatigue

Some hypotheses have already been proposed concerning the generation mechanisms of central fatigue. The most well known of these is the serotonin hypothesis [1]. Serotonin (5-hydroxy tryptamine) is abundant in the digestive system. In addition, this substance functions as a neurotransmitter in the central nervous system. The serotonergic nervous system is known to have many important roles in the brain. The precursor of serotonin is tryptophan, a type of amino acid. The rate-limiting step of serotonin synthesis in the brain is a supply of tryptophan into the brain. Serum albumin is a carrier of hydrophobic substances in the blood. Tryptophan is associated with, and transported by, serum albumin. Nonesterified fatty acids are also carried by serum albumin. With endurance exercise, fatty acids are recruited from fat tissues, their concentrations increase, and more fatty acids bind to serum albumin. Consequently, tryptophan molecules are excluded from the albumin, and the concentrations of "free" tryptophan in the blood increase. During similar exercise, branched-chain amino acids are utilized as energy sources and their concentrations decrease. The uptake of branched-chain amino acids into the brain is mediated by the L-system, one of the amino acid transporter systems. The uptake system for serotonin is the same L-system, and therefore the incorporations of these amino acids are in competition with one another. The increase in the concentration of free tryptophan and decrease in branched-chain amino acids will facilitate the synthesis rate of serotonin in the brain. The serotonin hypothesis ascribes the manifestation of a feeling of fatigue to the increase in serotonin synthesis and consequent elevation of the activities of serotonergic neurons [2,3]. Another hypothesis is based on ammonia. During an endurance exercise, which causes depletion of the energy store in the body, proteins in the body will be degraded and utilized as energy sources in the form of amino acids. Ammonia produced by the deamination of amino acids is toxic to neurons [4,5], and this will cause a feeling of fatigue. These two hypotheses are based on the substances derived from peripheral tissues. However, exercise which causes an increase in the concentrations of free fatty acids and ammonia would be long and strenuous. Therefore, this hypothesis may not be adequate to explain the mechanism of a manifestation of a feeling of fatigue in normal people who are not engaged in such strenuous exercise.

Many cytokines, e.g., interferon and interleukin, are used in cancer therapy. Serious tiredness is known to be a side effect caused by the administration of these cytokines. These cytokines are members of the defense system of the body, and are thought to be involved with fatigue during a cold or during an influenza virus infection. Because some cytokines are reported to be released during exercise [6], further elucidation is necessary about the contribution of cytokines to the manifestation of fatigue during exercise. The relation between proinflammatory cytokines and a feeling of fatigue is described in the chapter by T. Katafuchi in this volume.

Manifestation of Central Fatigue and TGF-β in the Brain

The mechanisms of the generation of a feeling of fatigue described above are based on an extended period of exercise or an infection. Therefore, a different mechanism could be assumed in the feeling of "ordinary" fatigue which is felt in daily life without intense exercise or infection.

The Presence of a Factor that Generates Central Fatigue

An experiment for the detection of a factor which causes central fatigue was conducted according to the working hypothesis described below.

1. The factor is produced in the brain, acts on the brain, and generates a feeling of fatigue.
2. The chemical activity in the brain is reflected to a certain extent in the cerebrospinal fluid (CSF). Therefore, the factor which generates a feeling of fatigue might be detected in the CSF.
3. Physical exercise could be used to generate a feeling of fatigue. Physical (peripheral) fatigue and central fatigue are inseparable, and both types of fatigue occur simultaneously in a certain ratio from any kind of load. When we exercise, we usually feel fatigue some time before reaching our physical limitations, and then we stop the exercise. This type of sensation is assumed to be a component of central fatigue.
4. When we are tired, we are unwilling to do anything voluntarily. A similar sensation can be reconstructed in experimental animals, and could be estimated by measuring their spontaneous motor activities.

Therefore, CSF was collected from rats which were exhausted by swimming. One period of exercise consisted of swimming for 15 min in a continuous-current pool and 5 min rest. Eight periods of exercise were recorded. The CSF collected was administered to the cisterna magna of a mouse. The spontaneous motor activities of mice which were given CSF from exercise-fatigued rats gradually decreased, and were significantly lower than those of mice given CSF from sedentary rats as a control (Fig. 1). This indicates the presence of a factor in the CSF from rats which

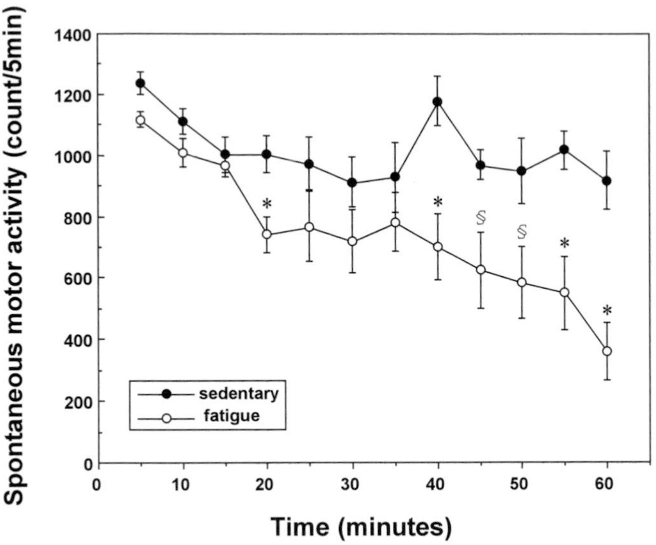

Fig. 1. Depression of spontaneous motor activity of mice by intracisternal administration of cerebrospinal fluid (CSF) from exercise-fatigued rats. The changes in spontaneous motor activity of mice which were administered CSF from exercise-fatigued rats (Fatigued) and mice administered CSF from sedentary control rats (Sedentary) are shown. Significant decreases are seen in the Fatigue group. Values are means ± SEM. Number of mice in each group, 11. §, $P < 0.05$; *, $P < 0.01$

were fatigued by exercise which depresses the spontaneous motor activity of mice [7]. This factor was heat-inactivated and had a relatively high molecular mass, as determined from the study using ultrafiltration. These results indicate that the factor we found was not caused by a classical neurotransmitter.

Identification of the Activities Which Cause Central Fatigue

Hydra Bioassay

We tried to identify the factor which depresses the spontaneous motor activity of mice. However, a standard identification by the usual protein–chemical methods was difficult for this sample because CSF is a dilute solution and its volume is limited. Therefore, a bioassay system using hydra, a fresh water coelenterate, was adopted for the detection and identification of trace amounts of bioactive substances. This system has been shown to be suitable, especially for the detection of bioactive peptides and proteins [8–10]. A hydra catches plankton for food with its tentacles, swallows the plankton, and then changes into a ball-like shape designated a tentacle ball. Tentacle ball formation is a reaction to food intake by hydra, and they take in only live plankton. They discover whether what they catch with their tentacles is edible or not by detecting a reduced form of glutathione, which is contained only in living cells.

Tentacle-ball formation can be induced by adding the reduced form of glutathione to the medium where hydra are cultured. Interestingly, the simultaneous addition of bioactive peptides inhibits tentacle-ball formation under these artificial feeding conditions. Individual bioactive peptides show the strongest inhibition of tentacle-ball formation at a specific concentration of glutathione. Therefore, determination of the inhibitory pattern of tentacle-ball formation at 0.1, 0.3, 3.0, 10, and 50 μM glutathione could detect, and at least partially identify, the presence of a certain peptide in an unknown sample by checking the profile against those which have already been determined. In addition, the inhibition usually occurs with trace amounts of bioactive peptide, and therefore this assay was suitable for the identification of a substance in a dilute sample such as CSF. CSF from exercise-fatigued rats showed a characteristic pattern which inhibits tentacle-ball formation at all concentrations of glutathione in a hydra bioassay. This reaction was known to be caused by transforming growth factor-β (TGF-β). The reaction pattern of the CSF from sedentary rats added with purified TGF-β was similar to that of the CSF from exercise-fatigued rats. This result suggested that there was an increase in the concentration of TGF-β in the CSF from exercise-fatigued rats (Fig. 2) [11–14].

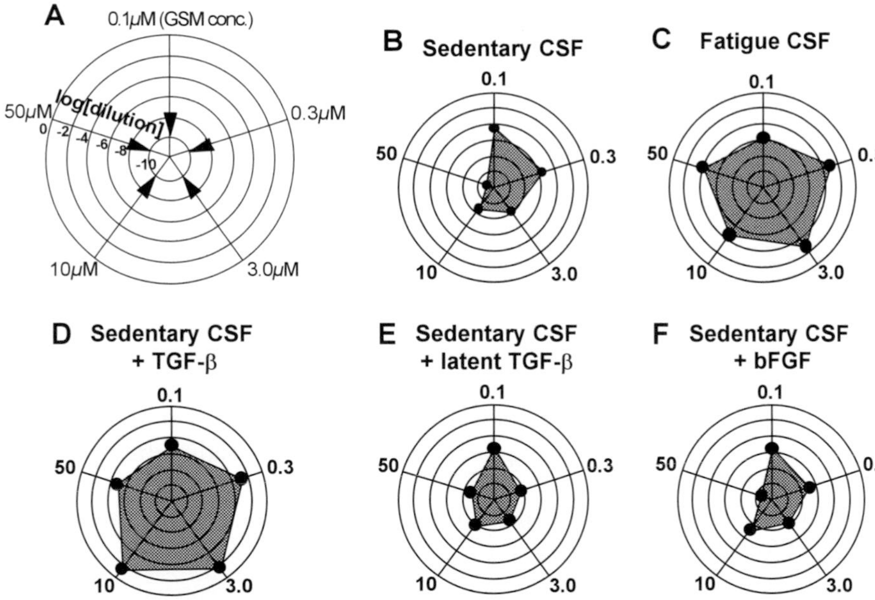

Fig. 2. Response patterns of the hydra bioassay. The patterns of hydra response are shown as the concentrations of reduced glutathione indicated. Higher values in the inner concentric circle mean a stronger inhibitory effect on the hydra feeding response by a substance in the sample. The patterns of **C** (CSF from fatigued rats) and **D** (CSF from sedentary rats with added TGF-β) are similar

Transforming Growth Factor-β (TGF-β)

TGF-β was found to be a factor which transforms certain types of cells and promotes their proliferation. Further studies elucidated that this factor not only promotes cell growth but also inhibits cell growth, depending on the type of cell and the stage of differentiation, and is a multifunctional factor which has a variety of effects. In addition, TGF-β is considered to be a type of cytokine which has a role in information transmission among cells. In the course of the biosynthesis of TGF-β, it is synthesized as a preproprotein, cleaved in the molecule, and secreted in an associated form, which is a complex of an N-terminal fragment and a C-terminal fragment. The N-terminal fragment masks the bioactive C-terminal fragment, which is TGF-β itself, and functions to retain the molecule in an inactive latent form. Therefore, the N-terminal part is called a latency-associated protein (LAP).

TGF-β is a homodimer and is covalently bonded by intermolecular disulfide. In addition, it forms a conformation with intramolecular disulfide, which is called a cysteine knot.

The activity of TGF-β is regulated at two steps, i.e., the level of protein expression and the activation of the latent form. The latent form of TGF-β is activated by the elimination of LAP by certain mechanisms. Five isoforms of TGF-β have been reported, and TGF-β1, 2, and 3 are present in mammals. The similarity of the amino acid sequences of these isoforms is relatively high (70%–80%) and their bioactivities are considered to be almost the same. TGF-β has an important role in morphogenesis during development, and gene-targeted mice of each isoform each show a specific characteristic phenotype [15–17].

Measurement of the Concentration of TGF-β in CSF

After the hydra bioassay, the concentrations of TGF-β in the CSF from exercise-fatigued rats and from sedentary control rats were determined. The determination was based on the inhibitory activity of TGF-β on the proliferation of mink lung epithelial cells (Mv1Lu), which is measured by the incorporation of tritium-labeled thymidine into the DNA. The concentration of the active form of TGF-β in the CSF from fatigued rats was significantly higher than that from sedentary rats (Table 1). However, the concentrations of total TGF-β which is the sum of the active and latent forms of TGF-β from both groups, were not significantly different. These data suggest that the increase in the concentration of active TGF-β in the CSF from fatigued rats was not the result of protein synthesis, but the activation of an existing but latent form of TGF-β [11].

Immunoneutralization of TGF-β in CSF

The responsibility of TGF-β for the depression of spontaneous motor activity in animals was then investigated. Immunoneutralization was conducted by treating

Table 1. Concentration of TGF-β in cerebrospinal fluid (CSF) from sedentary and exercise-fatigued rats

	Sedentary	Fatigued
Active TGF-β (pg/ml)	145.8 ± 11.1	270.5 ± 7.3*
Total TGF-β (pg/ml)	1028 ± 46.1	1123 ± 60.7

The concentration of the active form of TGF-β in the CSF is shown as active TGF-β. The sum of the concentrations of active and latent TGF-β was determined after the activation of latent form by a temporal acidification of CSF, and is shown as total TGF-β
Fatigued, CSF from exercise-fatigued rats; sedentary, CSF from sedentary control rats
Values are means ± SEM
Number of rats in each group, 12

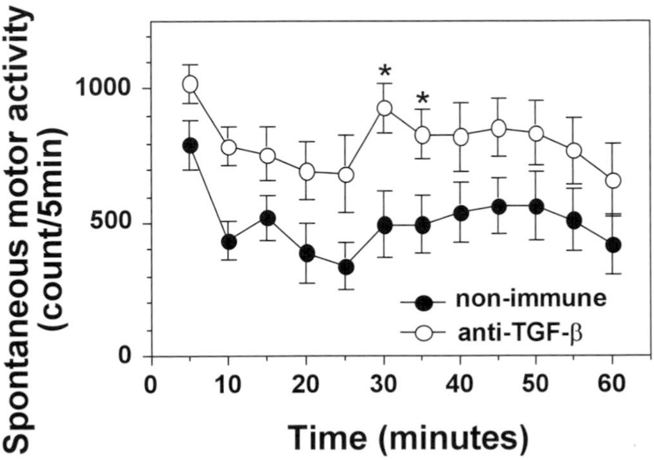

Fig. 3. Elimination of the inhibitory effect on spontaneous motor activity by treatment with anti-TGF-β antibody. A substance which depressed the spontaneous motor activities of mice was eliminated by treating CSF from fatigued rats with anti-TGF-β antibody. The depressive effects on the spontaneous motor activities of mice were retained when the same procedure was followed with preimmune antibody. Values are means ± SEM. Number of mice in each group, 14. §, $P < 0.05$; *, $P < 0.01$

the CSF from fatigued rats with anti-TGF-β antibody. The CSF from fatigued rats was pooled and divided into two fractions. One fraction was treated with preimmune antibody and the other was treated with anti-TGF-β antibody. This treated CSF was intracisternally administered to mice, and the depressive effect on their spontaneous motor activity was determined. The CSF treated with preimmune antibody retained its depressive effect on spontaneous motor activity, but the spontaneous motor activities of mice which were administered the CSF treated with anti-TGF-β antibody were significantly higher than those of mice administered preimmune antibody. The depressive effect which the CSF originally possessed was eliminated by treatment with anti-TGF-β antibody (Fig. 3). This result demonstrates that the substance in the CSF from fatigued rats which is responsible for

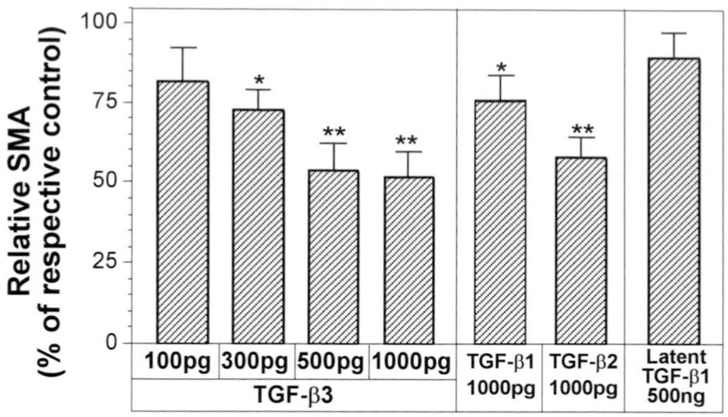

Fig. 4. Dose-dependent depression of spontaneous motor activity (*SMA*) by TGF-β. The relation between the inhibitory effect on spontaneous motor activity and the dosage of TGF-β was examined by intracisternal administration of TGF-β to mice. The spontaneous motor activities were expressed as a percentage of those in the control group, which was administered with vehicle. Spontaneous motor activity was depressed in a dose-dependent manner. Each isoform of TGF-β showed a depressive effect on spontaneous motor activity, but latent TGF-β had no such effect

the depression of spontaneous motor activity is TGF-β [11]. The intracisternal administration of purified TGF-β also caused dose-dependent depression of the spontaneous motor activities of mice (Fig. 4).

Correlation with Exercise Intensity

The relationship between the intensity of the exercise taken by rats and the concentrations of TGF-β in their CSF, and the effects of that CSF on the spontaneous motor activities of mice were investigated. Thus the positive correlation between exercise intensity and the concentration of active TGF-β in the CSF was demonstrated. In addition, a similar positive correlation between the concentration of TGF-β in the CSF and the depressive effect on the spontaneous motor activities of mice was also confirmed when the mice were intracisternally administered CSF (Fig. 5). These results also support the involvement of TGF-β in the CSF in the decrease in spontaneous motor activities, probably because TGF-β would generate a sensation of fatigue [11].

Involvement with Fatigue Caused by Loads Other than Exercise

The involvement of TGF-β with the manifestation of a feeling of fatigue caused by loads other than exercise was then investigated. As described in the section on the cytokine hypothesis, central fatigue can also be caused by infection. An administration of double-stranded RNA (poly I:C) was used for the animal model of

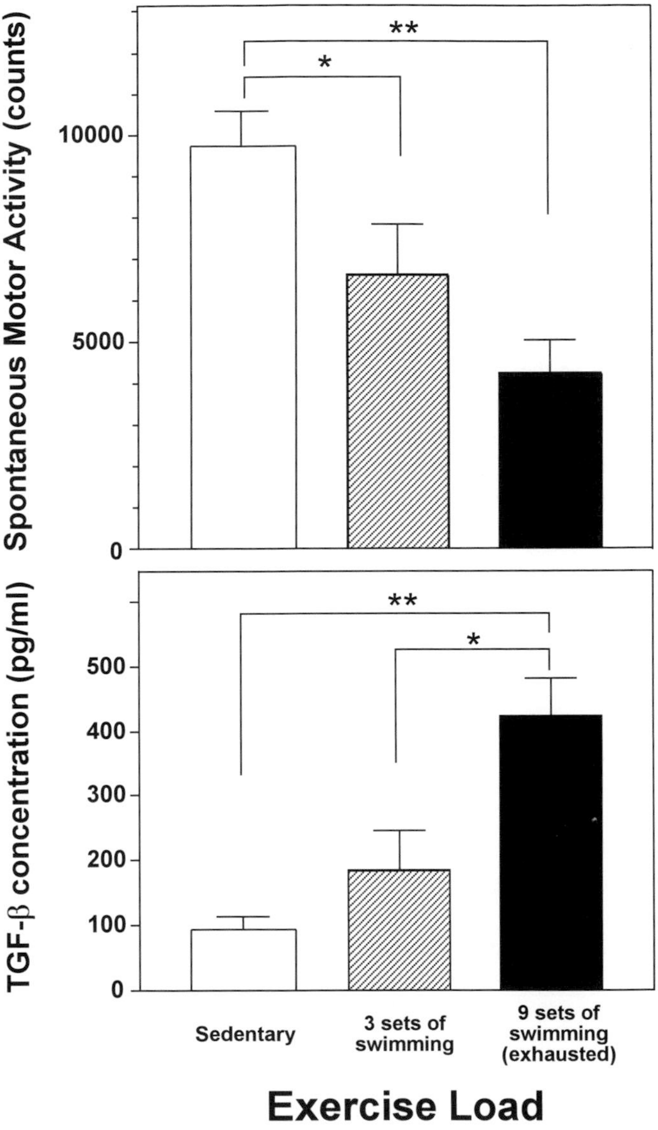

Fig. 5. Correlation between the intensity of the exercise load and the concentration of TGF-β in CSF, and its depressive effect on spontaneous motor activity. A correlation was observed between the intensity of the exercise load and the concentration of active TGF-β in the CSF of rats. The intracisternal administration of CSF with a high concentration of active TGF-β to mice showed a similar relation. The CSF from rats which had carried out intense exercise had a more depressive effect on the spontaneous motor activity of mice. Values are means ± SEM. **, $P < 0.05$; *, $P < 0.01$

infection. Poly I:C, which is administered intraperitoneally, is recognized as a virus and causes a series of defense responses, including fever and a decrease in spontaneous motor activity. An administration of poly I:C to a rat caused a decrease in its spontaneous motor activity about 2 h later, and a rise in body temperature which peaked 2–3 h after that. In this condition, the concentration of TGF-β in the CSF had increased significantly 1 h after the administration of poly I:C (data not shown; Matsumura et al., in preparation). This indicates the possibility of the involvement of TGF-β with the manifestation of a feeling of fatigue with infection. If the body is in an infected condition, a decrease in physical activity would be advantageous for recovery, and for this reason spontaneous motor activity would be suppressed and the appetite would also be inhibited. It is of interest that TGF-β in the brain might be related to these physiological responses. In addition, an increase in the concentration of TGF-β in the CSF was observed in the constraint stress of rats (Ishikawa et al., unpublished results 2004). This suggests that the generation of central fatigue by TGF-β in the brain may relate not only to the manifestation of a feeling of fatigue during exercise, but also to those feelings caused by loads other than physical exercise.

Demonstrations of the Effects of TGF-β on the Activities of the Brain

There has been no report that TGF-β modulates the activities of the brain and affects the behavior of animals except for our data. After the intracisternal administration of TGF-β, the effect causing the fatigue-like behavior has a relatively short duration. This may not imply that this response is associated with gene expression and protein synthesis. A sensation like central fatigue could be generated through changes in brain activity. Therefore, the actual effect of TGF-β on the brain was investigated neurochemically. When the activity of a neuronal cell (neuron) changes, the release of neurotransmitters from that neuron will change. After the release of neurotransmitters, most of them will be recycled by their specific transporters, but some of them will leak from the synaptic cleft into extracellular space. The modulation of neuronal activities can be determined by measuring the changes in the extracellular concentrations of neurotransmitters. Microdialysis is a method that utilizes a probe equipped with a very small dialysis membrane at its tip. A microdialysis probe is implanted in the location of interest in the brain, and dialysate from a free-moving animal is collected and analyzed with respect to changes in the concentration of neurotransmitters. Changes in the concentrations of serotonin, dopamine, and noradrenaline in some locations in the brain after the intracisternal administration of TGF-β were investigated by microdialysis. The intracisternal administration of TGF-β was shown to cause an increase in the concentration of serotonin in the hippocampus, an increase in the concentrations of serotonin and noradrenaline (Fig. 6) in the ventromedial nucleus of the hypothalamus, and a decrease in the concentration of serotonin in the lateral hypothalamic area

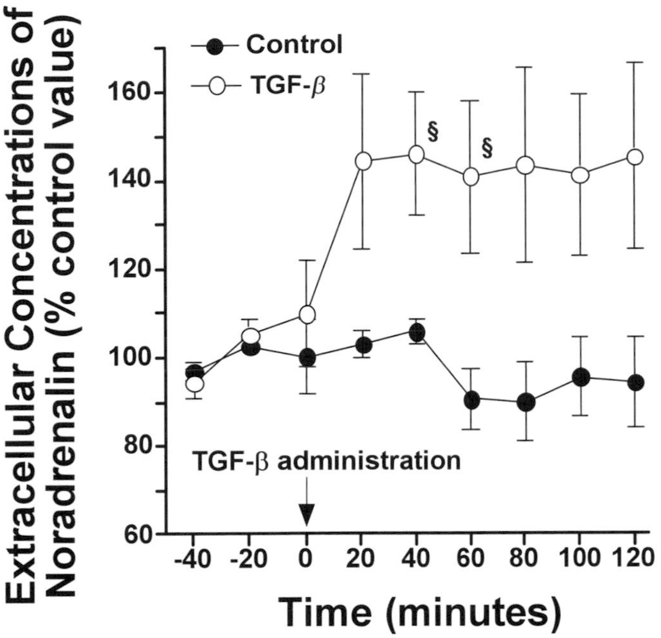

Fig. 6. An example of the effect of TGF-β on the brain: modulation of noradrenergic neurons in the ventromedial nucleus of the hypothalamus (VMH). The extracellular concentration of noradrenaline in the VMH was determined by microdialysis. A significant increase in noradrenaline was observed after the intracisternal administration of TGF-β to rats. Values are means ± SEM. Number of rats in each group, 10. §, $P < 0.05$

(Fujikawa et al., in preparation). In addition to the data from microdialysis, the effects of the intracisternal administration of TGF-β on the changes in the turnover rate of neurotransmitters in brain tissues and on an electroencephalogram [18] were demonstrated. These results clearly indicate that TGF-β in the brain acts on neurons and modulates brain activity.

Effect of TGF-β in the Brain on Energy Metabolism

Central Fatigue and Energy Metabolism

In conditions where central fatigue occurs, the activity of the substance causing it cannot always be stopped at will. In the case of a wild animal, when it is being chased by a predator, a cessation of escape behavior by reason of a manifestation of the feeling of fatigue will lead to a life disaster. When a feeling of fatigue manifests itself, stopping the physical exercise ought to be less hazardous for the body. If an animal cannot stop the exercise for any reason, it is natural that its body will respond in a way that will minimize the impairment. If the exercise is expected to persist for a long time, it is advantageous to change the body's metabolism to a rate which is suitable for endurance exercise. It is reasonable, and most likely, that the factor which causes central fatigue is also a metabolic modulator.

Effect of Intracisternal Administration of TGF-β on Energy Metabolism

A determination of the respiratory exchange ratio (RER, also known as the respiratory quotient, RQ) was used to estimate the whole body metabolism. RER is the ratio of oxygen consumption from inspiration to carbon dioxide production in expiration. This value shows what metabolic fuels are being oxidized in the body. The intracisternal administration of TGF-β to sedentary rats decreased their RER (Fig. 7), and the ratio of fat oxidization was increased (Fig. 8) [19]. There was no significant change in the oxygen consumption, which meant no change in the energy expenditure. This result indicates that intracisternal administrations of TGF-β not only depress spontaneous motor activity, but also enhance fat metabolism [19].

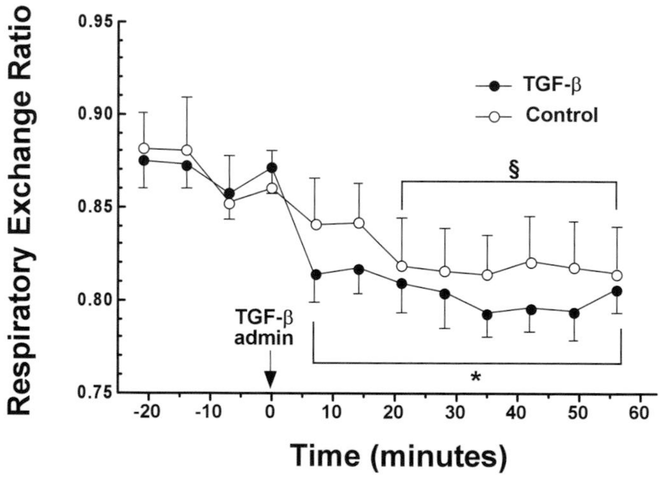

Fig. 7. The decrease in the respiratory exchange ratio (RER) after the intracisternal administration of TGF-β to rats. Changes in RER and oxygen consumption were measured after the intracisternal administration of TGF-β to rats. Although the RER gradually decreased in the control group because of food deprivation during the measurements, a greater decrease was observed shortly after the intracisternal administration of TGF-β. Values are means ± SEM. Number of rats in the control group, 10; number of rats in the TGF-β group, 11. *, $P < 0.01$; §, $P < 0.05$

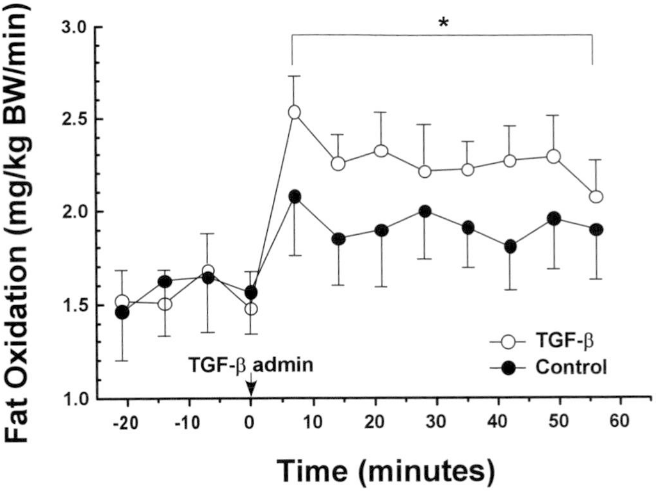

Fig. 8. The increase in fatty acid oxidization by the intracisternal administration of TGF-β to rats. The value of fatty acid oxidization was calculated from measurements of RER and oxygen consumption. Significant increases in fatty acid oxidization were observed after the intracisternal administration of TGF-β, even in a sedentary condition. Values are means ± SEM. Number of rats in the control group, 10; number of rats in the TGF-β group, 11. *, $P < 0.01$

Mechanism of Enhancing Fatty Acid Oxidization

A determination of the concentration of energy substrates in the blood was conducted on rats administered TGF-β. An increase in the concentration of nonesterified fatty acids was observed in the group intracisternally administered TGF-β, but there was no significant difference in the concentration of glucose between the control group and the TGF-β-administered group. In addition, no changes were observed in the concentrations of hormones such as insulin and adrenalin in the blood. Therefore, the effects of intracisternal administration of TGF-β were considered to be caused via the autonomic nervous system [19]. Organs such as skeletal muscles and liver are important for the execution of physical exercise. To elucidate the mechanism of the enhancement of fat metabolism by the intracisternal administration of TGF-β, its effect on the concentration of malonyl-CoA, which is a key substance for fat metabolism in these organs, was investigated. The intracisternal administration of TGF-β to rats caused a decrease in the concentration of malonyl-CoA in the hind leg muscles and the liver, and this partially explained the mechanism of TGF-β in the brain increasing the fat metabolism in the whole body (Shibakusa et al., in preparation).

Conclusion

Central fatigue is considered to be a sensation that alarms the body to the possibility of impairment as well as a sensation of pain. A manifestation of the feeling of fatigue has been considered to be caused by an increase in the concentration of serotonin in the brain. We found a mechanism which causes central fatigue by the presence of TGF-β in the brain, and which seems to be independent from the mechanism causing an increase in brain serotonin. The increase in the concentration of TGF-β in the brain was observed not only during physical exercise, but also during infection and from stress caused by constraint. In addition, a similar increase in TGF-β in CSF from patients with chronic fatigue syndrome has been reported [20,21]. These data strongly suggest a relationship between TGF-β in the brain and the generation of central fatigue. It is also of interest, and considered to be reasonable, that a substance which causes central fatigue is simultaneously involved with modulation of the energy metabolism of the whole body. This suggests the regulation of the energy metabolism during exercise by the central nervous system, and is considered to be part of the integrated regulation of the overall energy metabolism.

Acknowledgments. This work is a collaboration between the members of the Laboratory of Nutrition Chemistry, Kyoto University, Chiaki Fukuda, Hanae Aketa-Yamazaki, Yasuko Manabe, Masanao Arai, Muneo Nagoya, Seiko Uesaki, Shigenobu Matsumura, Teturo Shibakusa, Yuki Okabe, Wataru Mizunoya, Teppei Fujikawa, Toma Ishikawa, Prof. Kazumitsu Hanai of Kyoto Prefectural University of Medicine, and Prof. Toshihiko Iwanaga of Hokkaido University Faculty of Medicine, and the authors express sincere gratitude to them.

References

1. Newsholme EA, Acworth IN, Blomstrand E (1987) Amino acids, brain neurotransmitters and a functional link between muscle and brain that is important in sustained exercise. In: Benzi G (ed) Advances in myochemistry. John Libbey Eurotext, London, pp 127–133
2. Blomstrand E, Perrett D, Parry-Billings M, Newsholme EA (1989) Effect of sustained exercise on plasma amino acid concentrations and on 5-hydroxytryptamine metabolism in six different brain regions in the rat. Acta Physiol Scand 136:473–481
3. Yamamoto T, Newsholme EA (2000) Diminished central fatigue by inhibition of the L-system transporter for the uptake of tryptophan. Brain Res Bull 52:35–38
4. Lin S, Raabe W (1985) Ammonia intoxication: effects on cerebral cortex and spinal cord. J Neurochem 44:1252–1258
5. Raabe W, Lin S (1985) Pathophysiology of ammonia intoxication. Exp Neurol 87:519–532
6. Inoue K, Fushiki T (2003) Exercise and central fatigue. Korean J Exercise Nutr 7:227–233
7. Inoue K, Yamazaki H, Manabe Y, Fukuda C, Fushiki T (1998) Release of a substance that suppresses spontaneous motor activity in the brain by physical exercise. Physiol Behav 64:185–190
8. Hanai K, Kato H, Matsuhashi S, Morita H, Raines EW, Ross R (1987) Platelet proteins, including platelet-derived growth factor, specifically depress a subset of the multiple components of the response elicited by glutathione in hydra. J Cell Biol 104:1675–1681

9. Hanai K, Oomura Y, Kai Y, Nishikawa K, Shimizu N, Morita H, Plata-Salaman CR (1989) Central action of acidic fibroblast growth factor in feeding regulation. Am J Physiol 256: R217–R223
10. Hanai K (1995) Potentiation of tentacle ball formation by a trypsin-like protease and accompanying augmented ingestion in glutathione-induced feeding in hydra. Zool Sci 12:185–193
11. Inoue K, Yamazaki H, Manabe Y, Fukuda C, Hanai K, Fushiki T (1999) Transforming growth factor-beta activated during exercise in brain depresses spontaneous motor activity of animals. Relevance to central fatigue. Brain Res 846:145–153
12. Manabe Y, Yamazaki H, Fukuda C, Inoue K, Fushiki T, Hanai K (2000) Determination of TGF-β-like activity in the rat cerebrospinal fluid after exhaustive exercise using anti-TGF-β IgG and the hydra bioassay. Biomed Res 21:191–196
13. Manabe Y, Yamazaki H, Fukuda C, Inoue K, Fushiki T, Hanai K (2000) Hydra biological detection of biologically active peptides in rat cerebrospinal fluid. Brain Res Protcol 5:312–317
14. Manabe Y, Yamazaki H, Fukuda C, Inoue K, Fushiki T, Hanai K (2000) Suppression of S-methylglutathione-induced tentacle ball formation by peptides and nullification of the suppression by TGF-beta in hydra. Chem Senses 25:173–180
15. Massagué J (1990) The transforming growth factor-β. Annu Rev Cell Biol 6:597–641
16. Derynck R, Feng X-H (1997) TGF-β receptor signaling. Biochim Biophys Acta 1333: F105–F150
17. Massagué J, Chen Y-G (2000) Controlling TGF-β signaling. Genes Dev 14:627–644
18. Arai M, Yamazaki H, Inoue K, Fushiki T (2002) Effects of intracranial injection of transforming growth factor-beta relevant to central fatigue on the waking electroencephalogram of rats. Comparison with effects of exercise. Prog Neuro-Psychopharmacol Biol Psychiatr 26: 307–312
19. Yamazaki H, Arai M, Matsumura S, Inoue K, Fushiki T (2002) Intracranial administration of transforming growth factor-beta 3 increases fat oxidation in rats. Am J Physiol Endocrinol Metab 283:E536–E544
20. Bennett AL, Chao CC, Hu S, Buchwald D, Fagioli LR, Schur PH, Peterson PK, Komaroff AL (1997) Elevation of bioactive transforming growth factor-beta in serum from patients with chronic fatigue syndrome. J Clin Immunol 17:160–166
21. Chao CC, Janoff EN, Hu S, Thomas K, Gallagher M, Tsang M, Peterson PK (1991) Altered cytokine release in peripheral blood mononuclear cell cultures from patients with the chronic fatigue syndrome. Cytokine 3:292–298

Mechanism of Fatigue Studied in a Newly Developed Animal Model of Combined (Mental and Physical) Fatigue

Masaaki Tanaka and Yasuyoshi Watanabe

Summary

Recently, we established an animal model of combined (mental and physical) fatigue. To make this model, we kept rats for 5 days in a cage filled with water (23 ± 1°C) to a height of 1.5 cm, and for an evaluation of the extent of fatigue, a weight-loaded forced swimming test was used. The fatigued animals showed reduced brain energy utilization as compared with the controls. Although acutely stressed rats showed increased turnover of serotonin and dopamine in the brain, the fatigued rats did not show any change in the levels of these neurotransmitters and the metabolites in the brain regions in which the synaptic terminals are abundant. Hence, decreased energy utilization induced by prolonged deprivation of rest may introduce a vicious cycle of fatigue and lead to insufficient activation of the serotonin and dopamine systems in the brain. Since the serotonin and dopamine systems are not activated properly under the condition of fatigue, the fatigue sensation and physical activity may become insufficient, and in the terminal stage, long-term deprivation of rest may lead to death (*Karoshi*). We also found that by using this animal model of fatigue, we could screen for candidates for antifatigue substances for human use.

Introduction

Recently, much attention has been paid to the phenomenon known as fatigue. However, the molecular and neuronal mechanisms of fatigue still remain unclear. One of the reasons that it is difficult to investigate the mechanisms of fatigue has

---

Department of Physiology, Osaka City University Graduate School of Medicine, 1-4-3 Asahimachi, Abeno-ku, Osaka 545-8585, Japan

been the lack of adequate animal models of fatigue except for those of acute-exercise fatigue. Another was that there have been no proper scales to evaluate the fatigue level objectively and quantitatively. Therefore, we sought to establish an animal model of fatigue, and a quantitative and objective fatigue scale, and use them to reveal the mechanism of fatigue by investigating the energy state, and also the monoamine activities in the central nervous system which have been assumed to be associated with fatigue. In addition, we tested whether this animal model could be used to screen for candidates for antifatigue substances for human use.

Establishment of an Animal Model of Fatigue

We used 7-week-old male Sprague–Dawley rats, which were housed in a controlled environment (temperature 23 ± 1°C, humidity 50% ± 5%, lights on at 08:00 hours and off at 20:00 hours). Food and water were provided ad libitum. This fatigue experiment was approved by the Animal Ethics Committee of Osaka City University (approval number 00093), and was carried out in accordance with the guidelines laid down by the National Institute of Health (NIH) in the United States regarding the care and use of animals for experimental procedures.

It is essential for the establishment of an animal model of fatigue to develop an objective and quantitative fatigue scale, and it is also necessary for the establishment of a fatigue scale to develop an animal model of fatigue. Thus, it might be difficult to establish both concomitantly. We hypothesized that animals subjected to an environment in which it was impossible to rest mentally and physically would progressively become fatigued unless they could adapt to that situation. Therefore, we previously established a rat model of fatigue in which rats were kept for several days in a cage filled with water (23 ± 1°C) to a height of 1.5 cm [1], because under such conditions they would try to avoid the water, and therefore they could not assume a resting position or sleep soundly. In practice, at best they only took a short sleep with their shoulders pressed against the side of the cage.

In order to evaluate the extent of their fatigue, the previously described weight-loaded forced swimming test was used [2], with some modifications. The rats swam with a load of steel rings that weighed approximately 8% of their body weight and were attached to their tails. The swimming time was measured from the beginning of swimming with the weights until the point at which the rats could not again return to the surface of the water 10 s after sinking. Then the animals were helped out of the water and returned to their home cage for recovery. When kept in water for various periods of time and then tested, the animals showed a significantly (except the 1-day group) and progressively shorter swimming time (Fig. 1). Thus, the swimming time with

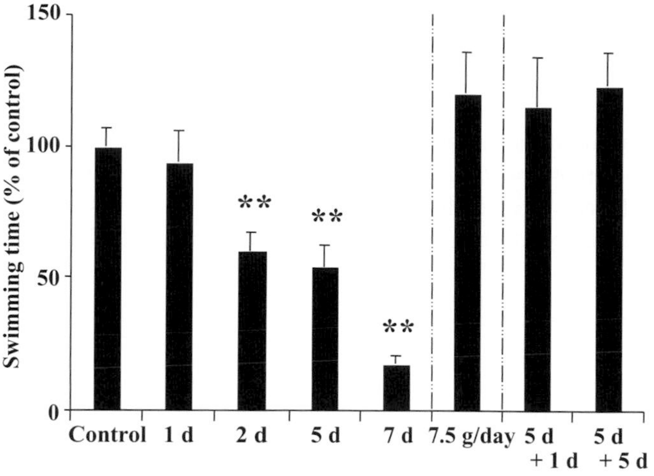

Fig. 1. Swimming time of animals. Rats were kept for 1 (*1 d*), 2 (*2 d*), 5 (*5 d*), or 7 (*7 d*) days or in a cage filled with water to a height of 1.5 cm in their home cage (*Control*). In addition to these groups, two other groups of rats were allowed to return to their home cages for 1 (*5 d + 1 d*) or 5 (*5 d + 5 d*) days after a session in water for 5 days. In addition, one group of rats was food-restricted (*7.5 g/day*) in their home cage for 5 days. The swimming time is shown as a percentage of the value for the control group. The values are mean and SEM ($n = 5$–7). $^{**}P < 0.01$ indicates significantly different from the control. (From [1], with permission)

a weight load was considered to be an appropriate scale to measure the fatigue level objectively and quantitatively. It was hard for the rats that had been immersed in water for 7 days to recover. We therefore proceeded with experiments on rats kept in water for 5 days, since these animals showed the shortest swimming time (excluding the 7-day group) and could recover. In rats, C-reactive protein is present in normal serum, and its level increases during infection. In our experiments, all rats immersed in water for 5 days showed normal values of serum C-reactive protein, indicating that no infection was present, and they did not exhibit any change in rectal temperature as compared with the corresponding control value. In addition, the 5-day sessions did not produce any gastric ulcers. The animals kept in water showed a significant decrease in body weight as compared with the control rats. As a control, food-restricted (7.5 g per day) rats showed almost the same time-course of change in body weight, but showed a significantly lower blood glucose level and almost the same serum ketone body level as the water-immersed rats (glucose, 115.5 ± 4.5 mg/dl and 143.2 ± 8.2 mg/dl (mean ± SD), respectively, $P = 0.029$; ketone, 969 ± 122 μmol/l and 643 ± 177 μmol/l (mean ± SD), respectively, $P = 0.195$). Although the food-restricted rats were at a greater disadvantage than the water-immersed rats, at least in terms of their blood level of energy substrates, they showed almost the same swimming time as the control rats. This fact indicates that the water-immersed rats were not just a model of starved animals. Also, as the rats which were immersed in water for 5 days and then returned to their home cages for 1 or 5 days showed the same swimming time as the control rats, recovery from fatigue was demonstrated, indicating that this animal model of fatigue was reversible. Hence, we established an animal model of combined (mental and physical) fatigue by keeping rats for 5 days in a cage filled with water (at 23 ± 1°C) to a height of 1.5 cm.

Brain Energy State

Fatigue can be defined physiologically as the inability to maintain power output. In order to sustain power output, it seems to be essential to maintain a sufficient energy level. The maintenance of synaptic transmission during recurrent activity involves the mobilization and recycling of synaptic vesicles [3]. These processes require ATP for their continual operation [4,5], and inhibitors of oxidative ATP production promote synaptic fatigue in crayfish motor neurons [6], indicating that reduced ATP utilization can lead to synaptic fatigue. We hypothesized that reduced energy utilization in the brain is a feature of central fatigue.

Brain glucose uptake was dramatically reduced in the fatigued rats (the glucose uptake values of the fatigued animals in the frontal cortex, hippocampus, striatum, thalamus, hypothalamus, midbrain, brainstem, and cerebellum were approximately 40% of the corresponding control values) (Table 1). Since glucose uptake into the brain was reduced, we assumed that the ATP level

Table 1. 2-[^{18}F]fluoro-2-deoxy-D-Glucose uptake (PSL/mm^2) of the control and fatigued groups (From [1], with permission)

Brain region	Control	Fatigued
Frontal cortex	1335 ± 38	489 ± 29**
Hippocampus	1003 ± 91	355 ± 52**
Striatum	1291 ± 53	492 ± 30**
Thalamus	1249 ± 50	485 ± 33**
Hypothalamus	896 ± 29	340 ± 23**
Midbrain	1063 ± 40	401 ± 24**
Brainstem	833 ± 31	330 ± 23**
Cerebellum	888 ± 46	352 ± 28**

Rats were kept for 5 days in their home cage (control) or in a cage filled with water to a height of 1.5 cm (fatigued)
Values are the mean ± SEM ($n = 5 - 6$)
** $P < 0.01$, significantly different from the control

in the brain would also be reduced in the fatigued rats. Surprisingly, however, the fatigued rats showed a slight increase in the ATP level in their brain (control, 16.9 ± 2.6 nmol/protein; fatigued, 20.0 ± 2.9 nmol/protein (mean ± SD), $P = 0.031$) [7]. In addition, cerebral blood flow was not different between the fatigued and control rats in any of the brain regions [7]. There are two possible explanations for these results. One possibility is that energy production is increased, and another is that energy utilization is reduced in the brain under the condition of fatigue.

To determine which was the case, we examined the ability of mitochondria in the brain of the fatigued rats to produce ATP. We used a novel method, "bioradiography," in which the dynamic process could be followed in living slices of the brain by use of positron-emitter labeled compounds and imaging plates. We studied the incorporation of 2-[^{18}F]fluoro-2-deoxy-D-glucose (FDG) into rat brain slices incubated in oxygenated Krebs–Ringer solution. Respiration within mitochondria occurs with 2,4-dinitrophenol (DNP) loading, but ATP is not produced, so glucose uptake increases until it compensates for the ATP production in the mitochondria, thereby reflecting the ability of mitochondria to produce ATP [8,9]. The net influx constant values of FDG were no different at the baseline, but these values were increased by DNP loading in the control and fatigued rats, and the increments of these values after DNP loading were almost equal in all the brain regions in both the fatigued and control groups [7]. These findings suggest that the glucose transporters were not functionally impaired in the fatigued rats, and that the ability of mitochondria to produce ATP was no different between the two groups. Taken together, these results suggest that energy utilization in the brain was decreased under the condition of fatigue.

Brain Monoamine Activities

In addition to the brain energy state, monoamine activities in the central nervous system are thought to be associated with central fatigue. An increase in the turnover of serotonin and dopamine in the brain has been reported to occur following exercise [10]. Quipazine (a 5-hydroxytryptamine (5-HT) agonist) caused reduced endurance performance in rats running on a treadmill, whereas LY-53,857 (a 5-HT antagonist) increased it [11]. It was also found that the swimming endurance of rats improved following the administration of amphetamine [12], and that their endurance performance was impaired following the destruction of dopaminergic neurons by 6-hydroxydopamine [13]. Thus, increased serotonin turnover has been thought to be the cause of the fatigue sensation, and endurance performance seems to depend on dopaminergic neuronal activity [14].

Although acutely stressed rats showed increased serotonin and dopamine turnover in their brain, the fatigued rats did not show any change in the levels of these neurotransmitters in the brain regions rich in serotonergic and dopaminergic

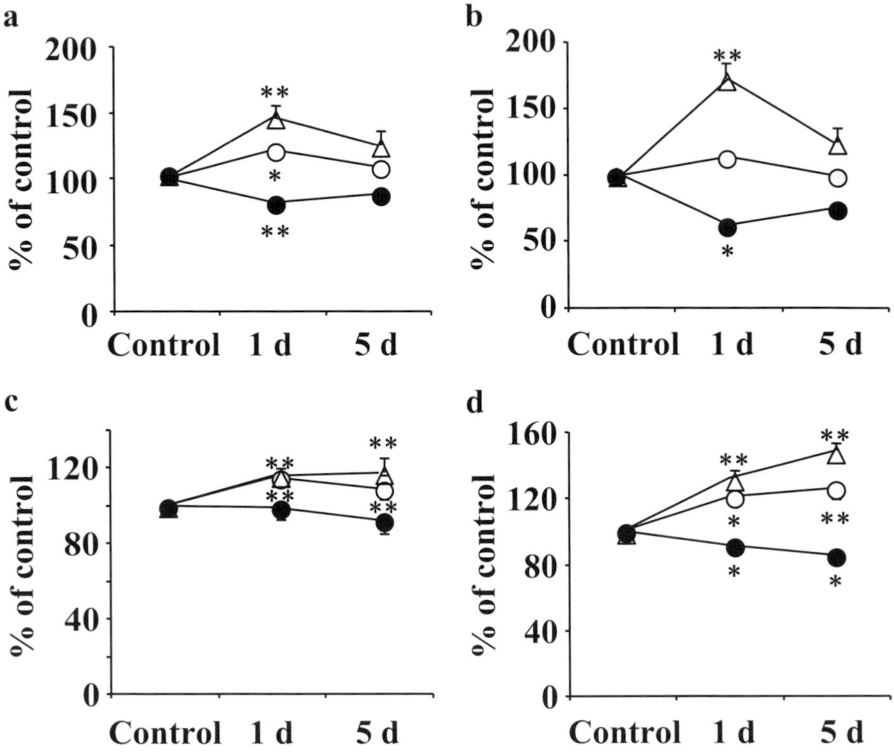

Fig. 2. Effects of fatigue on 5-HIAA and 5-HT concentrations and on the 5-HIAA/5-HT ratio in the hippocampus (**a**), hypothalamus (**b**), midbrain (**c**), and brainstem (**d**). 5-HIAA, 5-hydroxyindoleacetic acid; 5-HT, 5-hydroxytryptamine. Concentrations of 5-HIAA (*open circles*), 5-HT (*closed circles*), and 5-HIAA/5-HT ratio (*open triangles*) are shown as a percentage of the corresponding values of the control group. The values are mean and SEM ($n = 8$). $^{*}P < 0.05$, $^{**}P < 0.01$, significantly different from the control. (From [1], with permission)

synaptic terminals (Figs. 2 and 3). However, the fatigued animals did not show increased serotonin and dopamine turnover in the midbrain and brainstem, which are regions rich in the cell bodies (Figs. 2 and 3). Under the condition of fatigue, serotonin and dopamine turnover in the synaptic terminals may not be properly activated, and thus the fatigue sensation and physical activity may be insufficient. Since the maintenance of synaptic transmission requires energy [4,5], and stimulation of synaptic release and recycling of synaptic vesicles is induced through ATP receptors in the presynaptic aminergic terminals [15], insufficient serotonin and dopamine turnover in the synaptic terminals might be a consequence of the reduced energy utilization in the brain of the rest-deprived, fatigued rats.

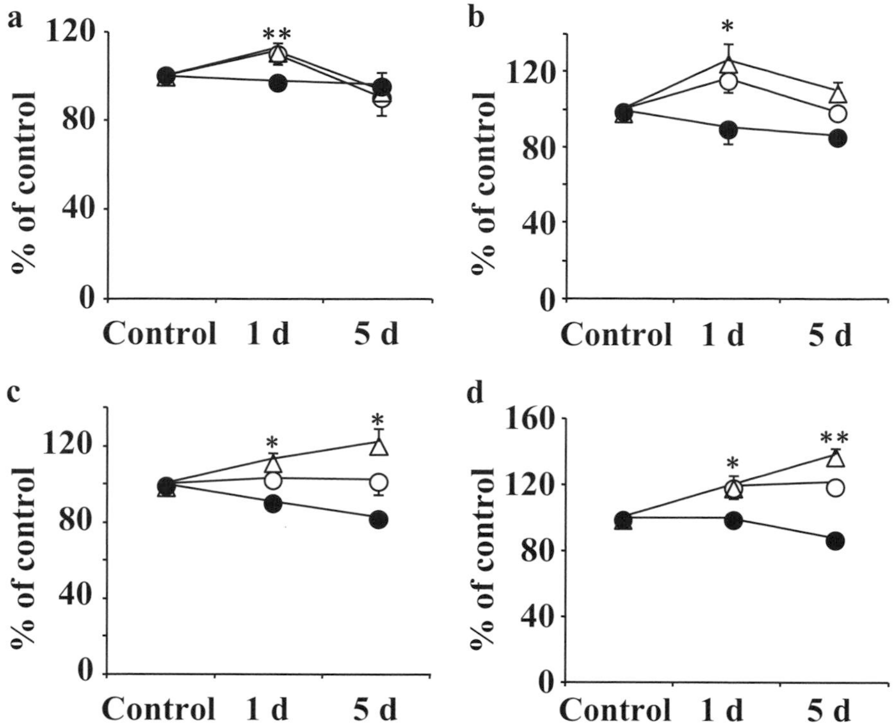

Fig. 3. Effects of fatigue on DOPAC, HVA, and DA concentrations and on the (DOPAC + HVA)/DA ratio in the striatum (**a**), hypothalamus (**b**), midbrain (**c**), and brainstem (**d**). DOPAC, 3,4-dihydroxyphenylacetic acid; HVA, homovanillic acid; DA, dopamine. Concentrations of DOPAC + HVA (*open circles*), DA (*closed circles*), and (DOPAC + HVA)/DA ratio (*open triangles*) are shown as a percentage of the corresponding values of the control group. The values are mean and SEM ($n = 8$). $^{*}P < 0.05$, $^{**}P < 0.01$, significantly different from the control. (From [1], with permission)

Hypothesis of Central Fatigue

Our hypothesis of the mechanism which is responsible for central fatigue is shown in Fig. 4. First, in the acutely stressed stage, the serotonin and dopamine systems are activated in the central nervous system. Second, in the late stage of severe fatigue, reduced neuronal activities and energy utilization induced by prolonged deprivation of rest elicit a vicious cycle of central fatigue and lead to insufficient activation of the serotonin and dopamine systems in the brain. Since the serotonin and dopamine systems are not activated properly, the fatigue sensation and physical activity are insufficient. Cytokines (e.g., transforming growth factor-β (TGF-β)) may also be correlated with central fatigue, since exercise increases active TGF-β in the brain and an intracranial injection of active TGF-β suppresses spontaneous

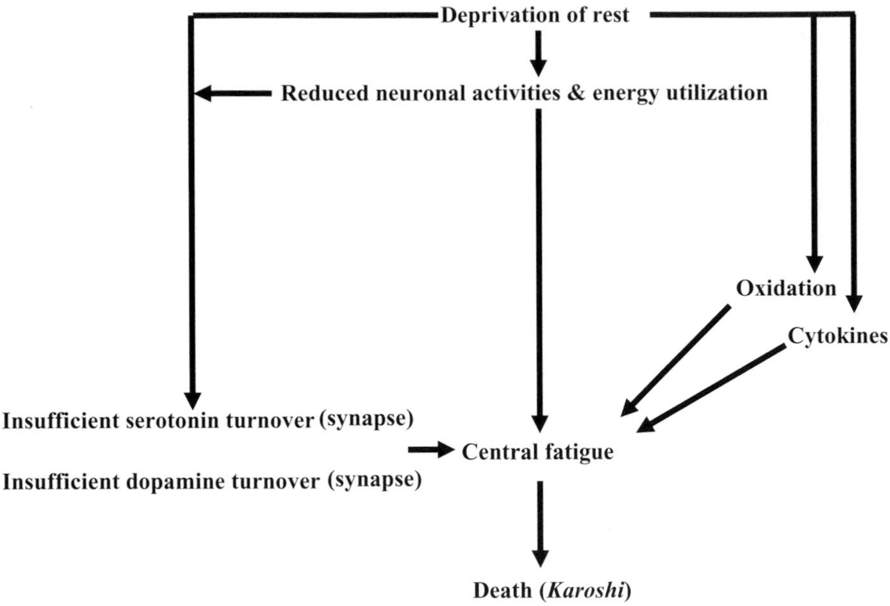

Fig. 4. Hypothesis of central fatigue. Details are given in the text

motor activity in the mouse [16]. Moreover, since stress causes oxidation in many regions of the brain [17], oxidation in the brain can be related to central fatigue. Eventually, in the terminal stage, prolonged deprivation of rest leads to death (*Karoshi*).

Antifatigue Substances

Finally, we tested the effects of various substances on fatigue by using our animal model of fatigue. Rats were injected with vehicle (saline), ascorbic acid (AsA, 300 mg/kg), dehydroepiandrosterone sulfate (DHEA-S, 10 mg/kg), or acetyl-L-carnitine (AcC, 100 mg/kg) intraperitoneally once a day for 5 days at 1000 hours. In order to evaluate the extent of fatigue, we used the weight-loaded forced swimming test. Fatigued rats injected with AsA, DHEA-S, or AcC showed longer swimming times as compared with the saline-injected, fatigued animals (Fig. 5). Therefore, AsA, DHEA-S, and AcC were useful in attenuating the level of fatigue in these animals. It has been reported that AsA [18,19], DHEA-S [20–22], and AcC [23] may be useful for the treatment of patients with chronic fatigue syndrome, a human model of severe fatigue. Therefore, by using this animal model of fatigue, we can screen for other candidates for antifatigue substances for human use.

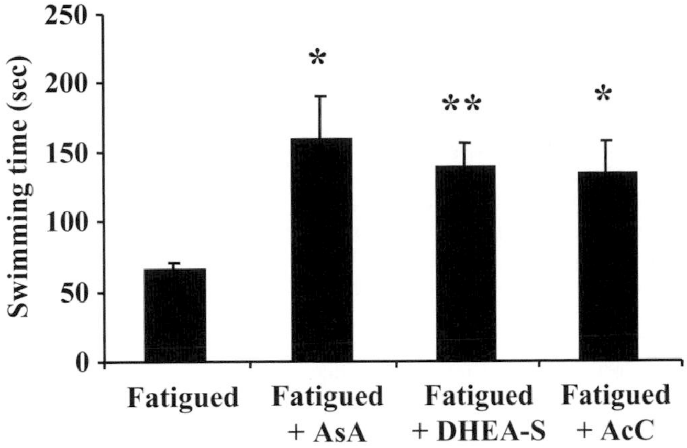

Fig. 5. Effects of ascorbic acid (AsA, 300 mg/kg), dehydroepiandrosterone sulfate (DHEA-S, 10 mg/kg), or acetyl-L-carnitine (AcC, 100 mg/kg) on the swimming time. Rats were kept in a cage filled with water to a height of 1.5 cm and injected with saline (*Fatigued*), AsA (*Fatigued + AsA*), DHEA-S (*Fatigued + DHEA-S*), or AcC (*Fatigued + AcC*) intraperitoneally once a day for 5 days. The values are mean and SEM ($n = 5$–6). *$P < 0.05$, **$P < 0.01$, significantly different from the fatigued group

Conclusions

We established an animal model of combined (mental and physical) fatigue and a fatigue scale, and clarified the mechanism (in terms of energy state and monoamine systems in the brain) that might be related to central fatigue. In addition, we demonstrated that we can screen for candidates for antifatigue substances for human use by using our animal model of fatigue.

Acknowledgments. This work was supported in part by Special Coordination Funds for Promoting Science and Technology and by the 21st Century COE Program "Base to Overcome Fatigue," from the Ministry of Education, Culture, Sports, Science and Technology, the Japanese government.

References

1. Tanaka M, Nakamura F, Mizokawa S, Matsumura A, Nozaki S, Watanabe Y (2003) Establishment and assessment of a rat model of fatigue. Neurosci Lett 352:159–162
2. Moriura T, Matsuda H, Kubo M (1996) Pharmacological study on Agkistrodon blomhoffii blomhoffii BOIE. V. anti-fatigue effect of the 50% ethanol extract in acute weight-loaded forced swimming-treated rats. Biol Pharm Bull 19:62–66
3. Heuser JE, Reese TS (1973) Evidence for recycling of synaptic vesicle membrane during transmitter release at the frog neuromuscular junction. J Cell Biol 57:315–344

4. Atwood HL, Lang F, Morin WA (1972) Synaptic vesicles: selective depletion in crayfish excitatory and inhibitory axons. Science 176:1353–1355
5. Nguyen PV, Marin L, Atwood HL (1997) Synaptic physiology and mitochondrial function in crayfish tonic and phasic motor neurons. J Neurophysiol 78:281–294
6. Llinas R, Sugimori M, Lin JWL, Leopold PL, Brady ST (1989) ATP-dependent directional movement of rat synaptic vesicles injected into the presynaptic terminal of squid giant synapse. Proc Natl Acad Sci USA 86:5656–5660
7. Tanaka M, Watanabe Y (2008) Reduced energy utilization in the brain is a feature of an animal model of fatigue. Int J Neurosci (in press)
8. Nakahara H, Kanno T, Inai Y, Utsumi K, Hiramatsu M, Mori A, Packer L (1998) Mitochondrial dysfunction in the senescence-accelerated mouse (SAM). Free Radic Biol Med 24:85–92
9. Sibille B, Ronot X, Filippi C, Nogueira V, Keriel C, Leverve X (1988) 2,4-dinitrophenol uncoupling effect on delta psi in living hepatocytes depends on reducing equivalent supply. Cytometry 32:102–108
10. Meeusen R, De-Meirleir K (1995) Exercise and brain neurotransmission. Sports Med 20:160–188
11. Bailey SP, Davis JM (1993) Serotonergic agonists and antagonists affect endurance performance in the rat. Int J Sports Med 14:330–333
12. Bhagat B, Wheeler N (1973) Effect of amphetamine on the swimming endurance of rats. Neuropharmacology 12:711–713
13. Heyes MP, Garnett ES, Coates G (1988) Nigrostriatal dopaminergic activity is increased during exhaustive exercise stress in rats. Life Sci 42:1537–1542
14. Davis LM, Bailey SP (1997) Possible mechanisms of central nervous system fatigue during exercise. Med Sci Sports Exerc 29:45–57
15. Giraldez L, Diaz-Hernandez M, Gomez-Villafuertes R, Pintor J, Castro E, Miras-Portugal MT (2001) Adenosine triphosphate and diadenosine pentaphosphate induce [Ca(2+)](i) increase in rat basal ganglia aminergic terminals. J Neurosci Res 64:174–182
16. Inoue K, Yamazaki H, Manabe Y, Fukuda C, Hanai K, Fushiki T (1999) Transforming growth factor-beta activated during exercise in brain depresses spontaneous motor activity of animals. Relevance to central fatigue. Brain Res 846:145–153
17. Liu J, Wang X, Shigenaga MK, Yeo HC, Mori A, Ames BN (1996) Immobilization stress causes oxidative damage to lipid, protein, and DNA in the brain of rats. FASEB J 10:1532–1538
18. Kodama M, Kodama T, Murakami M (1996) The value of the dehydroepiandrosterone-annexed vitamin C infusion treatment in the clinical control of chronic fatigue syndrome (CFS). II. Characterization of CFS patients with special reference to their response to a new vitamin C infusion treatment. In Vivo 10:585–596
19. Kodama M, Kodama T, Murakami M (1996) The value of the dehydroepiandrosterone-annexed vitamin C infusion treatment in the clinical control of chronic fatigue syndrome (CFS). I. A pilot study of the new vitamin C infusion treatment with a volunteer CFS patient. In Vivo 10:575–584
20. Cleare AJ, O'Keane V, Miell JP (2004) Levels of DHEA and DHEAS and responses to CRH stimulation and hydrocortisone treatment in chronic fatigue syndrome. Psychoneuroendocrinology 29:724–732
21. Scott LV, Salahuddin F, Cooney J, Svec F, Dinan TG (1999) Differences in adrenal steroid profile in chronic fatigue syndrome, in depression and in health. J Affect Disord 54:129–137
22. Kuratsune H, Yamaguti K, Sawada M, Kodate S, Machii T, Kanakura Y, Kitani T (1998) Dehydroepiandrosterone sulfate deficiency in chronic fatigue syndrome. Int J Mol Med 1:143–146
23. Vermeulen RC, Scholte HR (2004) Exploratory open label, randomized study of acetyl- and propionylcarnitine in chronic fatigue syndrome. Psychosom Med 66:276–282

Lactate Is Not a Cause of Fatigue

Masaaki Tanaka and Yasuyoshi Watanabe

Summary

For many years, it has generally been believed that the accumulations of lactate (lactic acid) in muscles and in the central nervous system are associated with peripheral and central nervous system fatigue, respectively. We conducted an overview of the roles of lactate, which have recently been clarified, under the condition of fatigue. First, the intracellular acidification of muscle caused by an accumulation of lactate has protective effects during muscle fatigue. The excitation-induced accumulation of extracellular K^+ leads action potentials to be a less effective trigger of Ca^{2+} release in working muscles, and acidification by the accumulation of lactate reduces this effect by decreasing the contribution of Cl^- channels, which act to keep the membrane potential near the Cl^- reversal potential. Since the Cl^- reversal potential is near the resting membrane potential, the effect of Cl^- channel activity is to increase the Na^+ current necessary to generate an action potential, which triggers Ca^{2+} release. Second, in the central nervous system, lactate generated in astrocytes contributes to the activity-dependent fuelling of the neuronal energy demands associated with synaptic transmission, and administered lactate can also be utilized as energy substrates. Finally, an increased blood lactate level during muscle fatigue is not associated with central fatigue. From these results, we can conclude that lactate is a favorable substrate rather than the cause of fatigue.

Introduction

For many years, it was generally believed that the accumulations of lactate (lactic acid) in muscles and in the central nervous system were associated with peripheral and central nervous system fatigue, respectively. However, the protective effects

Department of Physiology, Osaka City University Graduate School of Medicine, 1-4-3 Asahimachi, Abeno-ku, Osaka 545-8585, Japan

of lactate in muscle fatigue have now been shown. Moreover, in the brain, lactate is utilized in order to sustain the neuronal energy metabolism. Therefore, it is necessary for fatigue scientists to dismiss the false charge that lactate is a major cause of fatigue. This chapter gives an overview of the roles of lactate, which have recently been clarified, under the condition of fatigue.

Roles of Lactate During Muscle Fatigue

Fatigue can be defined as the failure to maintain the required or expected power output, and intense muscle activity leads to a decline in mechanical performance, which is known as muscle fatigue [1–4]. Contraction in a twitch skeletal muscle fiber in response to a nerve impulse is the result of a complex series of events known as excitation–contraction coupling [1]. Excitation–contraction coupling consists of (1) the initiation and propagation of an action potential along the surface membrane and into the T system, (2) activation of the voltage sensors in the tubular wall, (3) signal transmission to the sarcoplasmic reticulum from which the activation by Ca^{2+} is released, and (4) activation by Ca^{2+} of the Ca^{2+} regulatory system associated with the contractile apparatus. Therefore, muscle fatigue is caused by a decline in excitation–contraction coupling.

Hill and Kupalov [5] suggested that the accumulation of lactate in muscles leads to muscle fatigue. They showed that during electrical stimulation of isolated frog muscle, mechanical performance gradually declined in parallel with the accumulation of lactate in the muscle cells. When the muscle was moved to a saline solution, muscle mechanical performance was improved. These results suggested that an accumulation of lactate might be a cause of muscle fatigue.

As reviewed by Fitts [2], since intracellular acidification reduces the sensitivity of the contractile apparatus to Ca^{2+} and the maximum Ca^{2+}-activated force, the intracellular acidification of muscle caused by an accumulation of lactate has been thought to lead to muscle fatigue. However, the effects of intracellular acidification were too small to account for muscle fatigue [6,7]. Another factor in muscle fatigue is the reduced ability of the T system to conduct action potentials through excitation-induced accumulation of K^+ in the T system [3,4]. The accumulation of K^+ in the T system causes depolarization, which inactivates the Na^+ channels [2,8].

Nielsen et al. [9] argued that the accumulation of K^+ is a major cause of muscle fatigue. Elevated extracellular K^+ was of less importance in fatigue than had been indicated by previous studies on isolated muscles. In addition, intracellular acidification counteracts the depressing effects of elevated extracellular K^+ on muscle performance. Since intense exercise is associated with increased extracellular K^+, this suggests that, in contrast to the generally accepted role of acidification as a cause of muscle fatigue, intracellular acidification may protect against fatigue. Moreover, it also indicates that when the muscle is rendered acidic, much of the decline in force is reversed, and is accompanied by the recovery of action potential generation.

Finally, Pederson et al. [10] demonstrated that lactate has beneficial effects on performance during muscle fatigue. They showed that in a rat muscle fiber preparation, lactate influenced the activity of Cl^- channels, which sustain the action potentials that are necessary for muscle contractions. This process might be mediated by decreased Cl^- permeability, which enables action potentials to be propagated along the internal network of the T system despite muscle depolarization. These results suggest that the intracellular acidification of muscle has protective effects during muscle fatigue. A central feature of this new mechanism was reported by Allen and Westerblad [11]: the accumulation of extracellular K^+ leads action potentials to be a less effective trigger of Ca^{2+} release in working muscles. Acidification by the accumulation of lactate reduces this effect by decreasing the contribution of Cl^- channels, which act to keep the membrane potential near the Cl^- reversal potential. Since the Cl^- reversal potential is near the resting membrane potential, the effect of Cl^- channel activity is to increase the Na^+ current necessary to produce an action potential, which triggers Ca^{2+} release.

Utilization of Lactate in the Central Nervous System

Until the 1960s, it had been believed that the brain was exclusively dependent on glucose to fuel its metabolism and support neural function. However, transport mechanisms and enzyme systems exist in the brain that allow the potential metabolism of nonglucose fuels. An efficient and saturable transport mechanism for the uptake of lactate has been identified in cultured neurons [12,13]. The function of lactate as a nonglucose fuel in neurons is further indicated by the findings that lactate maintains synaptic function in the absence of glucose in rat hippocampal slices [14], and that synaptic utilization of monocarboxylates sustains hypoglycemic synaptic adaptation in guinea pig hippocampal slices [15]. Moreover, we have clarified that exogenous (or administrated) lactate could be a substitute for glucose in the energy metabolism in brain slices by using a novel method, *bioradiography*, in which the dynamic process could be followed in living slices by the use of positron-emitter labeled compounds and imaging plates [16]. In vivo studies of humans support these findings: lactate injection sustained cognitive function during hypoglycemia in humans [17], and the addition of lactate reduced cerebral glucose utilization in humans with normal blood glucose level [18].

Glycogen is stored in glia, and little is present in neurons [19–21], and it has been suggested that astrocytic glycogen plays a dynamic role both as an energy source supporting basal neuronal function and as an emergency energy reservoir [22]. In addition, lactate in astrocytes formed from glycogen or glucose has been suggested as the substrate for astrocyte-neuronal energy buffering in the retina and the brain [22,23]. Immunohistochemical studies on the human brain revealed that astrocytes contain the lactate dehydrogenase 5 (LDH_5) isoform, which efficiently favors lactate production, as the LDH_5 isoform exhibits a greater maximal velocity and a higher Michaelis constant (Km value) than the LDH_1 isoform, whereas neurons express the LDH_1 isoform, which favors lactate utilization [24,25]. Although the requirement of oxidative metabolism may be disadvantageous under certain circumstances, such as hypoxia, lactate use, in contrast to glycolysis, does not require an initial energy expenditure to drive ATP production, and functions when glycolysis is inhibited. While aerobic metabolism yields 17 or 18 ATP molecules per lactate molecule, anaerobic glycolysis only yields 2 ATP molecules per glucose molecule. Moreover, anaerobic glycolysis is time-wasting and needs a lot of metabolic processes. Thus, lactate use is more concise, and therefore effective, than glucose in the brain energy metabolism under aerobic conditions. Endogenous lactate (or lactate generated in astrocytes) maintained synaptic function during glucose deprivation in rat brain slices [26]. In addition, we also showed that endogenous lactate could be a substitute for glucose in the energy metabolism in living brain slices by using the bioradiography method [16]. As reported in the review by Magistretti [27], astrocytes play a major role in neurometabolic coupling, and the basic mechanism includes glutamate-stimulated aerobic glycolysis. The Na^+-coupled re-uptake of glutamate by astrocytes and the ensuing activation of the Na^+–K^+–ATPase triggers glucose uptake and processing via glycolysis, resulting in the release of lactate from astrocytes. Lactate can then contribute to the activity-dependent fuelling of the neuronal energy demands associated with synaptic transmission. Therefore, lactate produced in astrocytes from anaerobic glycolysis might continuously sustain neuronal energy metabolism.

Roles of Lactate During Central Fatigue

Lactate produced in muscles is removed and transferred to other tissues. This is not an exception for the central nervous system. Lactate generated from the anaerobic breakdown of glycogen in muscles was moved into the brain across the blood–

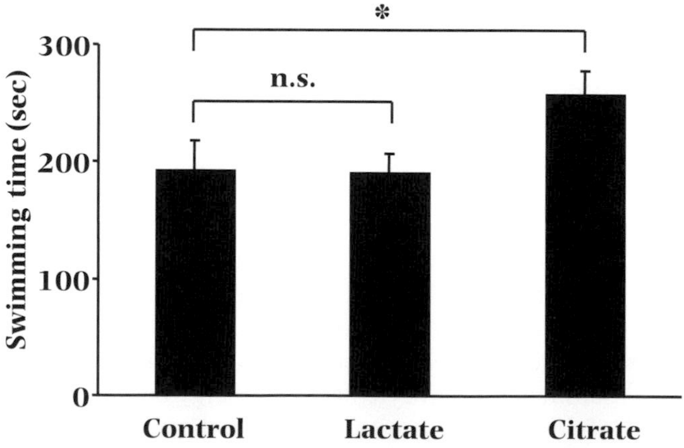

Fig. 1. Effects of lactate (50 mg/kg) or citrate (100 mg/kg) on swimming time with a weight load (8% of body weight). Rats were injected with saline (*Control*), lactate (*Lactate*), or citrate (*Citrate*) into their tail vein. The values are mean and SD (n = 3–5). *P < 0.05, significantly different from the control group; n.s., not significantly different from the control group

brain barrier. Even now, it is generally believed that lactate produced in the muscle during exercise is the cause of central fatigue or of the sensation of fatigue. However, a large amount of experimental evidence denies that theory. For example, Nakamura et al. [28] reported that after forced swimming for 30 min for 5 days, although rats gradually needed a shorter period to recover from fatigue, their blood lactate level after swimming did not change during the 5 days, suggesting that blood lactate level is not associated with fatigue. In addition, the administration of lactate did not affect the endurance performance of rats during weight-loaded forced swimming (Fig. 1). As mentioned in the previous section, lactate is utilized as a precious energy substrate and sustains neuronal energy metabolism, and therefore an increased blood lactate level is not associated with central fatigue.

Conclusions

Even now, there is a wide misunderstanding that the accumulation of lactate is a major cause of muscle fatigue, and that the lactate produced from the anaerobic breakdown of glycogen in the muscle is the cause of central fatigue or the sensation of fatigue. However, a large amount of experimental evidence has discounted this theory; the intracellular acidification of muscle caused by an accumulation of lactate actually has protective effects during muscle fatigue. Exogenous and endogenous lactate is utilized as an important energy substrate and sustains neuronal energy metabolism. Finally, an increased blood lactate level during muscle fatigue is not associated with central fatigue. From these results, we can conclude that lactate is a favorable substance rather than a cause of fatigue.

Acknowledgments. This work was supported in part by Special Coordination Funds for Promoting Science and Technology and by the 21st Century COE Program "Base to Overcome Fatigue," from the Ministry of Education, Culture, Sports, Science and Technology, the Japanese government.

References

1. Stephenson DG, Lamb GD, Stephenson GM (1998) Events of the excitation–contraction–relaxation (E–C–R) cycle in fast- and slow-twitch mammalian muscle fibres relevant to muscle fatigue. Acta Physiol Scand 162:229–245
2. Fitts RH (1994) Cellular mechanisms of muscle fatigue. Physiol Rev 74:49–94
3. Sjogaard G (1988) Muscle energy metabolism and electrolyte shifts during low-level prolonged static contraction in man. Acta Physiol Scand 134:181–187
4. Sejersted OM, Sjogaard G (2000) Dynamics and consequences of potassium shifts in skeletal muscle and heart during exercise. Physiol Rev 80:1411–1481
5. Hill AV, Kupalov P (1929) Proc R Soc London Ser 105:313
6. Lamb GD, Stephenson DG (1994) Effects of intracellular pH and [Mg2+] on excitation–contraction coupling in skeletal muscle fibres of the rat. J Physiol 478:331–339

7. Westerblad H, Allen DG, Lannergren J (2002) Muscle fatigue: lactic acid or inorganic phosphate the major cause? News Physiol Sci 17:17–21
8. Ruff RL (1996) Sodium channel slow inactivation and the distribution of sodium channels on skeletal muscle fibres enable the performance properties of different skeletal muscle fibre types. Acta Physiol Scand 156:159–168
9. Nielsen OB, de Paoli F, Overgaard K (2001) Protective effects of lactic acid on force production in rat skeletal muscle. J Physiol 536:161–166
10. Pedersen TH, Nielsen OB, Lamb GD, Stephenson DG (2004) Intracellular acidosis enhances the excitability of working muscle. Science 305:1144–1147
11. Allen D, Westerblad H (2004) Lactic acid: the latest performance-enhancing drug. Science 305:1112–1113
12. Dringen R, Wiesinge H, Hamprecht B (1993) Uptake of L-lactate by cultured rat brain neurons. Neurosci Lett 163:5–7
13. Nedergaard M, Goldman SA (1993) Carrier-mediated transport of lactic acid in cultured neurons and astrocytes. Am J Physiol 265:282–289
14. Schurr A, West CA, Rigor BM (1988) Lactate-supported synaptic function in the rat hippocampal slice preparation. Science 240:1326–1328
15. Sakurai T, Yang B, Takata T, Yokono K (2002) Synaptic adaptation to repeated hypoglycemia depends on the utilization of monocarboxylates in guinea pig hippocampal slices. Diabetes 51:430–438
16. Tanaka M, Nakamura F, Mizokawa S, Matsumura A, Matsumura K, Murata T, Shigematsu M, Kageyama K, Ochi H, Watanabe Y (2004) Role of lactate in the brain energy metabolism: revealed by bioradiography. Neurosci Res 48:13–20
17. Maran A, Cranston I, Lomas J, Macdonald I, Amiel SA (1994) Protection by lactate of cerebral function during hypoglycaemia. Lancet 343:16–20
18. Smith D, Pernet A, Hallett WA, Bingham E, Marsden PK, Amiel SA (2003) Lactate: a preferred fuel for human brain metabolism in vivo. J Cereb Blood Flow Metab 23:658–664
19. Rosenberg PA, Dichter MA (1985) Glycogen accumulation in rat cerebral cortex in dissociated cell culture. J Neurosci Methods 15:101-112
20. Kato K, Shimizu A, Kurobe N, Takashi M, Koshikawa T (1989) Human brain-type glycogen phosphorylase: quantitative localization in human tissues determined with an immunoassay system. J Neurochem 52:1425–1432
21. Ignacio PC, Baldwin BA, Vijayan VK, Tait RC, Gorin FA (1990) Brain isozyme of glycogen phosphorylase: immunohistological localization within the central nervous system. Brain Res 529:42–49
22. Swanson RA (1992) Physiologic coupling of glial glycogen metabolism to neuronal activity in brain. Can J Physiol Pharmacol 70:138–144
23. Tsacopoulos M, Magistretti PJ (1996) Metabolic coupling between glia and neurons. J Neurosci 16:877–885
24. Gehardt Hansen W (1968) Lactate dehydrogenase isoenzymes in the central nervous system. Dan Med Bull 15:111–112
25. Bishop MJ, Everse J, Kaplan NO (1972) Identification of lactate dehydrogenase isoenzymes by rapid kinetics. Proc Natl Acad Sci USA 69:1761–1765
26. Izumi Y, Benz AM, Katsuki H, Zorumski CF (1981) Endogenous monocarboxylates sustain hippocampal synaptic function and morphological integrity during energy deprivation. J Neurosci 17:9448–9457
27. Magistretti PJ (2006) Neuron-glia metabolic coupling and plasticity. J Exp Biol 209: 2304–2311
28. Nakamura F, Tanaka M, Matsumura A, Mizokawa S, Watanabe Y(1994) Biochemical adaptations of rats from fatigue by modified forced swim. 32nd Annual Meeting Society for Neuroscience 385:18

Brain Mechanisms of Poly I:C-Induced Fatigue in Rats

Toshihiko Katafuchi

Summary

The clinical symptoms of chronic fatigue syndrome (CFS) have been shown to include disorders in the neuroendocrine, autonomic, and immune systems. On the other hand, it has been demonstrated that cytokines produced in the brain play significant roles in neural–immune interactions through their various central actions, such as activation of the hypothalamo-pituitary axis and sympathetic nervous system. We have recently developed an animal model for fatigue induced by intraperitoneal (i.p.) injection of synthetic double-stranded RNAs, polyriboinosinic: polyribocytidylic acid (poly I:C, 3 mg/kg), in rats, and shown a decrease in the daily amounts of spontaneous running-wheel activity to about 60% of the preinjection level for more than 1 week. Simultaneously, mRNAs for interferon-α (IFN-α) and serotonin transporter (5-HTT), which is known to be induced by IFN-α, increased for more than a week following poly I:C injection in the same hypothalamic nuclei and cortex. The increased 5-HTT had a functional significance, since in vivo brain microdialysis revealed that an i.p. injection of poly I:C induced a decrease in the extracellular concentration of 5-HT in the prefrontal cortex, which was blocked by a local perfusion with the selective 5-HT re-uptake inhibitor, fluoxetine. Finally the poly I:C-induced fatigue was attenuated by 5-HT_{1A} receptor agonist, but not by 5-HT_2, 5-HT_3, or dopamine D_3 agonists. These findings suggested that the decrease in 5-HT actions on 5-HT_{1A} receptors may at least partly contribute to the poly I:C-induced fatigue.

Introduction

Chronic fatigue syndrome (CFS) is characterized not only by severe fatigue, but also by the impairment of autonomic, neuroendocrine, cognitive, and immune functions, suggesting an involvement of the disorders in the neuronal–endocrine–

Department of Integrative Physiology, Graduate School of Medical Sciences, Kyushu University, 3-1-1 Maidashi, Higashi-ku, Fukuoka 812-8582, Japan

immune interactions [1–5]. It is well known that cytokines produced in the brain exert various central actions, including activation of the sympathetic nervous system and hypothalamic pituitary axis, impairment of learning memory, and suppression of peripheral cellular immunity [6,7]. Therefore it is possible that brain cytokines may play a role in the pathogenesis of the CFS.

It is considered that experimental fatigue can be divided into four categories: (1) physical fatigue caused by such things as forced exercise or swimming; (2) mental fatigue; (3) environmental fatigue caused by such things as heat exposure; (4) immunologically induced fatigue. Among these models, immunologically induced fatigue [8] is thought to be most closely associated with the neuronal–endocrine–immune interactions [2]. Although the administration of lipopolysaccharide (LPS), which is commonly used as a model for bacterial infection, induces sickness behavior, including lowered locomotor activity, recovery usually takes place within 2–3 days in rats as well as in mice [9]. Since it is suggested that an infection and/or reactivation of a latent virus may have a contributory role in a subset of CFS cases [2], we decided to inject polyriboinosinic:polyribocytidylic acid (poly I:C) (synthetic double-stranded RNAs that are known to mimic viral infection) into rats to establish an immunologically induced fatigue model. To investigate the brain mechanisms of the fatigue, we measured the expression of mRNAs for cytokines and their related molecules in the brain using a real-time capillary reverse transcriptase–polymerase chain reaction (RT–PCR) method such as interferon-α (IFN-α), interleukin-1β (IL-1β), IL-6, an inhibitor of nuclear factor κB (IκB)-β, and p38 mitogen-activated protein kinase (p38 MAPK). In addition, the possible involvement of the brain 5-hydroxytryptamine (serotonin, 5-HT) system was also examined since 5-HT was implicated in the mechanisms of central fatigue after exhaustive exercise [10].

Fatigue Induced by Poly I:C

Male Wistar rats (8–10 weeks old) were housed individually in plastic cages with free access to food and water. Each cage contained a 30-cm-diameter running wheel, and the rats could enter the wheel any time (Fig. 1). Fatigue was assessed by the decrease in the total running-wheel activity of each animal after the i.p. administration of poly I:C (1.0 or 3.0 mg/ml/kg) or vehicle (saline), given between 09:00 and 10:00 hours [11].

The average of the total running-wheel activity before treatment was about 800–1000 wheel turns/day. The animals that were injected with poly I:C (3.0 mg/kg) showed a marked decrease in running-wheel activity to about 40% of the baseline levels on day 1 compared with the saline group (Fig. 2). The reduction in activity (to 60%–70% of the baseline level) lasted until day 9, and then gradually recovered until day 14. In addition to the poly I:C-injected groups, some animals were given heat exposure (36°C) for 1 h in the 3 days following this experiment, since we thought that heat stress might reduce the running-wheel activity, and

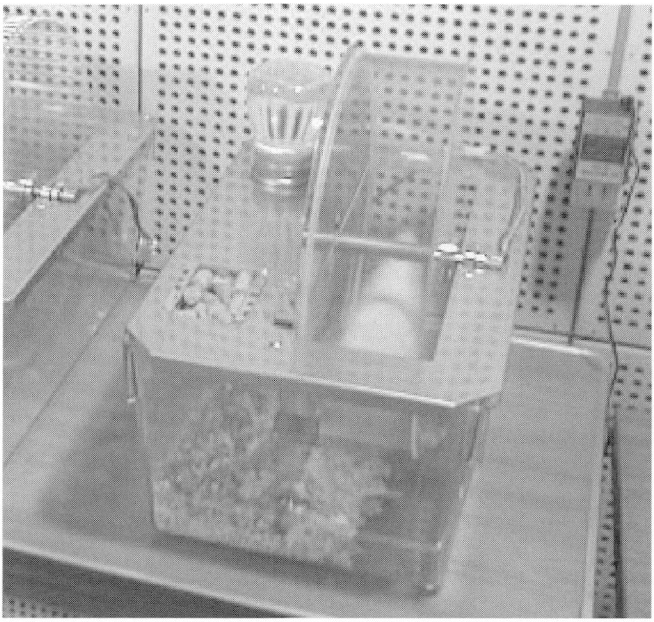

Fig. 1. Home cage equipped with running wheel (diameter 30 cm). Rats were housed individually with a 12-h light/dark cycle and had free access to food and water. They could enter the running wheel at any time, and the number of wheel turns per minute was counted continuously using an analog/digital interface and computer software

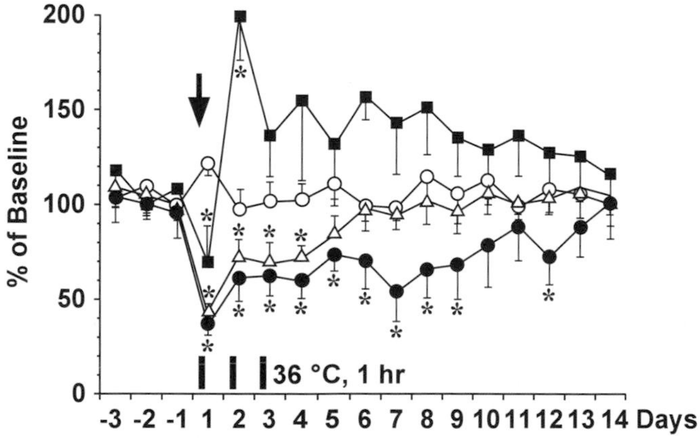

Fig. 2. Changes in total running-wheel activity after a poly I:C injection and heat exposure for three consecutive days. Total daily activity was expressed as a percentage of the baseline levels (averages from day −3 to day −1 in each group). *Open circles*, saline group ($n = 8$); *open triangles*, 1.0 mg/kg poly I:C ($n = 4$); *filled circles*, 3.0 mg/kg poly I:C ($n = 9$); *filled squares*, heat exposure (36°C for 1 h, $n = 9$). Poly I:C or saline was injected between 09:00 and 10:00 hours on day 1 (*arrow*), and heat exposure was given on days 1–3 (*filled bars*). *, $P < 0.05$ vs. saline group, Fisher's PLSD test. (From [11], with permission)

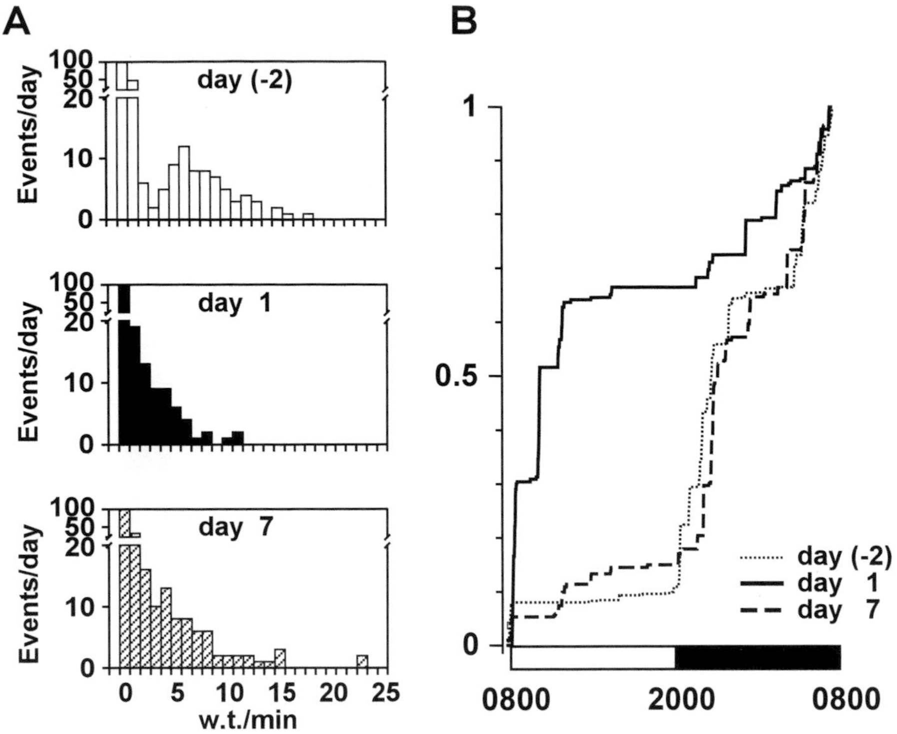

Fig. 3. Running-wheel activity histogram (**A**) and normalized cumulative curve of activity (**B**) in a day. **A** Activity histogram on day −2 (*top*), day 1 (*middle*), and day 7 (*bottom*). Note the absence of a peak of 6 wheel turns per min (w.t./min) on days 1 and 7. **B** Normalized cumulative curves based on the total number of events in a day. *Dotted line*, on day −2; *solid line*, on day 1; *thick broken line*, on day 7. Note the absence of a circadian rhythm on day 1 and its reappearance on day 7. (From [11], with permission)

possibly serve as a positive control. However, as shown in Fig. 2, the heat-exposure group showed a transient but significant increase in total running-wheel activity on day 2 following a slight decrease on day 1. These findings suggest that a transient rise in body temperature, induced either by heat exposure or by poly I:C injection, is not necessarily the cause of a decrease in running-wheel activity. Since animals are known to demonstrate increased behavioral activation in response to either novelty or mild stress, it is suggested that repeated exposure to a hot environment may serve as a stressor that induces an activation of the arousal system, resulting in an increase in running-wheel activity.

To further analyze the pattern of running activity, histograms for the number of wheel turns in 1 min (w.t./min) were made from data recorded on days −2, 1, and 7. As shown in Fig. 3A top, there were two peaks of 6 and 1 w.t./min before poly I:C on day −2. The raw data indicated that the events of 1 w.t./min occurred mostly in the light period, while those of 6 w.t./min occurred in the dark period. Thus the cumulative curve based on the total events in a day showed a very slow increase in the light period and a rapid increase in the dark period on day −2 (Fig. 3B). After the administration of poly I:C, on days 1 and 7 (the middle and lower panels, respectively, of Fig. 3A), the peak of 6 w.t./min did not occur. However, the circadian rhythm of running-wheel activity was present on day 7, as shown in the normalized cumulative curve of the activity (Fig. 3B). The long-term depression of voluntary running in the wheel was not directly associated with the acute-phase responses, since the rise in body temperature, serum ACTH, and catecholamine levels returned to the baseline level 24 h after the injection [11]. Furthermore, an open-field test, which can evaluate locomotor activity in a novel situation as well as anxiety, showed no differences in total distance moved, number of instances of rearing up, and length of time staying in the center of the field between the poly I:C and control (saline) groups when performed on day 7. Thus it is strongly suggested that the decrease in running-wheel activity is produced by central fatigue, but not by anxiety-induced suppression or peripheral problems such as muscle and/or joint pain.

Poly I:C-Induced Expression of mRNAs for Cytokines and Related Molecules

Messenger RNAs (mRNAs) for IFN-α, Il-1β, IL-6, and TNF-α in a discrete region of hypothalamic nuclei such as the medial preoptic area (MPO), lateral preoptic area (LPO), paraventricular hypothalamic nucleus (PVN), and lateral hypothalamic area (LHA), cortex, hippocampus, and cerebellum were measured quantitatively using a real-time capillary RT–PCR method on days 1 and 8 in poly I:C-injected rats [12]. We found that the amount of both IL-1β (Fig. 4A) and IFN-α (Fig. 4B) mRNAs increased significantly in the cortex and in some hypothalamic nuclei such as MPO and LPO on day 1. Although Il-1β mRNA returned to the baseline level on day 8, an increase in IFN-α mRNA in the cortex, cerebellum, MPO, LPO, and PVN was still found on day 8. The amounts of TNF-α and IL-6 mRNAs were not affected by poly I:C. These findings suggest that the changes in expression of IFN-α are more closely associated with the behavioral effects of poly I:C than the changes in expression of IL-1β if cytokine production in the brain is involved in the mechanisms of fatigue.

The quantitative measurement of mRNAs for cytokine-related molecules such as an inhibitor of nuclear factor κB (IκB)-β and p38 mitogen-activated protein kinase (MAPK), which are one of the IL-1β- and IFN-α-activated transcriptional factors, respectively, was also performed on days 1 and 8 after poly I:C injection [12]. As expected, IκB-β mRNA increased only on day 1, while p38 MAPK mRNA increased on both days 1 and 8 in almost the same regions where IL-1β and IFN-α mRNAs increased, indicating that the expression patterns of IκB-β and p38 MAPK mRNAs are very similar to those of IL-1β and IFN-α, respectively.

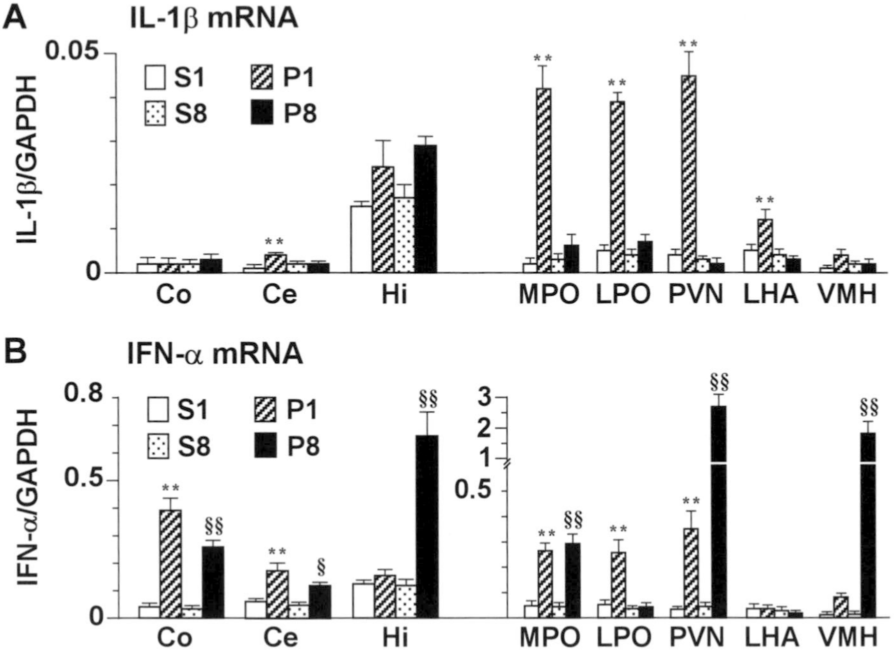

Fig. 4. Effects of poly I:C on brain IL-1β (**A**) and IFN-α (**B**) mRNA expression. *Open bars*, S1 group ($n = 5$); *hatched bars*, P1 ($n = 5$); *dotted bars*, S8 ($n = 5$); *filled bars*, P8 ($n = 5$). Each value was normalized to the mRNA levels of glyceraldehydes 3-phosphate dehydrogenase (GAPDH), one of the housekeeping genes, obtained by the same method. *Co*, parietal cortex; *Ce*, cerebellum; *Hi*, hippocampus; *MPO*, medial preoptic area; *LPO*, lateral preoptic area; *PVN*, paraventricular nucleus; *LHA*, lateral hypothalamic area; *VMH*, ventromedial nucleus. **, $P < 0.01$, P1 vs. S1; §, $P < 0.05$, and §§, $P < 0.01$, P8 vs. S8, Bonferroni's test. No significant difference was found between the S1 and S8 groups. (From [12], with permission)

Possible Mechanisms of IFN-α Expression in the Brain

Since we measured the amounts of mRNA in the total RNA from brain tissues, the cellular origin of IFN-α is not clear. Previous studies have shown that IFN-α is detected in neurons and microglia in human brain tissues from control and neurological cases [13,14], while astrocytes of rats and mice in vitro produce IFN-α/β in response to poly I:C [15]. It is also not known how peripheral poly I:C signals the brain to induce IFN-α. Systemic injection of LPS can induce fever, one of the central effects of the immune activators, through LPS itself, or through peripherally and/or centrally produced cytokines by multiple routes, including (1) cerebral endothelial cells and perivascular microglial cells, (2) cells in circumventricular organs such as the organum vasculosum of the lamina terminalis and the area postrema, which lack a functional blood–brain barrier, and (3) visceral vagal afferent nerves [16]. It has been reported that double-stranded RNAs, including poly I:C, are recognized by Toll-like receptor (TLR) 3, that is present in the periphery and brain, to induce IFNs [17]. It is possible that the peripheral poly I:C- and LPS-induced expression of cytokines in the brain may share common pathways.

Poly I:C-Induced Changes in 5-HTT Expression

We also found that transcription of 5-HT transporter (5-HTT) increased in the hypothalamic nuclei and cortex where IFN-α mRNA increased for more than a week after poly I:C injection (Fig. 5A). Immunoblot analysis also revealed that expression of 5-HTT increased in membrane extracts from prefrontal cortex (Fig. 5B) [12]. Although in situ hybridization studies of 5-HTT labeled only the serotonergic cell bodies in the rat and human midbrain [18,19], the functional expression of 5-HTT mRNA in astrocytes [20] and endothelial cells [21] has been demonstrated in the rat brain by means of a RT–PCR method. Since IFN-α has been shown to up-regulate the transcription of 5-HTT in cultured cells [22], it is suggested that the expression of 5-HTT is enhanced by the poly I:C-induced IFN-α through its actions on astrocytes and/or endothelial cells in the respective brain regions. It has been reported that the activity of 5-HTT is elevated by p38 MAPK, and this activation is abolished by the suppression of p38 MAPK expression [23]. These findings are in accordance with the present results, which show a similar expression pattern of mRNAs for IFN-α, p38 MAPK, and 5-HTT in the brain.

In order to examine whether the poly I:C-induced 5-HTTs have a functional significance, the effects of poly I:C on extracellular 5-HT levels in the prefrontal cortex were examined using an in vivo microdialysis technique [12]. Within a few hours after the poly I:C injection, 5-HT levels started to decrease in the prefrontal cortex. A local administration of imipramine, an inhibitor of monoamine transporters, through a dialysis probe completely blocked the poly I:C-induced decrease in the 5-HT level (Fig. 6). We have observed that fluoxetine, a selective 5-HT reuptake inhibitor (SSRI), also has the same effect. It has been reported that 5-HTT induced in astrocytes can be a target of antidepressant drugs including SSRI, thus contributing to the control of the extracellular 5-HT fraction. Furthermore, 5-HT taken-up by glial or endothelial 5-HTTs is not re-used as a neurotransmitter, but scavenged into the blood or cerebrospinal fluid after being metabolized to 5-hydroxyindoleacetic acid (5-HIAA) [24]. Since poly I:C injection did not affect the extracellular concentration of 5-HIAA in the prefrontal cortex (unpublished data), the poly I:C-induced decrease in 5-HT levels (Fig. 6) was not due to either an enhancement of 5-HT turnover or a reduction of 5-HT release, which might result in an increase or decrease in 5-HIAA, respectively. It is thus possible that 5-HT released from nerve terminals is taken up by the poly I:C-induced 5-HTTs of glial and/or endothelial cells and scavenged immediately, thereby resulting in the decrease in 5-HT.

Recently, we have found that microinjection of IFN-α into the prefrontal cortex also produced a decrease in 5-HT levels, which was again blocked by SSRI

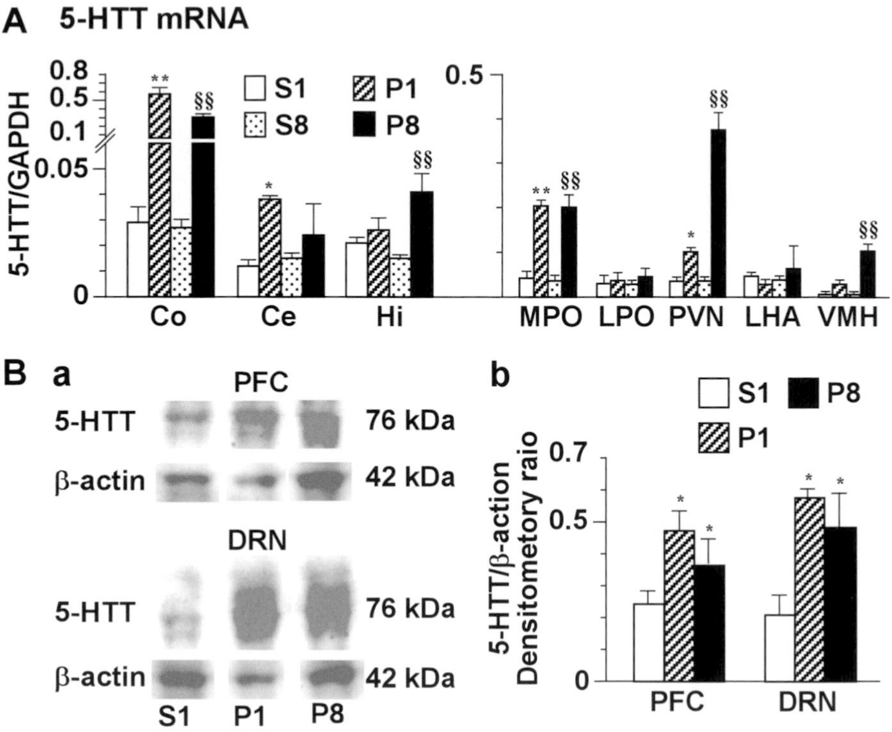

Fig. 5. Effects of poly I:C on brain 5-HTT mRNA (**A**) and 5-HTT protein (**B**). **A** *Open bar*, S1 group; *hatched bar*, P1; *dotted bar*, S8; *filled bar*, P8 (each group, $n = 5$). Each value was normalized to the corresponding GAPDH mRNA level obtained by the same method. *Co*, parietal cortex; *Ce*, cerebellum; *Hi*, hippocampus; *MPO*, medial preoptic area; *LPO*, lateral preoptic area; *PVN*, paraventricular nucleus; *LHA*, lateral hypothalamic area; *VMH*, ventromedial nucleus. *, $P < 0.05$, **, $P < 0.01$, P1 vs. S1; §§, $P < 0.01$, P8 vs. S8, Bonferroni's test. No significant difference was found between the S1 and S8 groups. **B** 5-HTT protein expression following poly I:C injection. **B**, *a*, Western blot analysis in the prefrontal cortex (*PFC, upper bands*) and dorsal raphe nucleus (*DRN, lower bands*) in S1, P1, and P8 rats. Note a marked increase in immunostaining on days 1 and 8 in both regions. **B**, *b*, summary of the Western blot experiment. Each group, $n = 3$. *, $P < 0.05$, vs. S1, Bonferroni's test. (From [12], with permission)

(unpublished data). It has been shown that an intracerebroventricular injection of IFN-α decreases 5-HT levels in dissected blocks of the rat frontal cortex 2 h after the injection [25]. These findings strongly suggest an involvement of 5-HTT in the IFN-α-induced decrease in 5-HT. As mentioned previously, IFN-α can induce 5-HTT in cultured cells and in the mouse brain in vivo [22], while poly I:C evokes an increased expression of 5-HTT in the same brain regions where IFN-α mRNA increases (Fig. 5) [12]. These findings suggest that the IFN-α-induced decrease in 5-HT levels in the prefrontal cortex is mediated by the enhanced expression of 5-HTT.

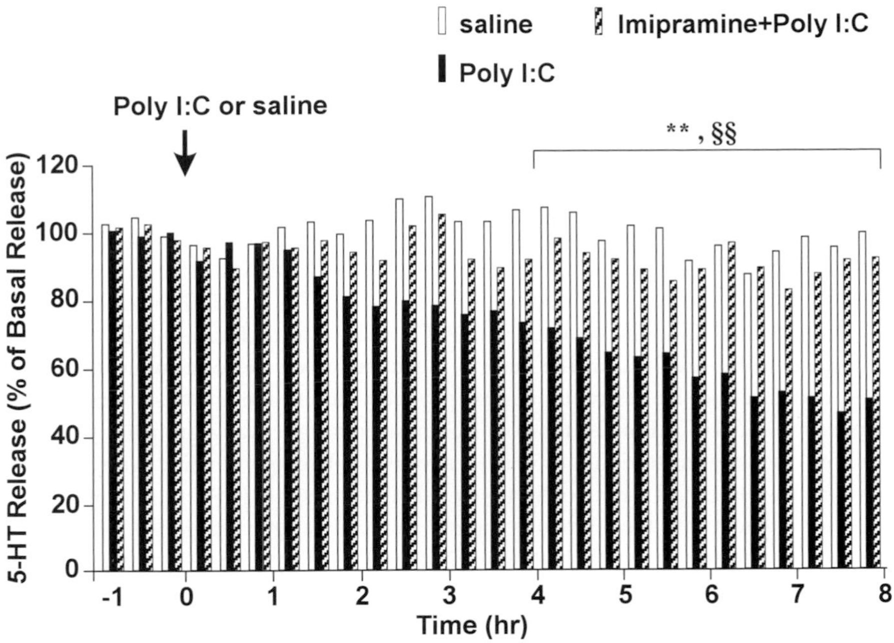

Fig. 6. Effects of poly I:C with or without local perfusion of imipramine on 5-HT levels in the prefrontal cortex measured by in vivo microdialysis. 5-HT levels are expressed as a percentage of each basal level measured before the poly I:C (3 mg/kg, i.p.) or saline injection (*arrow*). The poly I:C injection produced a significant decrease in 5-HT levels (*filled bars*, $n = 4$) from 4 to 8 h after the injection compared with the saline group (*open bars*, $n = 4$). Local perfusion with imipramine (10 μM) through the dialysis probe blocked the poly I:C-induced decrease in 5-HT levels (*hatched bars*, $n = 4$). Error bars are omitted. **, $P < 0.01$, poly I:C vs. saline group; §§, $P < 0.01$, poly I:C vs. imipramine + poly I:C group, Bonferroni's test. (From [12], with permission)

Brain IFN-α and Fatigue

Since poly I:C is a strong inducer of IFN-α, it is likely that the plasma IFN-α level may be elevated at least in the acute phase of poly I:C treatment. In IFN-α-therapy-associated fatigue that is often the dominant dose-limiting side effect, and one of the causes of the fatigue is suggested to be neuromuscular fatigue, similar to that observed in patients with postpolio syndrome [26]. Since the reduction of the treadmill run time to fatigue following poly I:C injection was significantly attenuated by the peripheral administration of anti-IFN-α/β antibody, early fatigue induced by poly I:C may, at least partially, result from an increase in peripheral IFNs [27]. However, the persistent fatigue observed until a week after poly I:C seems to involve the central mechanisms rather than the peripheral ones for the reasons described below.

First, although a decrease in running-wheel activity on day 1 may be due to acute sickness following poly I:C, the open-field test performed on day 7 suggests that a motivated activity, but not locomotor activity, has been suppressed by poly I:C. Second, it has been reported that CFS is often accompanied by low levels of natural killer (NK) cell activity [2,3]. We have shown that the central, but not peripheral, administration of IFN-α produces a significant suppression of splenic NK cell activity through the activation of the splenic sympathetic nerve in rats [28,29]. In addition, the action site of IFN-α to induce the suppression of NK activity was the MPO [30,31], where expression of IFN-α mRNA increased on day 7 after poly I:C. It has been reported that IFN-α, but not IL-1β and TNF-α, is elevated in cerebrospinal fluid in patients with CFS [32]. Third, brain 5-HT, which is suggested to be involved in the central mechanisms of exercise-induced fatigue [10], decreased in the prefrontal cortex, probably due to the IFN-α-induced overexpression of 5-HTT. Finally, the poly I:C-induced fatigue was significantly attenuated by the administration of 5-HT_{1A} agonist, 8-hydroxy-2-(di-*n*-propylamino) tetraline (8-OH DPAT), but not 5-HT_2 or 5-HT_3 agonist [12]. These findings taken together suggest that the immunologically induced fatigue by poly I:C involves central mechanisms in which the brain IFN-α and 5-HT system may play an important role.

It has recently been reported that in 5-HTT gene promoter polymorphism studies, CFS patients had a significant increase in longer (L and XL) alleic variants [33], which retain higher transcriptional activity than the short (S) allele. In addition, Narita et al. [33] described their preliminary observation that a selective serotonin re-uptake inhibitor, fluvoxamine, was effective enough for about one-third of the CFS patients to return to work. These findings suggest that poly I:C-induced fatigue is a useful animal model for studying the central mechanisms of fatigue.

Acknowledgments. This work was performed through Special Coordination Funds for Promoting Science and Technology, and Grants-in-Aid for Scientific Research (19603004) to T. K. from the Ministry of Education, Culture, Sports, Science and Technology of the Japanese government.

References

1. Freeman R, Komaroff AL (1997) Does chronic fatigue syndrome involve the autonomic nervous system? 102:357–364
2. Glaser R, Kiecolt-Glaser JK (1998) Stress-associated immune modulation: relevance to viral infections and chronic fatigue syndrome. Am J Med 105:35S–42S
3. Whiteside TL, Friberg D (1998) Natural killer cells and natural killer cell activity in chronic fatigue syndrome. Am J Med 105:27S–34S
4. Komaroff AL (2000) The biology of chronic fatigue syndrome [comment]. Am J Med 108:169–171
5. Joyce E, Blumenthal S, Wessely S (1996) Memory, attention, and executive function in chronic fatigue syndrome. J Neurol Neurosurg Psychiatr 60:495–503

6. Hori T, Katafuchi T, Oka T (2001) Central cytokines: effects on peripheral immunity, inflammation and nociception. In: Ader R, Felten DL, Cohen N (eds) Psychoneuroimmunology. Academic Press, San Diego, pp 517–545
7. Rothwell NJ, Hopkins SJ (1995) Cytokines and the nervous system. II. Actions and mechanisms of action. Trends Neurosci 18:130–136
8. Chao CC, DeLaHunt M, Hu S, Close K, Peterson PK (1992) Immunologically mediated fatigue: a murine model. Clin Immunol Immunopathol 64:161–165
9. Kozak W, Conn CA, Kluger MJ (1994) Lipopolysaccharide induces fever and depresses locomotor activity in unrestrained mice. Am J Physiol 266:R125–R135
10. Yamamoto T, Newsholme EA (2000) Diminished central fatigue by inhibition of the L-system transporter for the uptake of tryptophan. Brain Res Bull 52:35–38
11. Katafuchi T, Kondo T, Yasaka T, Kubo K, Take S, Yoshimura M (2003) Prolonged effects of polyriboinosinic:polyribocytidylic acid on spontaneous running-wheel activity and brain interferon-α mRNA in rats: a model for immunologically induced fatigue. Neuroscience 120:837–845
12. Katafuchi T, Kondo T, Take S, Yoshimura M (2005) Enhanced expression of brain interferon-α and serotonin transporter in immunologically induced fatigue in rats. Eur J Neurosci 22:2817–2826
13. Akiyama H, Ikeda K, Katoh M, McGeer EG, McGeer PL (1994) Expression of MRP14, 27E10, interferon-α and leukocyte common antigen by reactive microglia in postmortem human brain tissue. J Neuroimmunol 50:195–201
14. Yamada T, Horisberger MA, Kawaguchi N, Moroo I, Toyoda T (1994) Immunohistochemistry using antibodies to α-interferon and its induced protein, MxA, in Alzheimer's and Parkinson's disease brain tissues. Neurosci Lett 181:61–64
15. Tedeschi B, Barrett JN, Keane RW (1986) Astrocytes produce interferon that enhances the expression of H-2 antigens on a subpopulation of brain cells. J Cell Biol 102:2244–2253
16. Ledeboer A, Binnekade R, Breve JJ, Bol JG, Tilders FJ, Van Dam AM (2002) Site-specific modulation of LPS-induced fever and interleukin-1β expression in rats by interleukin-10. Am J Physiol 282:R1762–R1772
17. Alexopoulou L, Holt AC, Medzhitov R, Flavell RA (2001) Recognition of double-stranded RNA and activation of NF-κB by Toll-like receptor 3. Nature 413:732–738
18. Blakely RD, Berson HE, Fremeau RT Jr, Caron MG, Peek MM, Prince HK, Bradley CC (1991) Cloning and expression of a functional serotonin transporter from rat brain. Nature 354:66–70
19. Austin MC, Bradley CC, Mann JJ, Blakely RD (1994) Expression of serotonin transporter messenger RNA in the human brain. J Neurochem 62:2362–2367
20. Hirst WD, Price GW, Rattray M, Wilkin GP (1998) Serotonin transporters in adult rat brain astrocytes revealed by [^{3}H]5-HT uptake into glial plasmalemmal vesicles. Neurochem Int 33:11–22
21. Brust P, Friedrich A, Krizbai IA, Bergmann R, Roux F, Ganapathy V, Johannsen B (2000) Functional expression of the serotonin transporter in immortalized rat brain microvessel endothelial cells. J Neurochem 74:1241–1248
22. Morikawa O, Sakai N, Obara H, Saito N (1998) Effects of interferon-α, interferon-γ and cAMP on the transcriptional regulation of the serotonin transporter. Eur J Pharmacol 349:317–324
23. Zhu CB, Carneiro AM, Dostmann WR, Hewlett WA, Blakely RD (2005) p38 MAPK activation elevates serotonin transport activity via a trafficking-independent, protein phosphatase 2A-dependent process. J Biol Chem 280:15649–15658
24. Bel N, Figueras G, Vilaro MT, Sunol C, Artigas F (1997) Antidepressant drugs inhibit a glial 5-hydroxytryptamine transporter in rat brain. 9:1728–1738
25. Kamata M, Higuchi H, Yoshimoto M, Yoshida K, Shimizu T (2000) Effect of single intracerebroventricular injection of α-interferon on monoamine concentrations in the rat brain. Eur Neuropsychopharmacol 10:129–132

26. Patarca R (2001) Cytokines and chronic fatigue syndrome. Ann NY Acad Sci 933:185–200
27. Davis JM, Weaver JA, Kohut ML, Colbert LH, Ghaffar A, Mayer EP (1998) Immune system activation and fatigue during treadmill running: role of interferon. Med Sci Sports Exerc 30:863–868
28. Katafuchi T, Take S, Hori T (1993) Roles of sympathetic nervous system in the suppression of cytotoxicity of splenic natural killer cells in the rat. J Physiol 465:343–357
29. Take S, Mori T, Katafuchi T, Hori T (1993) Central interferon-α inhibits natural killer cytotoxicity through sympathetic innervation. Am J Physiol 265:R453–R459
30. Katafuchi T, Ichijo T, Take S, Hori T (1993) Hypothalamic modulation of splenic natural killer cell activity in rats. J Physiol 471:209–221
31. Take S, Uchimura D, Kanemitsu Y, Katafuchi T, Hori T (1995) Interferon-α acts at the preoptic hypothalamus to reduce natural killer cytotoxicity in rats. Am J Physiol 268: R-1406–R1410
32. Lloyd A, Hickie I, Brockman A, Dwyer J, Wakefield D (1991) Cytokine levels in serum and cerebrospinal fluid in patients with chronic fatigue syndrome and control subjects. J Infect Dis 164:1023–1024
33. Narita M, Nishibami N, Narita N, Yamaguti K, Okado N, Watanabe Y, Kuratsune H (2003) Association between serotonin transporter gene polymorphism and chronic fatigue syndrome. Biochem Biophys Res Commun 311:264–266

Index